Emergency Nursing Examination

R·E·V·I·E·W

Emergency Nursing Examination
R·E·V·I·E·W

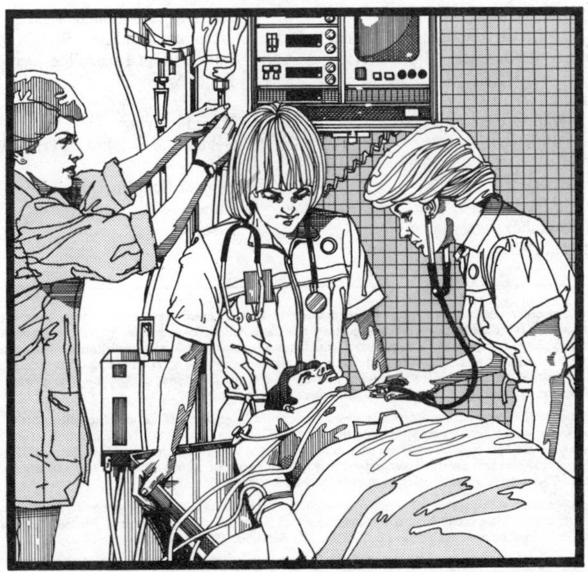

Laura Gasparis, RN, MA, CCRN, CEN
Joanne Noone, RN, MSN, CCRN, CEN

Springhouse Corporation
Springhouse, Pennsylvania

STAFF FOR THIS VOLUME

CLINICAL STAFF

Clinical Director
Barbara McVan, RN

Clinical Editors
Joanne Patzek DaCunha, RN
Joan E. Mason, RN, EdM
Diane Schweisguth, RN, BSN

PUBLICATION STAFF

Executive Director, Editorial
Stanley Loeb

Executive Director, Creative Services
Jean Robinson

Design
John Hubbard (art director), Stephanie Peters (associate art director), Maria Errico

Editing
Regina Ford (project manager), Patricia McKeown

Copy Editing
Edith McMahon (supervisor), Nick Anastasio, Keith de Pinho, Diane Labus, Doris Weinstock, Debra Young

Art Production
Robert Perry (manager), Anna Brindisi, Loretta Caruso, Donald Knauss, Christina McKinley, Robert Wieder

Typography
David Kosten (manager), Diane Paluba (assistant manager), Brenda Mayer, Robin Rantz, Brent Rinedoller, Joyce Rossi Biletz, Nancy Wirs

Manufacturing
Deborah Meiris (manager), T.A. Landis

Project Coordination
Aline S. Miller (supervisor), Elizabeth B. Kiselev

The clinical procedures described and recommended in this publication are based on research and consultation with nursing, medical, and legal authorities. To the best of our knowledge, these procedures reflect currently accepted practice; nevertheless, they can't be considered absolute and universal recommendations. For individual application, all recommendations must be considered in light of the patient's clinical condition and, before administration of new or infrequently used drugs, in light of latest package-insert information. The authors and the publisher disclaim responsibility for any adverse effects resulting directly or indirectly from the suggested procedures, from any undetected errors, or from the reader's misunderstanding of the text.

Library of Congress Cataloging-in-Publication Data
Gasparis, Laura, 1952-
Emergency nursing examination review.
Includes bibliographies and index.
1. Emergency nursing—Examinations, questions, etc.
I. Noone, Joanne, 1956— . II. Title. [DNLM: 1. Critical Care—examination questions. 2. Emergencies—examination questions. 3. Emergency Service, Hospital—examination questions. 4. Nursing—examination questions. WY 18 G249e]
RT120.E4G37 1988 610.73'61 88-2157
ISBN 0-87434-129-9

Contents

Contributors

Chapter 1—Fluid, Electrolyte, and Acid-Base Alterations
Marcia Downs, RN, CEN
Educational Coordinator, Life Flight,
Baptist Medical Center, Jacksonville, Florida

David Unkle, RN, CCRN, CEN
Clinical Research Coordinator, Division of Trauma and Emergency Services,
Cooper Hospital/University Medical Center, Camden, New Jersey

Charles T. Vonfrolio, MD (consultant)
Chief of Anesthesia, Staten Island Hospital
New York, New York

Chapter 2—Shock
Laura Gasparis, RN, MA, CCRN, CEN
Assistant Professor of Nursing
College of Staten Island
New York, New York

Charles T. Vonfrolio, MD
Chief of Anesthesia
Staten Island Hospital
New York, New York

Chapter 3—Cardiovascular Emergencies
Laura Gasparis, RN, MA, CCRN, CEN
Assistant Professor of Nursing, College of Staten Island
New York, New York

Linda Anne Laner, RN, MSN, CS, CCRN, CEN
Staff Nurse, Emergency Department, Staten Island Hospital
New York, New York

Eva Scripps, RN, BSN, CCRN, CEN
Nurse Care Coordinator, Emergency Department, Staten Island Hospital
New York, New York

Chapter 4—Respiratory Emergencies
Mary Blum, RN, MSN
Instructor of Nursing, Rutgers—The State University
Newark, New Jersey

Deborah S. Gough, RN, MSN, CCRN, CEN
Clinical Education Coordinator, Bayley Seton Hospital
New York, New York

Marilyn McDonald, RN, MA
Assistant Professor of Nursing, College of Staten Island
New York, New York

Janet A. Neff, RN, MN, CCRN, CEN
Editorial Board, *Journal of Emergency Nursing*
Instructor of Nursing, University of Arizona
Tucson, Arizona

Chapter 5—Neurologic Emergencies

Kathy Daly, RN, CCRN, CEN
Staff Nurse II, Emergency Department, Beth Israel Medical Center
New York, New York

Laura Gasparis, RN, MA, CCRN, CEN
Assistant Professor of Nursing, College of Staten Island
New York, New York

Maureen Sheehy, RN, CCRN, CEN
Staff Nurse, Emergency Department
Bayley Seton Hospital
Health Coordinator
Ellis Island Restoration Project
New York, New York

Chapter 6—Metabolic/Endocrine Emergencies

Patrice Case, RN, MA
Adjunct Faculty, College of Staten Island
New York, New York

Laura Gasparis, RN, MA, CCRN, CEN
Assistant Professor of Nursing
College of Staten Island
New York, New York

Joanne Noone, RN, MSN, CCRN, CEN
Nursing Instructor, Kauai Community College
Lihue, Hawaii

Debra Toth, RN, BSN, MA Candidate
Transplant Coordinator
New Jersey Organ and Tissue Network
Springfield, New Jersey

Chapter 7—Renal/Genitourinary Emergencies

Joanne Noone, RN, MSN, CCRN, CEN
Nursing Instructor, Kauai Community College
Lihue, Hawaii

Catherine Paradiso, RN, MSN, CCRN, CEN
Clinical Nurse Specialist for Critical Care
Veterans Administration Hospital
Instructor of Nursing
Kingsborough Community College
New York, New York

Chapter 8—Musculoskeletal/Skin Emergencies

Alice Belcher, RN, BSN, CCRN
Critical Care Educator
Dover General Hospital
Dover, New Jersey

Deborah Reilly, RN, MSN, CEN
Nurse Care Coordinator
Emergency Department
Staten Island Hospital
New York, New York

John P. Reilly, MD
Fellow, Orthopedic Traumatology
Maryland Institute for Emergency Medical Services
Baltimore, Maryland

Chapter 9—Gynecologic Emergencies

Vincent J. Ferragano, MD (consultant)
Attending Physician, Obstetrics & Gynecology
Staten Island Hospital
Assistant Clinical Professor
State University of New York Health Sciences Center
New York, New York

Joanne Lapidus-Graham, RN, MA
Instructor, Maternal/Child Nursing
Molloy College
Rockville Centre, New York

Lisa Mayercik, RN, BSN
Assistant Head Nurse, Maternity
Staten Island Hospital
New York, New York

Theresa Nauta, RN, MSN
Obstetrical Inservice Clinician
Maimonides Medical Center
New York, New York

Chapter 10—Eye/Ear/Nose/Throat Emergencies

Laura Gasparis, RN, MA, CCRN, CEN
Assistant Professor of Nursing
College of Staten Island
New York, New York

Patricia Murphy, MD
Attending Physician, EENT
Long Island College Hospital
New York, New York

Neil Nepola, MD
Family Physician
Attending Physician, Emergency Department
Bayley Seton Hospital
New York, New York

Chapter 11—Systemic Emergencies
Alice Belcher, RN, BSN, CCRN
Critical Care Educator, Dover General Hospital
Dover, New Jersey

Kathleen McMahon, RN, MSN, CEN
Assistant Director of Nurses
Treat and Release Center
New York, New York

Joanne Scotto, RN, BSN
Clinic Nurse-Ambulatory Care
Staten Island Hospital
President, Health Awareness, Inc.
New York, New York

Chapter 12—Gastrointestinal Emergencies
Stephanie Higie, RN, BSN, CEN
Trauma Nurse Coordinator
University Medical Center
Tucson, Arizona

Joanne Noone, RN, MSN, CCRN, CEN
Nursing Instructor, Kauai Community College
Lihue, Hawaii

Patricia Tooker, RN, MSN, CCRN
Supervisor, Critical Care
Bayley Seton Hospital
New York, New York

Chapter 13—Hematologic Emergencies
Patricia Robertazza, RN, MSN, CCRN
Critical Care Educator
Kimball Medical Center
Lakewood, New Jersey

Susan Weaver, RN, MSN, CCRN, CEN
Critical Care Educator
St. Claire's Medical Center
Denville, New Jersey

Chapter 14—Behavioral Emergencies
Linda Reese, RN, MA
Assistant Professor of Nursing
College of Staten Island
New York, New York

Nancy C. Seddio, RN, CS, PhD
Clinical Nurse Specialist in Psychiatry
Interfaith Medical Center
Brooklyn, New York
Psychotherapist, Private Practice
New York, New York

Chapter 15—Abuse/Neglect/Sexual Assault
Mary Blum, RN, MSN
Instructor of Nursing
Rutgers—The State University
Newark, New Jersey

Catherine T. Kelly, RN, MSN, EMT-P, CCRN, CEN
Clinical Nurse Specialist/Chief Flight Nurse
Emergency Department
St. Francis Hospital
Poughkeepsie, New York

Chapter 16—Roles and Responsibilities of the Emergency Nurse
Carol A. Bottin, RN
Lecturer/Consultant
Procurement Coordinator
Organ Retrieval Program
Department of Surgery
University of Florida
Jacksonville, Florida

Joanne Noone, RN, MSN, CCRN, CEN
Nursing Instructor
Kauai Community College
Lihue, Hawaii

Susan Schulmerich, RN, MS, MBA, CNA, CEN
Administrator, Emergency Department
North Central Bronx Hospital
New York, New York

Joanne Scotto, RN, BSN
Clinic Nurse
Staten Island Hospital
President, Health Awareness, Inc.
New York, New York

David Weaver, Esq. (consultant)
Trapasso, Dolan, & Hollander
Newton, New Jersey

Chapter 17—Challenges in Dosage Calculations
Laura Gasparis, RN, MA, CCRN, CEN
Assistant Professor of Nursing
College of Staten Island
New York, New York

June L. Olsen, RN, MS
Deputy Chairperson
College of Staten Island
New York, New York

Acknowledgments

We would like to express our heartfelt gratitude to many people. First, we owe our deepest thanks to our contributing authors for their inspiring commitment to the creation of this book.

Secondly, we want to thank Fay Gasparis, who demonstrated a nearly psychic ability to decipher reams of handwritten material accompanied by complicated format directions. From these piles of scribbled sheets, she consistently produced beautiful manuscript pages in time for every deadline, all the while enthusiastically responding to the material she was typing.

Special thanks to Louise DeVito and Eugenia Borgia Murray, RN, BA. It is for her many helpful suggestions that we are indebted to our personal editorial consultant, Mrs. Murray, who seemed to have an extraordinary gift using words correctly. Thanks for helping this book become reality.

And lastly, thank you to our special friends at Springhouse—Marie Connor, editorial assistant, and Regina Ford, our editor. They remained energetic and positively encouraging, tactfully delivering valuable feedback, helpful suggestions, and ever-so-gentle criticisms of the work in progress. Their guiding support served ultimately to make this book as responsive as possible to the needs of our readers.

These people believed in this book before it was a reality, and we are grateful to them for their dedication.

L.G. and J.N.

To my mom, Fay Gasparis, whose continuous encouragement and endless assistance brighten my life.

L.G.

To my son, Jesse Noone.

J.N.

Foreword

Emergency Nursing Examination Review presents a structured study guide that allows you to update your clinical knowledge as you prepare for the Emergency Nursing Certification examination. Successful completion of this examination qualifies you as a Certified Emergency Nurse (CEN), ready to take your place on the multidisciplinary emergency medical service provider team.

As you know, death and disability are reduced significantly when skilled professional personnel are immediately available to provide specialized emergency care. This care must be delivered by a competent multidisciplinary professional team in an emergency care facility.

To provide effective emergency care, you, as a team member, must possess the basic and advanced theoretical knowledge and practical skills that will enable you to work with other professionals without compromising your own professional identity.

Passing the state boards is only the first step in the professional development of a CEN. Interdisciplinary cooperation and understanding is also required because of cost containment, increased consumer awareness, and the threat of malpractice suits. The complexities of today's health care technology mandate specialization.

Recognizing the need for quality emergency nursing care, the Emergency Nurses Association (ENA) developed *Standards of Emergency Nursing Practice* (ENA, 1983) and published the *Emergency Nursing Core Curriculum* (ENA, 3rd edition, 1987). The core curriculum, based on emergency nursing standards, defines the basic knowledge and practical skills needed to practice emergency nursing.

The Board of Certification of Emergency Nursing developed the certification process to measure the attainment and application of this knowledge and to certify the competency of the CEN. Since emergency nursing practice is constantly changing and evolving, the CEN must validate this certification by achieving a passing score on the CEN examination every 5 years.

You'll find this book valuable and challenging, as the contributors are not only experts, but also clinically active in their respective content areas. This book serves as a thorough resource for the specified knowledge that underlies emergency nursing practice. Using it allows you to review your mastery of the *Emergency Nursing Core Curriculum.*

Emergency Nursing Examination Review is packed with information that will foster professional development and clinical competence; it is an excellent way to prepare for the CEN examination. Best of luck in the examination—you have chosen a dynamic, challenging nursing specialty.

MAUREEN V. O'BRIEN, RN, MA
Assistant Vice-President, Ambulatory Services,
Richmond Memorial Hospital, New York;
Nurse Consultant, New York State Nurses Association
Emergency Medical Services
New York State EMT Association;
Director, Irish/American Emergency Care Conference

Introduction

Unlike many specialities, emergency health care, with its many nurses, physicians, emergency medical technicians, and paramedics, has demonstrated how important it is to maintain and perfect the team concept. The ultimate goal of every member of the emergency health care team is to provide immediate, competent emergency care.

This book is a learning and teaching tool designed to increase your self-confidence and effectiveness in an emergency. The multiple choice question-and-answer format allows you to test your knowledge of assessment and intervention skills.

Through education and certification, the Emergency Nurses Association actively promotes the practice of emergency nursing as a specialty. We believe that all emergency nurses should seek further clinical knowledge and demonstrate competency through the certification process.

About the CEN Examination

The emergency certification examination was first offered in July 1980. Each nurse who passes this test is recognized as a Certified Emergency Nurse (CEN). The purpose of the certification examination is to help you measure your knowledge of emergency nursing practices.

The Emergency Nursing Certification examination contains a maximum of 250 multiple-choice, objective questions. The total testing time is 4 hours. The test is weighted as follows:

I. Nursing Practice	
Assessment	30.5%
Analysis/Nursing Diagnosis	15.0%
Planning/Intervention	30.0%
Evaluation	14.5%
II. Professional Issues	10.0%
	100%

Although the test begins at 9:00 a.m., you are expected to be at the test center by 8:00 a.m. Test-takers are seated alphabetically in various rooms. Be sure to bring two forms of identification to the examination, for example, any photo I.D. and your hospital admission ticket.

Two proctors usually are present in each room.

Immediately before the test, you'll have time to review the instructions for filling out the answer sheet. This sheet has a grid format that should be filled out in pencil. Make sure you bring at least two #2 pencils. However, if you forget, the proctors usually have extras. Bring calipers with you if you feel you need them to decipher a rhythm. However, there are usually only a few rhythm strips on the CEN examination. A nonprinting calculator is also allowed.

Carefully follow the instructions for filling out the grid, as your test results may be delayed if there is an error. The test comes in a sealed booklet. Do not break the seal before you are told to do so. When the test begins, the proctors periodically will let you know how much time remains by writing it on a blackboard.

Test-Taking Tips

1. Take a vacation from studying a few days before the test. Too much studying may tire you so much that you may not do well on the test. Resting a few days will help you get things in perspective. If possible, take the day before the test off.

2. Get a good night's sleep the night before the test. Being rested will give you an edge that you may not have if you're exhausted.

3. When you see the test for the first time, scan the first page for a question you can easily answer. This will give you the confidence you need to approach the test without panic.

4. Check the answer sheet frequently during the test to make sure you aren't making small but serious errors, such as answering Question #2 in Question #3's box. Such an error will affect your entire test score.

5. Our best advice is to keep the first answer you choose. It is probably right. The more you fret over which answer to select, the more indecisive you can become. If you don't know an answer, come back to it later. Try to narrow down your choices to the point where your guess has greater odds of being correct. For example, if you can narrow your choices down to two answers and then guess, you have a 50% chance of being correct.

6. Try to relax. Remember, overwhelming anxiety will hamper you. Don't let this test intimidate you, even though it's important for you to pass. Also remember, you've prepared well for this test; you will have studied our book.

7. If you've taken the test before, you've already had a valuable test-taking experience. This experience plus the help you'll receive from this book will give you that extra edge you need to pass the test this time.

Good luck! We hope our efforts will prove helpful to you. Let us hear from you. We look forward to comments from our readers on our book.

Laura Gasparis
Joanne Noone

Chapter 1

Fluid, Electrolyte, and Acid-Base Alterations Questions and Answers

You must begin with Question 1 of this chapter and progress in sequence. **Do not skip around.** Subsequent answers build on previous ones.

Marcia Downs, RN, CEN
David Unkle, RN, CCRN, CEN
Consultant: Charles T. Vonfrolio, MD

SITUATION

A 17-year-old female model comes to your emergency department (ED) complaining of generalized cramps and numbness in her fingers. Medical history is noncontributory. When questioned, she tells you that she has been on a high-protein diet for "about 6 weeks." An I.V. line is started and blood is drawn for laboratory studies. Her serum calcium level is 5.5 mg/dl.

Questions 1 to 4 refer to the above situation.

1 In assessing this patient for hypocalcemia, Chvostek's sign is elicited by:

A. Applying a blood pressure (BP) cuff to the upper arm, inflating it, and observing for carpopedal spasm
B. Tapping a finger on the skin above the supramandibular portion of the parotid gland and observing for twitching of the upper lip on side opposite stimulation
C. Tapping a finger on the skin above the supramandibular portion of the parotid gland and observing for twitching of the upper lip on same side as stimulation
D. Having the patient hyperventilate (more than 30 breaths/minute) to produce carpopedal spasm resulting from respiratory alkalosis

2 Trousseau's sign can be elicited in the hypocalcemic patient by:

A. Applying a BP cuff to upper arm, inflating it, and observing for carpopedal spasm
B. Tapping a finger on the supramandibular portion of the parotid gland and observing for twitching of the upper lip on the side opposite to the stimulation
C. Tapping a finger on the supramandibular portion of the parotid gland and observing for twitching of the upper lip on the same side as stimulation
D. Having the patient hyperventilate (more than 30 breaths/minute) to produce carpopedal spasm resulting from respiratory acidosis

3 Patients with hypocalcemia demonstrate which of the following EKG changes?

A. Shortened PR interval
B. Prolonged PR interval
C. Prolonged QT interval
D. U wave

4 Complications that may develop in the hypocalcemic patient include all of the following *except*:

A. Seizures or twitching
B. Oliguria or anuria
C. Laryngeal stridor
D. Bleeding abnormalities

SITUATION

A 71-year-old woman is transported to the ED because of fatigue and a change in mental status. On physical examination, her temperature is 96.8° F. (36° C.) rectally. Her BP is 110/74 mm Hg; pulse, 48 beats/minute; respirations, 12 breaths/minute; periorbital edema is present, and a yellowish skin pigmentation is noted. Her daughter relates a history of "thyroid problem" and noncompliance with medical therapy. The diagnosis of myxedema coma is made.

Questions 5 to 8 refer to the above situation.

5 The patient admitted with hypothyroid crisis (myxedema coma) would most likely have which of the following electrolyte abnormalities?

A. Hyponatremia
B. Hypernatremia
C. Hyperglycemia
D. Hypocalcemia

6 Which of the following acid-base imbalances is most likely to occur in this patient?

A. Respiratory acidosis
B. Respiratory alkalosis without compensation
C. Metabolic alkalosis
D. Respiratory alkalosis with compensation

7 Which of the following signs and symptoms are likely to be seen in this patient?

A. Increased urine output and hyperactive bowel sounds
B. Oliguria and abdominal distention
C. Diarrhea and polydipsia
D. Polycythemia and hypothermia

8 Which of the following I.V. fluids is most likely to be used in caring for this patient?

A. 5% dextrose in water (D_5W)
B. 10% dextrose in water
C. 5% dextrose in 0.9% sodium chloride (D_5NS)
D. 0.3% sodium chloride

SITUATION

A 78-year-old woman presents herself to your ED with the chief complaint of abdominal cramping. She states that she has had "diarrhea and has felt tired for about a week." She has a history of diabetes mellitus and chronic renal failure. An I.V. line is established and blood is drawn for laboratory studies. Her serum potassium level (K^+) is 6 mEq/liter. The diagnosis of hyperkalemia is made.

Questions 9 to 12 refer to the above situation.

9 The nurse would anticipate pharmacologic management of hyperkalemia to include all of the following *except*:

A. Lactulose enemas
B. 50% dextrose and regular insulin
C. Sodium bicarbonate
D. Calcium chloride

10 Patients with hyperkalemia need to be monitored for which of the following EKG changes?

A. Prolonged QT interval
B. Peaked T waves
C. Prominent U waves
D. Shortened PR interval

11 When performing the physical assessment on the patient with hyperkalemia, which of the following signs and symptoms can the nurse expect to find?

A. Apathy, oliguria, and absent bowel sounds
B. Ascending muscle weakness and bradycardia
C. Descending muscle weakness and tachycardia
D. Hyperactive bowel sounds and polyuria

12 Which of the following acid-base imbalances is commonly associated with hyperkalemia?

A. Respiratory acidosis
B. Metabolic alkalosis
C. Respiratory alkalosis
D. Metabolic acidosis

SITUATION

A 52-year-old man with newly diagnosed multiple myeloma is admitted to your ED with back pain. He states that he fell against a bookcase at home. X-rays reveal a rib fracture. Electrolyte measurements reveal a serum calcium level of 12.7 mg/dl. The diagnosis of hypercalcemia is made.

Questions 13 to 16 refer to the above situation.

13 Hypercalcemia occurs in multiple myeloma as a result of:

A. Calcium being mobilized from intestines, teeth, and bones
B. "Lesions" releasing calcium into plasma
C. Increased tubular reabsorption of calcium
D. Increased intestinal reabsorption of calcium, secondary to excessive vitamin D intake

14 The nurse should be aware that the complications of hypercalcemia may include:

A. Flank or thigh pain and polyuria
B. Anuria or oliguria and constipation
C. Diarrhea and metabolic alkalosis
D. Constipation and metabolic acidosis

15 Which of the following EKG changes occurs in the patient with hypercalcemia?

A. Prolonged PR interval
B. Prolonged QT interval
C. Shortened ST segment
D. U waves

16 Treatment modalities to correct hypercalcemia include:

A. Normal saline infusion and loop diuretics
B. Normal saline infusion and thiazide diuretics
C. Sodium polystyrene sulfonate (Kayexalate) enemas
D. Hemodialysis, glucose, and insulin

SITUATION

A 64-year-old man is admitted to the ED with altered mental status, jaundice, and increased abdominal girth. Medical history is significant for cirrhosis. An I.V. line is established and blood is drawn for laboratory studies. Liver enzyme levels (serum glutamic oxaloacetic transaminase [SGOT], serum glutamic pyruvic transaminase [SGPT], bilirubin) are elevated. The diagnosis of hepatic encephalopathy is made.

Questions 17 to 22 refer to the above situation.

17 The patient with hepatic failure should be monitored for which one of the following?

A. Hypercalcemia
B. Hyperproteinemia
C. Hypokalemia
D. Free water depletion

18 This patient also should be assessed for:

A. Decreased plasma protein level
B. Decreased serum aldosterone level
C. Decreased antidiuretic hormone (ADH) secretion
D. Movement of potassium into the intracellular space

19 Respiratory alkalosis, a common acid-base imbalance seen in hepatic failure, is a result of:

A. High blood ammonia levels, acting as a respiratory stimulant
B. Hypocalcemia, causing neuromuscular irritability
C. Hypokalemia, causing hyperventilation
D. Hypomagnesemia, causing hypoventilation

20 Aldosterone-blocking agents, such as spironolactone (Aldactone), may be administered to the patient who has hepatic failure. The mechanism of action of these agents involves:

A. Sodium retention and potassium excretion
B. Sodium excretion and potassium retention
C. Sodium excretion and magnesium retention
D. Sodium and potassium excretion

21 All of the following are used to treat hepatic failure *except*:

A. Sodium polystyrene sulfonate (Kayexalate) enemas to remove excess potassium
B. Limiting the administration of hypotonic solutions
C. Decreasing or eliminating dietary protein intake
D. Decreasing dietary sodium intake

22 Restricting the patient's water intake is based on:

A. An elevated plasma potassium level
B. An elevated plasma sodium level
C. A decreased plasma sodium level
D. A decreased magnesium level

SITUATION

A 28-year-old woman is admitted to your ED after a house fire. She has second- and third-degree burns over approximately 30% of her body surface area (BSA), including her face. Endotracheal intubation is performed, and I.V. lines are established.

Questions 23 to 27 refer to the above situation.

23 I.V. therapy for this patient is based on all of the following *except*:

A. Gender and medical history
B. Depth and percentage of burn
C. Urine output and urine specific gravity
D. Hemoglobin and hematocrit values

24 The parenteral solution most frequently used as fluid replacement for the patient with burns is:

A. D_5W
B. Lactated Ringer's solution
C. Hypotonic saline solution
D. 5% dextrose in 0.45% saline with 20 mEq potassium chloride

25 During initial treatment, fluid replacement at 4 ml/kg/ percent of burns is given over the first 24 hours. The calculated amount of solution is divided so that:

A. ⅓ of the solution is given every 8 hours
B. ½ of the solution is given in the initial 8 hours; ½ in the next 16 hours
C. ½ of the solution is given in the first 12 hours; ½ in the next 12 hours
D. ½ of the solution is given in the first 16 hours; ½ in the next 8 hours

26 In the *initial* stages (first 3 days) of burn injuries, which of the following fluid and electrolyte imbalances are likely to occur?

A. Interstitial-to-plasma fluid shift and sodium excess
B. Plasma-to-interstitial fluid shift and potassium excess
C. Interstitial-to-extracellular space fluid shift and sodium deficit
D. Intracellular-to-intravascular compartment fluid shift and potassium deficit

27 In the *later* stages (after 3 days) of burn injuries, which of the following fluid and electrolyte imbalances are likely to occur?

A. Interstitial-to-plasma fluid shift and potassium deficit
B. Plasma-to-interstitial fluid shift and potassium deficit
C. Plasma-to-intracellular fluid shift and potassium deficit
D. Intravascular-to-interstitial fluid shift and sodium deficit

SITUATION

A 40-year-old man is admitted to the ED with lethargy and tachypnea. His skin is dry and flushed, and he has a fruity breath odor. An I.V. line is started and blood is drawn for laboratory studies. His blood glucose level is 840 mg/dl, and his urinalysis reveals +3 glucose, +3 ketones. The diagnosis of diabetic ketoacidosis (DKA) is made.

Questions 28 to 31 refer to the above situation.

28 Physiologic abnormalities that are likely to occur in this patient include all of the following *except*:

A. Hypoosmolality
B. Hyperkalemia
C. Hypocapnia
D. Dehydration

29 The *first* priority in caring for this patient would be to:

A. Administer insulin I.V.
B. Administer insulin subcutaneously
C. Administer isotonic saline and insulin I.V.
D. Establish and monitor an airway

30 The I.V. solution most frequently used to treat a patient with DKA is:

A. Isotonic saline solution
B. Hypotonic saline solution
C. Hypertonic saline solution
D. Lactated Ringer's solution

31 Continuous evaluation of this patient's serum potassium level is likely to demonstrate:

A. Initial elevation, then gradual decrease
B. Initial decrease, then gradual elevation
C. Increase while generally remaining elevated
D. Decrease while generally remaining low

SITUATION

A 12-year-old boy is admitted to your ED complaining of difficulty in breathing. His parents say that he has "never been this bad before." The family has had a long history of asthma, and the boy has had wheezing in the past. Arterial blood gas (ABG) studies performed while the patient is breathing room air (21% oxygen) reveal pH, 7.21; PO_2*, 65 mm Hg;* PCO_2*, 62 mm Hg; and* HCO_3^-*, 24 mEq/liter.*

Questions 32 to 35 refer to the above situation.

32 This child's ABG measurements reflect:

A. Metabolic acidosis
B. Metabolic alkalosis
C. Respiratory acidosis
D. Respiratory alkalosis

33 The rationale for interpretation of this ABG measurement is supported by:

A. Low PO_2, low pH
B. Low PO_2, high PCO_2
C. Low PO_2, normal bicarbonate
D. High PCO_2, low pH

34 When caring for this patient, which of the following nursing actions holds the *lowest* priority?

A. Oxygen therapy
B. Inhaled bronchodilator therapy
C. Continuous cardiac monitoring
D. Preparation for possible tracheotomy

35 If immediate therapy is not implemented, which of the following complications is most likely to occur?

A. Respiratory arrest
B. Gastric aspiration
C. Adult respiratory distress syndrome (ARDS)
D. Acute renal failure

SITUATION

The patient stops breathing shortly after you have begun inhaled bronchodilator therapy. He is initially ventilated with a bag-valve-mask device, and good chest rise is achieved bilaterally. He is then intubated with an orotracheal tube, and ventilation is continued. A repeat ABG analysis shows the pH to be 7.12; PCO_2, 55 mm Hg; PO_2, 33 mm Hg; HCO_3^-, 25 mEq/liter. No loss of vital signs is noted. He is given 100 mEq of sodium bicarbonate. Ten minutes later, blood gas analysis shows pH, 7.55; PCO_2, 35 mm Hg; PO_2, 425 mm Hg; and HCO_3^-, 36.5 mEq/liter.

Questions 36 to 38 refer to the above situation.

36 Which of the following acid-base imbalances does this patient exhibit now?

A. Metabolic acidosis
B. Metabolic alkalosis
C. Respiratory acidosis
D. Respiratory alkalosis

37 The most likely cause for this imbalance is:

A. Respiratory arrest
B. Hyperventilation with bag-valve-mask device
C. Excessive bicarbonate administration
D. Excessive oxygen administration

38 The correct treatment in this situation should have been:

A. Hyperventilation with bag-valve-mask device
B. Sodium bicarbonate 1 mEq/kg I.V. push
C. 40% oxygen via Venturi mask
D. Epinephrine 0.5 to 1 mg I.V.

SITUATION

A 37-year-old woman comes to your ED having ingested 10 5-mg Valiums (diazepam) about 2 hours ago. She appears excited and nervous. Her blood pressure is 145/70 mm Hg; pulse, 124 beats/minute; respiratory rate, 44 breaths/minute; and temperature, 99.5° F. (37.5° C.). She complains of circumoral tingling and numbness, as well as tingling in her hands and feet. ABG studies, while the patient is receiving 28% O_2 by face mask, show pH, 7.60; PCO_2, 15 mm Hg; PO_2, 140 mm Hg; and HCO_3^-, 22 mEq/liter.

Questions 39 to 42 refer to the above situation.

39 This patient is in a state of:

A. Metabolic acidosis
B. Metabolic alkalosis
C. Respiratory acidosis
D. Respiratory alkalosis

40 The goal of treatment for this patient is to increase:

A. Oxygenation
B. Ventilation
C. HCO_3^-
D. CO_2 retention

41 Which of the following statements is *false* regarding the care of this patient?

A. After treatment in the ED, follow-up is necessary
B. The patient is having an anxiety attack
C. Treatment includes rebreathing exhaled CO_2
D. Treatment includes bicarbonate administration I.V.

42 The patient is experiencing numbness and tingling because:

A. Alkalosis causes vasodilation
B. Hypocapnia causes vasoconstriction
C. The pills the patient ingested are causing these symptoms
D. None of the above

SITUATION

A 78-year-old, 155-lb (70-kg) man was admitted to the ED about 4 hours ago, complaining of difficulty in voiding. He lives in a nursing home. Temperature upon arrival was 104.5° F. (40.2° C.). His respirations are labored, and he is tachycardic. ABG analysis reveals pH, 7.01; PO_2, 125 mm Hg (28% O_2); PCO_2, 42 mm Hg; and HCO_3^-, 2.3 mEq/liter.

Questions 43 to 46 refer to the above situation.

43 The correct interpretation of these data is:

A. Metabolic acidosis
B. Metabolic alkalosis
C. Respiratory acidosis
D. Respiratory alkalosis

44 In this situation, what is the bicarbonate deficit?

A. 2.3 mEq/liter
B. 10.7 mEq/liter
C. 21.7 mEq/liter
D. 39.7 mEq/liter

45 How many milliequivalents of sodium bicarbonate will be needed to correct this abnormality?

A. 70 mEq
B. 135 mEq
C. 250 mEq
D. 380 mEq

46 Which laboratory studies are likely to be of assistance in treating this patient?

A. Complete blood count (CBC) and reticulocyte count
B. Creatine phosphokinase (CPK) isoenzymes and serum amylase level
C. Lactate level and anion gap
D. Electrolyte studies and acetone level

SITUATION

You are in the midst of resuscitating a 45-year-old man. ABG measurements (obtained 5 minutes ago) show pH, 7.15; P_{O_2}, 55 mm Hg; P_{CO_2}, 60 mm Hg; and HCO_3^-, 18 mEq/liter.

Questions 47 to 49 refer to the above situation.

47 The correct interpretation of these data is:

A. Fully compensated respiratory acidosis
B. Fully compensated metabolic acidosis
C. Partially compensated respiratory alkalosis
D. Mixed metabolic and respiratory acidosis

48 The best initial therapy for this patient is:

A. Improved oxygenation and hyperventilation
B. Immediate defibrillation
C. Sodium bicarbonate administration
D. Epinephrine administration

49 What two blood gas parameters seriously compromise the myocardial function in this patient?

A. Hypoxemia and low bicarbonate level
B. Acidosis and hypoxemia
C. Acidosis and low bicarbonate level
D. Acidosis and hypercapnia

SITUATION

A family of five comes to a small, rural ED, complaining of headaches, malaise, nausea, and vomiting. This occurs during the winter, and toxic ingestion or inhalation is suspected. ABG measurements are pH, 7.25; PCO_2, 47 mm Hg; PO_2, 97 mm Hg; O_2 saturation, 75%; and HCO_3^-, 15 mEq/liter.

Questions 50 to 52 refer to the above situation.

50 This family's symptoms suggest:

A. Viral syndrome
B. CO_2 narcosis
C. Carbon monoxide poisoning
D. Radon poisoning

51 The initial treatment for this family should include:

A. Breathing into a paper bag
B. 100% O_2 via rebreather mask
C. Acetylcysteine (Mucomyst) inhalant therapy
D. I.V. bronchodilator therapy

52 Secondary treatment of this problem includes:

A. Hyperbaric therapy
B. Exploratory laparotomy
C. Cardiopulmonary bypass surgery
D. Hemodialysis

Answer Sheet

	A	B	C	D		A	B	C	D
1	○	○	○	○	31	○	○	○	○
2	○	○	○	○	32	○	○	○	○
3	○	○	○	○	33	○	○	○	○
4	○	○	○	○	34	○	○	○	○
5	○	○	○	○	35	○	○	○	○
6	○	○	○	○	36	○	○	○	○
7	○	○	○	○	37	○	○	○	○
8	○	○	○	○	38	○	○	○	○
9	○	○	○	○	39	○	○	○	○
10	○	○	○	○	40	○	○	○	○
11	○	○	○	○	41	○	○	○	○
12	○	○	○	○	42	○	○	○	○
13	○	○	○	○	43	○	○	○	○
14	○	○	○	○	44	○	○	○	○
15	○	○	○	○	45	○	○	○	○
16	○	○	○	○	46	○	○	○	○
17	○	○	○	○	47	○	○	○	○
18	○	○	○	○	48	○	○	○	○
19	○	○	○	○	49	○	○	○	○
20	○	○	○	○	50	○	○	○	○
21	○	○	○	○	51	○	○	○	○
22	○	○	○	○	52	○	○	○	○
23	○	○	○	○					
24	○	○	○	○					
25	○	○	○	○					
26	○	○	○	○					
27	○	○	○	○					
28	○	○	○	○					
29	○	○	○	○					
30	○	○	○	○					

Answer Sheet

	A	B	C	D		A	B	C	D
1	○	○	○	○	31	○	○	○	○
2	○	○	○	○	32	○	○	○	○
3	○	○	○	○	33	○	○	○	○
4	○	○	○	○	34	○	○	○	○
5	○	○	○	○	35	○	○	○	○
6	○	○	○	○	36	○	○	○	○
7	○	○	○	○	37	○	○	○	○
8	○	○	○	○	38	○	○	○	○
9	○	○	○	○	39	○	○	○	○
10	○	○	○	○	40	○	○	○	○
11	○	○	○	○	41	○	○	○	○
12	○	○	○	○	42	○	○	○	○
13	○	○	○	○	43	○	○	○	○
14	○	○	○	○	44	○	○	○	○
15	○	○	○	○	45	○	○	○	○
16	○	○	○	○	46	○	○	○	○
17	○	○	○	○	47	○	○	○	○
18	○	○	○	○	48	○	○	○	○
19	○	○	○	○	49	○	○	○	○
20	○	○	○	○	50	○	○	○	○
21	○	○	○	○	51	○	○	○	○
22	○	○	○	○	52	○	○	○	○
23	○	○	○	○					
24	○	○	○	○					
25	○	○	○	○					
26	○	○	○	○					
27	○	○	○	○					
28	○	○	○	○					
29	○	○	○	○					
30	○	○	○	○					

1 Correct answer—**C**

A decrease in ionized calcium causes an increase in neuromuscular excitability. Tapping over a branch of the facial nerve and observing for twitching of the upper lip on the ipsilateral (same) side as stimulation is considered a positive Chvostek's sign. Inflating a BP cuff on the upper arm or having the patient hyperventilate will both produce carpopedal spasm and are part of the diagnostic tests used to elicit Trousseau's sign.

2 Correct answer—**A**

Trousseau's sign is elicited by applying a BP cuff to the patient's arm, inflating to the patient's systolic pressure, and observing for carpopedal spasm. Another method for producing this phenomenon is hyperventilation, in which the alkalotic state decreases serum calcium levels.

3 Correct answer—**C**

Impairment of cardiac contractility results from hypocalcemia. This is demonstrated on the EKG as a prolonged QT interval, which predisposes the patient to a polymorphous ventricular tachycardia (Torsades de Pointes).

4 Correct answer—**B**

Bleeding abnormalities occur in hypocalcemia because calcium assists in converting prothrombin to thrombin in the coagulation cascade. Seizures result from the reduced calcium levels. Bronchospasm leading to laryngeal stridor results from neuromuscular irritability.

5 Correct answer—**A**

Patients with myxedema coma suffer from hyponatremia. This usually is a result of inappropriate secretion of antidiuretic hormone (ADH). Also, the myxedematous state results from the interstitial accumulation of a mucopolysaccharide substance that attracts water and produces water retention. Therefore, the hyponatremia is caused by dilution. Hypoglycemia is also seen in myxedema coma, owing to the hypometabolic state.

6 Correct answer—**A**

Respiratory acidosis and CO_2 narcosis are a result of lowered thyroxine (T_4) and tri-iodothyronine (T_3) levels. These hormones increase metabolic functions, such as respiration. Thus, a decrease in T_3 and T_4 levels depresses respiratory function, thereby causing hypoventilation. In addition, metabolic acidosis may develop as hypoxia increases serum lactate levels.

7 Correct answer—**B**

Patients with myxedema exhibit oliguria as a result of a decreased glomerular filtration rate (GFR) and decreased renal perfusion. Abdominal distention, a result of decreased peristalsis, may lead to paralytic ileus. A decrease in red blood cells (RBCs) is seen in myxedema.

8 Correct answer—**C**

Because patients with myxedema have a dilutional hyponatremia, fluid restriction is instituted initially, followed by administration of a hypertonic solution (D_5NS). A hypotonic solution such as D_5W or 0.3% sodium chloride would worsen the hyponatremia. Fluid therapy is aimed at correcting imbalances. In this case, D_5NS I.V. dextrose provides calories, and saline corrects hyponatremia.

9 Correct answer—**A**

Treatment of hyperkalemia consists of administration of calcium, glucose, insulin, and sodium bicarbonate. Glucose drives potassium into the cells, as does the administration of I.V. insulin. Sodium bicarbonate corrects the accompanying metabolic acidosis. I.V. calcium stimulates cardiac contractility. Lactulose is used in the treatment of hepatic failure.

10 Correct answer—**B**

An impairment of neuromuscular transmission produces intraventricular conduction disturbances. The predominant cardiac abnormalities are repolarization changes, reflected as a peaked T wave. This is seen in the initial states of hyperkalemia. As potassium levels increase, other changes occur, including prolongation of PR interval, absence of P waves, and widened QRS complex.

11 Correct answer—**B**

An *ascending* muscle weakness, usually originating in the lower extremities and traveling to the trunk, is seen in hyperkalemia. The diaphragm and intercostal muscles are usually spared; therefore, there is no impairment in respiratory function. Cardiac abnormalities include sinus bradycardia, prolonged PR interval, and widened QRS complex. Peristalsis is increased, and oliguria results from hyperkalemia. Apathy can be seen in both hypokalemic or hyperkalemic states.

12 Correct answer—**D**

Metabolic acidosis is the acid-base imbalance frequently seen with potassium excess. This occurs when potassium, rather than hydrogen, is exchanged for sodium in the kidney. Also, in an acidotic state, potassium is exchanged for hydrogen; thus, potassium shifts out of the cell.

13 Correct answer—**B**

In multiple myeloma, the calcium stores in the bone are released into the *extracellular* fluid, producing hypercalcemia. Hypercalcemia also results from the following: increased mobilization in primary hyperparathyroidism, increased intestinal reabsorption secondary to large dietary intake and excessive administration or intake of vitamin D, and altered renal tubular reabsorption.

14 Correct answer—**A**

Flank and thigh pain occurs as a result of renal calculi, which occur in approximately two thirds of patients with hypercalcemia. Polyuria is a result of inhibition of ADH by calcium in the distal tubules.

15 Correct answer—**C**

The increased extracellular levels of calcium predispose the patient to repolarization changes (shortening of ST segment) and ultimately cardiac arrest. If a patient is receiving digitalis therapy, hypercalcemia may cause an enhanced digitalis effect, which can contribute to dysrhythmias or arrest.

16 Correct answer—**A**

Normal saline solution is administered to increase the patient's GFR and calcium excretion. *Loop* diuretics are used to prevent tubular reabsorption of calcium. Other treatment modalities for hypercalcemia include corticosteroids to decrease gastrointestinal absorption of calcium, mythromycin therapy to stimulate bone uptake of calcium, and oral phosphates to bind calcium. Kayexalate therapy and glucose, insulin, and hemodialysis are used to treat hyperkalemia. Thiazide diuretics should be avoided, as they decrease calcium excretion.

17 Correct answer—**C**

In hepatic failure, hypokalemia occurs as a result of elevated aldosterone levels; aldosterone causes a loss of potassium. A *decreased* plasma protein level results from hypoalbuminemia. Calcium levels are decreased in hepatic failure because of inadequate storage of vitamin D. The patient with hepatic failure should be monitored for free water excess because of a plasma hyponatremia.

18 Correct answer—**A**

A decreased plasma protein level is a result of hypoalbuminemia. This loss mostly occurs in ascitic fluid (1 unit of blood contains as much albumin as 1 liter of ascitic fluid). This decreased protein level also allows intravascular fluid to enter the tissue, causing edema.

19 Correct answer—**A**

Respiratory alkalosis results from increased ammonia levels, which act to stimulate the respiratory drive and lead to hyperventilation. Hypermagnesemia will produce hypoventilation. Hypokalemia can result from metabolic alkalosis or renal tubular acidosis. Hypocalcemia is usually not associated with acid-base imbalances, except chronic renal failure (metabolic acidosis).

20 Correct answer—**B**

Aldosterone causes the body to retain both sodium and water and to excrete potassium. Spironolactone is an aldosterone-blocking agent that is used to enhance sodium excretion and potassium retention. Magnesium levels are decreased in hepatic failure.

21 Correct answer—**A**

Kayexalate enemas are not used in hepatic-failure treatment because potassium levels are already decreased. Lactulose enemas are used to eliminate intestinal ammonia. Limiting the administration of hypotonic solutions restricts free water intake. This is necessary to prevent further dilution of intravascular sodium, as a *plasma* hyponatremia is present in those patients with hepatic failure. Both dietary protein and sodium are restricted in the patient with hepatic failure.

22 Correct answer—**C**

A decreased *plasma* sodium level is usually an indication of dilutional hyponatremia; thus, water restriction should be enforced. The other values do not reflect changes in free water status.

23 Correct answer—**A**

Fluid resuscitation is a life-saving modality in the initial treatment of burns. Hemoconcentration, increased urine specific gravity, and oliguria are common sequelae in the early stages of burn injury. These are a result of intravascular depletion, as body fluids shift into the intracellular and interstitial compartments. Careful monitoring of urine specific gravity and urine output for signs of impending renal failure is necessary. The depth and percentage of burn injury (using the Rule of Nines) serve as the basis for determining the amount of fluid required.

24 Correct answer—**B**

The most common fluid used to manage the burn patient is lactated Ringer's solution. This isotonic solution assists in maintaining an adequate intravascular volume because large quantities of sodium and water are lost from the intravascular compartment during the initial postburn phase. Immediate fluid resuscitation protocol necessitates the rapid infusion of lactated Ringer's solution until the hemodynamic status of the patient is stable. Thereafter, resuscitation is solely with lactated Ringer's solution, usually at 4 ml/kg/percent of burn for the first 24 hours. Administering D_5W or a hypotonic saline solution is ineffective for fluid resuscitation because it does not correct electrolyte losses nor expand intravascular volume. Supplemental potassium replacement is usually not warranted since serum potassium levels are usually elevated from the existing cellular and muscle damage.

25 Correct answer—**B**

One half of the determined volume replacement is given in the first 8 hours, because this is the stage in which generalized dehydration and decreased circulating volume peak. The remaining fluid is administered over the next 16 hours. Vital signs, hourly urine output, and urine specific gravity must be monitored carefully to evaluate the patient's response to fluid resuscitation.

26 Correct answer—**B**

In the initial stages of burn injury, there is a *plasma*-to-*interstitial* fluid shift, causing a leakage through the capillaries, resulting in edema. Because of cellular trauma, a release of potassium to the extracellular space occurs, resulting in hyperkalemia. After the initial stage, usually after 36 hours, the body begins to mobilize burn edema; fluid shifts back into the intravascular space, thereby predisposing the patient to develop circulatory overload. At this time also, potassium is excreted in large amounts in the urine because of an increase in intravascular volume. Aldosterone, which reabsorbs sodium and excretes potassium, is released in large quantities in response to the dilutional hyponatremia that develops as intracellular and interstitial fluid shifts back into the intravascular compartment.

27 Correct answer—**A**

In the fluid remobilization phase (after 3 days) that follows burn injuries, there is an *interstitial*-to-*plasma* fluid shift into the intravascular compartment. A dilutional hyponatremia results. In response to a low serum sodium level, aldosterone is released. This results in reabsorption of sodium and excretion of potassium from the kidneys. Hypokalemia is further perpetuated as the expending intravascular volume fosters an increase in urine output with resultant potassium loss.

28 Correct answer—**A**

Initially, the hyperglycemic state shifts cellular fluid into the intravascular compartment, resulting in cellular dehydration. Glycosuria occurs and, as the glucose level exceeds tubular reabsorptive capacity, glucose remains in the renal tubules and acts as an osmotic diuretic. Circulatory insufficiency ensues; total fluid loss can average 8 to 10 liters. A serum hyperosmolality develops in response to elevated serum glucose level and intravascular fluid loss. Excessive ketone production leads to metabolic acidosis, which causes potassium to move from the cells into the intravascular fluid. Patients with DKA usually have depleted total-body potassium from renal losses. This effect of acidosis causes initial serum potassium levels to be elevated. Hypocapnia from hyperventilation also is present, as the body attempts to compensate in response to the metabolic acidosis.

29 Correct answer—**D**

The first priority in caring for *any* patient is to establish and maintain a patent airway. The patient with DKA should display Kussmaul's respirations (slow, deep, regular breathing) in response to the acidotic state. Frequent patient assessment and ABG studies are vital. Administrations of isotonic saline solution and I.V. insulin are secondary interventions in this situation.

30 Correct answer—**A**

The patient with DKA usually exhibits severe intravascular depletion and cellular dehydration. Efforts should be made to stabilize hemodynamic status initially by infusing isotonic saline solution to promote intravascular rehydration. Although isotonic, lactated Ringer's solution should be avoided in DKA because the lactate may cause a further increase in metabolic acidosis. If the circulatory system is stable but cellular dehydration is present, body fluid repletion can be achieved with a hypotonic solution, such as half normal saline solution. After fluid therapy and insulin administration have been initiated, careful monitoring of electrolyte and glucose levels is crucial. When the serum glucose level falls between 250 and 300 mg/dl, insulin is discontinued and fluid therapy is changed to a hypertonic solution containing glucose; for example, dextrose 5% in sodium chloride 0.45% (D_5½NS). This prevents the development of hypoglycemia, hypokalemia, and cerebral edema.

31 Correct answer—**A**

In DKA, serum potassium levels initially are elevated in response to the body's acidotic state, which causes shifting of cellular potassium into the intravascular space. However, in time, renal loss of potassium occurs from polyuria. Serum potassium is further depleted as potassium shifts into the intracellular compartment in response to insulin therapy and correction of acidosis.

32 Correct answer—**C**

Respiratory acidosis is an emergency situation in an asthmatic patient. During the early stages of an asthma attack, ABG measurements will reveal respiratory alkalosis from hyperventilation. As airway obstruction progresses, respiratory acidosis results.

33 Correct answer—**D**

The rationale for determining respiratory acidosis is that the PCO_2 is greater than 40 mm Hg (the respiratory component) and the pH is less than 7.35 (acidosis). The bicarbonate buffer is unchanged.

34 Correct answer—**D**

Preparing for possible tracheotomy is not a priority action, but it may be necessary to prepare for oral intubation if initial therapy is unsuccessful. Initial management includes O_2 administration, continuous cardiac monitoring, establishment of I.V. access, and delivery of inhaled bronchodilator therapy as ordered.

35 Correct answer—**A**

If this patient is not treated, respiratory arrest will occur as a result of airway obstruction, acidosis, and hypoxemia.

36 Correct answer—**B**

Metabolic alkalosis is indicated by a pH above 7.45 and an HCO_3^- level above 26 mEq/liter. The PCO_2 (respiratory component) is normal.

37 Correct answer—**C**

Metabolic alkalosis in this situation has resulted from overzealous administration of sodium bicarbonate. Respiratory arrest will result in a respiratory, and then metabolic, acidosis. Hyperventilation causes respiratory alkalosis. Excessive O_2 administration can cause O_2 toxicity and, in patients with obstructive lung disease, respiratory acidosis.

38 Correct answer—**A**

The patient's initial ABG measurements showed a respiratory acidosis, secondary to ineffective ventilation. Hyperventilating this patient with a bag-valve-mask device would have blown off CO_2, thus correcting the acidosis. Sodium bicarbonate is unnecessary because the HCO_3^- is normal. The patient's acid-base imbalance is unrelated to oxygen therapy. Epinephrine is not indicated because the patient did not lose pulse or blood pressure.

39 Correct answer—**D**

This patient is hyperventilating and, as a result, is in respiratory alkalosis. The pH is elevated above 7.45, and the PCO_2 (respiratory component) is low. The metabolic component of HCO_3^- is normal.

40 Correct answer—**D**

The goal of therapy for this patient is to increase CO_2 retention by helping the patient gain control of her respirations. That can be accomplished by using a paper bag to induce rebreathing of exhaled air, which will lead to CO_2 retention, breaking the cycle and slowing the respiratory rate.

41 Correct answer—**D**

The patient does not need sodium bicarbonate administration, which is indicated for metabolic acidosis. This woman had an anxiety attack and took an overdose of pills; she, therefore, requires either inpatient or outpatient follow-up.

42 Correct answer—**B**

This patient is experiencing numbness and tingling because hypocapnia produces vasoconstriction. CO_2 is a potent vasoactive agent. Hypocapnia leads to vasoconstriction of cerebral and peripheral vessels, which results in the paresthesias associated with hyperventilation.

43 Correct answer—**A**

The correct interpretation is metabolic acidosis. The pH is below 7.35, indicating acidosis; the respiratory component (PCO_2) is normal, but the metabolic component (HCO_3^-) is extremely low (normal, 22 to 26 mEq/liter), indicating an acid excess.

44 Correct answer—**C**

The bicarbonate deficit is 21.7 mEq/liter. The bicarbonate deficit is the amount of bicarbonate anion that would theoretically be necessary to fully correct the acid-base imbalance. It can be calculated by subtracting the measured bicarbonate (2.3) from the desired bicarbonate (average, 24).

45 Correct answer—**D**

A total of 380 mEq of sodium bicarbonate would be necessary to correct this acid-base imbalance. The calculation to correct this acidosis is: bicarbonate deficit × weight (in kg) × 0.25 = dose of sodium bicarbonate (in mEq). The amount 0.25 is a conversion factor that accounts for the bicarbonate space in the body. In this situation,

21.7 × 70 × 0.25 = 379.5 mEq of sodium bicarbonate. The patient may require a continuous infusion to receive this large amount of bicarbonate.

46 Correct answer—**C**

A lactate level and anion gap would help in treating this patient. An elevated lactate level (normal, 6 to 16 mg/dl) indicates lactic acidosis, usually a result of cardiogenic or septic shock or severe hypoxemia. An anion gap is calculated by subtracting serum anions from serum cations. The calculation is: anion gap = $(Na^+ + K^+)-(Cl^- + HCO_3^-)$. A normal anion gap is 12 mEq/liter. A metabolic acidosis with a normal anion gap results from a loss of HCO_3^-, such as with diarrhea or acute tubular necrosis or an excess of chloride, following the administration of calcium chloride or hydrochloric acid. A metabolic acidosis with an increased anion gap is seen in lactic acidosis, DKA, or uremia.

47 Correct answer—**D**

In this situation, the patient is in mixed metabolic and respiratory acidosis, a result of cardiopulmonary arrest. The pH is low; the respiratory component (PCO_2) is elevated, indicating CO_2 retention, and the metabolic component (HCO_3^-) is low, indicating excess systemic acids.

48 Correct answer—**A**

The initial therapy for this patient is to improve oxygenation and ventilation. If respiratory acidosis still exists after resuscitation measures have been instituted and the patient is intubated, some impediment to ventilation exists, such as pneumothorax, esophageal intubation, or pulmonary embolus. Improved oxygenation will prevent progression of metabolic acidosis. Sodium bicarbonate may then be required to reverse the metabolic acidosis. The patient's cardiac rhythm was not stated, so it is unclear whether defibrillation or epinephrine is indicated.

49 Correct answer—**B**

The two parameters that will cause a severe problem for this patient's myocardial function are acidosis and hypoxemia. Both depress contractility and reduce stroke volume. Myocardial contractility decreases dramatically as the pH falls below 7.24, a result of a dysfunction of calcium influx into the cell.

50 Correct answer—**C**

Carbon monoxide poisoning is suggested. An O_2 saturation of 75% in the presence of a PO_2 of 97 mm Hg suggests that a molecule other than oxygen is occupying the hemoglobin molecule. Diagnosis is confirmed by a high arterial carboxyhemoglobin level (normal, 0% to 2% in nonsmokers, 2% to 5% in smokers).

51 Correct answer—**B**

In an attempt to wash the carbon monoxide from the blood, the initial treatment for carbon monoxide poisoning is 100% O_2 by rebreather mask. This usually clears carbon monoxide in approximately 80 minutes.

52 Correct answer—**A**

Secondary treatment of carbon monoxide poisoning includes hyperbaric oxygen therapy. This family demonstrates carboxyhemoglobin levels above 20%, above which authorities recommend hyperbaric oxygen therapy. When carboxyhemoglobin levels approach 30%, permanent neurologic damage can occur if treatment is not begun.

Selected References

Alspach, J.G., and Williams, S.M. *Core Curriculum for Critical Care Nursing*, 3rd ed. Philadelphia: W.B. Saunders Co., 1985.

Felver, L. "Understanding the Electrolyte Maze." *American Journal of Nursing* 80:1591, September 1980.

Kee, J. *Fluids and Electrolytes with Clinical Applications: A Programmed Approach*. New York: John Wiley and Sons, 1982.

Linderman, R., and Papper, S. "Therapy of Fluid and Electrolyte Disorders." *Annals of Internal Medicine,* October 1980.

Maxwell, M., and Kleeman, C. *Clinical Disorders of Fluid and Electrolyte Metabolism*, 4th ed. New York: McGraw-Hill Book Co., 1986.

Metheny, N.M., and Snively, W.D., Jr. *Nurses Handbook of Fluid Balance*, 4th ed. Philadelphia: J.B. Lippincott Co., 1983.

Payne, N.R. "Emergency Care of the Patient with Myxedema Coma," *Journal of Emergency Nursing* 12:343, November/December 1986.

Rice, V. "The Role of Potassium in Health and Disease," *Critical Care Nurse* 2(3), May/June 1982.

Rose, Burton D. *Clinical Physiology of Acid-Base and Electrolyte Disorders*, 2nd ed. New York: McGraw-Hill Book Co., 1984

Sheehy, S.B., and Barber, J. *Emergency Nursing: Principles and Practice*, 2nd ed. St. Louis: C.V. Mosby Co., 1985.

Chapter 2

Shock
Questions and Answers

You must begin with Question 1 of this chapter and progress in sequence. **Do not skip around.** Subsequent answers build on previous ones.

Laura Gasparis, RN, MA, CCRN, CEN
Charles T. Vonfrolio, MD

SITUATION

A 26-year-old man was involved in an automobile accident. Approximately 20 minutes elapsed between the time of the accident and the arrival of the paramedics. He sustained severe abdominal injuries as well as multiple fractures. When he arrives in the emergency department (ED), his vital signs are: blood pressure (BP) 80/50 mm Hg; heart rate, 120 beats/minute; and respiratory rate, 30 breaths/minute.

Questions 1 to 6 refer to the above situation.

1 Which of the following nursing actions is *inappropriate* during the initial stabilization of this patient?

A. Administering oxygen therapy
B. Applying medical antishock trousers (MAST)
C. Placing the patient in the Trendelenburg (head-down) position
D. Infusing lactated Ringer's solution via a large-bore I.V. line

2 At the time of admission, the patient assessment findings most indicative of hypovolemic shock include:

A. Pulsus paradoxus
B. A hemoglobin value of 10/dl, hematocrit value of 38%
C. A widening pulse pressure
D. A central venous pressure (CVA) of 4 mm Hg

3 Patient assessment data that suggest hypovolemia as a cause of shock include:

A. Decreased central venous pressure (CVP) and distended neck veins only while the patient is prone
B. Increased urine sodium level, and a urine specific gravity of 1.010
C. A positive tilt-test result and a decreasing pulse pressure
D. Tachycardia with the presence of ventricular gallop (S_3)

4 Which of the following phrases best describes shock?

A. The inability of the body to excrete metabolic waste products
B. The collapse of the respiratory system
C. The collapse of the sympathetic nervous system
D. A state of inadequate tissue perfusion

5 Patients in early shock most likely have:

A. Metabolic acidosis
B. Metabolic alkalosis
C. Respiratory acidosis
D. Respiratory alkalosis

6 Patient integumentary assessment findings indicating that the compensatory response mechanisms for shock are failing include:

A. An increase in capillary refill time
B. Cool, clammy skin
C. Pale, moist skin
D. Mottled skin

7 Which of the following symptoms is a consequence of multiple transfusions?

A. Brudzinski's sign
B. Chvostek's sign
C. Cullen's sign
D. Babinski's sign

8 Administration of vasopressors such as dopamine (Intropin) is *least* beneficial for the patient in:

A. Cardiogenic shock
B. Distributive shock
C. Septic shock
D. Hypovolemic shock

9 The nurse should assess for hypovolemic shock in a patient admitted with:

A. A drug overdose
B. Postpartum fever
C. An intestinal obstruction
D. Cardiac tamponade

SITUATION

An 18-year-old man was injured when he lost control of his motorcycle and crashed into a tree. He was thrown from the motorcycle and sustained musculoskeletal and abdominal injuries. He is brought to the ED by paramedics. A MAST suit is in place.

Questions 10 to 13 refer to the above situation.

10 Which of the following statements regarding MAST suits is *false*?

A. It is a single-unit suit with three compartments
B. Each compartment may be pressurized and deflated individually or in combination
C. When inflated, it achieves pressures ranging from 0 to 160 mm Hg
D. Once optimal pressure is achieved, automatic release valves prevent further pressure increases

Shock Questions

11 The therapeutic effects of a MAST suit on the hypovolemic patient include:

A. Preload augmentation to increase stroke volume
B. Increased peripheral vascular resistance in those areas not under pressure
C. Decreased functional residual capacity and tidal volume
D. Decreased cerebral perfusion pressure

12 A MAST suit is *least* indicated for the patient with:

A. Spinal shock
B. Pelvic fractures
C. Severe intraabdominal bleeding
D. Bilateral hemothorax

13 Which of the following is the correct approach to using a MAST suit during patient stabilization?

A. Inflate to highest pressure then slowly deflate until desired response is obtained
B. When deflation is indicated, depressurize the leg segments, one at a time, then the abdominal segment
C. During deflation, if the patient's systolic blood pressure drops more than 5 mm Hg, stop and infuse fluids
D. If cyanosis of the feet occurs, even though dorsalis pedis pulses are palpable, decrease MAST pressure by 10 mm Hg

14 Which patient is *least* at risk for developing cardiogenic shock?

A. A 24-year-old patient with cardiac tamponade from a stab wound to the heart
B. A 72-year-old patient with a history of heart disease who has developed a dysrhythmia
C. A 55-year-old patient with acute pericarditis who underwent cardiac surgery 3 weeks ago
D. A 44-year-old patient with an anterolateral wall myocardial infarction (MI)

15 Clinical manifestations of cardiogenic shock include all of the following *except*:

A. Distended neck veins
B. Pulmonary congestion
C. Presence of an S_3
D. Low CVP

16 The management modality in cardiogenic shock that is *least* effective in protecting the myocardium from further damage is:

A. Decreasing peripheral vascular resistance
B. Decreasing ventricular preload
C. Increasing left ventricular afterload
D. Increasing cardiac output

17 When caring for the patient who has an acute MI, an early assessment finding that may indicate development of cardiogenic shock is:

A. Presence of an S_3
B. Bilateral crackles heard throughout inspiration
C. Warm, diaphoretic skin
D. Urine output of 30 ml in 1 hour

18 Evaluation of renal function in the patient with early circulatory failure does *not* reveal:

A. Increased blood urine nitrogen (BUN) level
B. Increased serum creatinine level
C. Decreased urine specific gravity
D. Decreased urine sodium level

19 For the patient in cardiogenic shock, the beneficial effect of vasodilator therapy is:

A. Increased systemic vascular pressure
B. Reduced preload and afterload
C. Increased pulmonary vascular pressure
D. Increased peripheral vascular resistance

20 The therapeutic outcome of inotropic agents used to manage the patient in cardiogenic shock is:

A. Vasodilation
B. Improved tissue perfusion
C. Increased heart rate
D. Decreased force of myocardial contractility

21 During assessment, your patient has a sharp decrease in systolic pressure and appears dyspneic. Crackles are heard bilaterally. A nursing priority at this time is to:

A. Begin a vasopressor drip
B. Rapidly infuse 0.45% saline solution to maintain BP
C. Place the patient in a supine position and elevate the legs to increase BP
D. Elevate the patient's head and administer oxygen

22 Considering the following admission histories, who is *least* at risk of developing septic shock?

A. A patient with multiple sclerosis who has an indwelling (Foley) catheter and a temperature of 100° F. (37.8° C.)
B. A patient with lung carcinoma who is receiving chemotherapy and radiation therapy
C. A patient with a permanent pacemaker that was inserted 1 week ago
D. A patient who severed two fingers while using garden machinery

23 When treatment is initiated for the patient with septic shock, which of the following actions receives the highest priority?

A. Obtaining an allergy history
B. Drawing blood for cultures, then administering antibiotic therapy
C. Initiating antibiotic therapy after obtaining urine culture results
D. Inserting a Foley catheter to monitor urine output

24 A patient admitted to the ED in the early stages of septic shock would present with the following symptoms:

A. Weak, thready pulses and low blood pressure
B. Decreased urine output and elevated serum creatinine level
C. Warm, flushed, moist skin
D. Hyperventilation and pulmonary congestion

25 During your assessment of the patient's respiratory system, which of the following findings indicates *early* septic shock?

A. Increased mucus production
B. Bilateral crackles
C. Hyperpnea
D. Respiratory acidosis

26 The nurse must know that patients with septic shock are depleted of intravascular fluid (hypovolemia). Which of the following factors does not cause hypovolemia in septic shock?

A. Leakage of fluid into tissues because of an increase in vessel permeability
B. Fluid loss associated with infections, such as sweating during fever, and respiratory losses during hyperventilation
C. Sequestering of plasma fluid in the extravascular spaces
D. Increased vascular resistance compromising blood flow to vital areas

27 Which of the following factors is *not* a likely explanation for the induction of the causative organisms of septic shock?

A. Bladder instrumentation
B. Childbirth
C. Appendectomy
D. A gingival abscess

28 Each of the following pharmacologic agents is an appropriate treatment for the management of septic shock *except*:

A. Beta-adrenergic blockers
B. Corticosteroids
C. Salicylates
D. Vasopressors

29 Which rationale is *not* responsible for the change in a patient's mental status during the early stages of septic shock?

A. Decreased cerebral perfusion because of the low flow state
B. Elevation of metabolic waste products such as BUN and creatinine because of decreased kidney perfusion
C. Alkalosis that results from hyperventilation, causing cerebral vascular constriction
D. Endotoxins acting directly on the central nervous system

SITUATION

Paramedics are transporting a 32-year-old woman with a severe anaphylactic reaction. Estimated time of arrival in the ED is 11 minutes.

Questions 30 to 36 refer to the above situation.

30 In most patients, anaphylaxis is precipitated by:

A. Insect venom
B. Food ingestion
C. Antibiotics
D. Blood transfusions

31 After exposure to an allergen, the patient usually develops the symptoms of anaphylaxis within:

A. 2 to 20 minutes
B. 20 to 60 minutes
C. 48 hours
D. 3 days

32 Which of the following clinical manifestations has the *lowest* priority for intervention:

A. Inspiratory wheezing
B. Stridor
C. Hoarseness
D. Angioneurotic edema

33 Which of the following symptoms is *not* considered a classic manifestation of anaphylaxis?

A. Urticaria or diffuse erythema
B. Laryngeal edema with bronchospasm
C. Hypotension
D. Paresthesias

34 Each of the following is a treatment used in the initial management of anaphylaxis *except*:

A. Corticosteroids
B. I.V. fluids
C. Epinephrine
D. Benadryl

35 The pharmacologic agent *least* likely to be used during the treatment of the patient with anaphylaxis is:

A. Hydrocortisone (Cortef)
B. Dobutamine (Dobutrex)
C. Aminophylline (Aminophyllin)
D. Antihistamines

36 Which of the following principles should hold the highest priority when caring for the patient with a history of allergies?

A. Avoid known allergens and unnecessary patient exposure by administering drugs only when indicated
B. Observe persons given penicillin in the ED for at least 30 minutes before discharge
C. Initiate current skin-testing procedures to identify allergen
D. Obtain an accurate, thorough drug history, identifying and describing previous drug reactions

37 Which of the following pathophysiologic alterations is responsible for the clinical manifestations of neurogenic shock?

A. Compression of the central nervous system within the spinal cord
B. Interruption of neural transmissions of the afferent spinal tracts
C. Inhibition of motor reflexes of the cerebral cortex
D. Disruption of transmission of the sympathetic nerve impulses from the vasomotor center

38 Which of the following conditions does *not* contribute to the development of neurogenic shock?

A. Encephalitis
B. General anesthesia
C. Head trauma
D. Spinal cord injury

39 Which of the following assessment findings indicates neurogenic shock?

A. Increased heart rate and low blood pressure
B. Shallow breathing and diaphoresis
C. Warm, dry skin and bradycardia
D. Weak, thready pulse and hypotension

40 During the management of a patient with neurogenic shock from a spinal cord injury, which of the following nursing actions is *inappropriate*?

A. Elevating the head of the bed 20 degrees to promote oxygenation
B. Inserting a nasogastric tube to prevent aspiration caused by paralytic ileus
C. Keeping the patient supine at all times
D. Inserting a Foley catheter to prevent urine retention

Answer Sheet

	A	B	C	D
1	○	○	○	○
2	○	○	○	○
3	○	○	○	○
4	○	○	○	○
5	○	○	○	○
6	○	○	○	○
7	○	○	○	○
8	○	○	○	○
9	○	○	○	○
10	○	○	○	○
11	○	○	○	○
12	○	○	○	○
13	○	○	○	○
14	○	○	○	○
15	○	○	○	○
16	○	○	○	○
17	○	○	○	○
18	○	○	○	○
19	○	○	○	○
20	○	○	○	○
21	○	○	○	○
22	○	○	○	○
23	○	○	○	○
24	○	○	○	○
25	○	○	○	○
26	○	○	○	○
27	○	○	○	○
28	○	○	○	○
29	○	○	○	○
30	○	○	○	○

	A	B	C	D
31	○	○	○	○
32	○	○	○	○
33	○	○	○	○
34	○	○	○	○
35	○	○	○	○
36	○	○	○	○
37	○	○	○	○
38	○	○	○	○
39	○	○	○	○
40	○	○	○	○

Answer Sheet

	A	B	C	D		A	B	C	D
1	○	○	○	○	31	○	○	○	○
2	○	○	○	○	32	○	○	○	○
3	○	○	○	○	33	○	○	○	○
4	○	○	○	○	34	○	○	○	○
5	○	○	○	○	35	○	○	○	○
6	○	○	○	○	36	○	○	○	○
7	○	○	○	○	37	○	○	○	○
8	○	○	○	○	38	○	○	○	○
9	○	○	○	○	39	○	○	○	○
10	○	○	○	○	40	○	○	○	○
11	○	○	○	○					
12	○	○	○	○					
13	○	○	○	○					
14	○	○	○	○					
15	○	○	○	○					
16	○	○	○	○					
17	○	○	○	○					
18	○	○	○	○					
19	○	○	○	○					
20	○	○	○	○					
21	○	○	○	○					
22	○	○	○	○					
23	○	○	○	○					
24	○	○	○	○					
25	○	○	○	○					
26	○	○	○	○					
27	○	○	○	○					
28	○	○	○	○					
29	○	○	○	○					
30	○	○	○	○					

1 Correct answer—**C**

The initial management of a patient in shock involves provisions for airway and ventilation; maintenance of blood volume, pressure, and circulation; and maintenance of cellular oxygen consumption. Specific measures would include oxygen therapy and administration of I.V. fluid, preferably lactated Ringer's solution via a large-bore I.V. line. A MAST suit can also be used in patients with lower-extremity or abdominal injuries who have signs and symptoms of hypovolemic shock. This will autotransfuse approximately 1,000 ml of blood, reduce blood loss by application of direct pressure, and immobilize injuries of the lower extremities. The patient in shock should be flat with only the legs elevated. The Trendelenburg position, once favored, has been abandoned because it allows the diaphragm to migrate upward, thus compromising ventilation. Also, this position may cause a reflex inhibition of the pressoreceptor activity, thereby decreasing sympathetic stimulation and further compromising arterial blood pressure.

2 Correct answer—**A**

Pulsus paradoxus may be present in patients with hypovolemic shock. Its cardinal sign is an abnormal fall (greater than 10 mm Hg) in systolic blood pressure during inspiration. The systolic sound disappears during inspiration because of pulmonary vascular pooling that is caused by increased lung expansion and increased intrathoracic negative pressure. When intravascular depletion is present, such as in hypovolemic shock, the fall of systolic blood pressure during inspiration is exaggerated when venous return to the heart is compromised. The patient may also demonstrate a narrowing pulse pressure, which indicates a fall in cardiac output, and a CVP reading below 4, indicative of intravascular depletion. Any single hematocrit or hemoglobin value is an unreliable indicator of the patient's condition. Either an increase or decrease in hemoglobin values may signal hypovolemia; dropping values suggest whole blood loss, whereas rising values suggest loss of plasma. Acute blood loss may cause a significant drop in hemoglobin over 1 to 2 hours; however, in older patients, acute blood loss may not cause a significant drop for at least 12 hours.

3 Correct answer—**C**

The patient assessment data that would suggest hypovolemia as the cause of shock include abnormal tilt-test findings and decreasing pulse pressure. The tilt test is an assessment tool that indicates circulating blood volume loss by measuring blood pressure and pulse rate changes during patient position changes. Abnormal tilt-test findings include improved blood pressure levels when the patient's legs are raised above heart level or a 10 mm Hg or greater drop in systolic blood pressure between supine and sitting positions. Pulse pressure is a far better indicator of early shock than is blood pressure. Pulse pressure is related to cardiac stroke volume; thus, changes provide a good indication of blood flow. During the early stages of shock, the systolic pressure usually drops faster than the diastolic pressure, thereby narrowing or decreasing the pulse pressure. The hypovolemic patient will have flat neck veins when prone, a low CVP, decreased urine sodium level, and a high urine specific gravity. An S_3 is heard when there is an increase in the left-ventricular end-diastolic pressure (LVEDP) as found in congestive heart failure (CHF) or in cardiogenic shock. Tachycardia is present in all forms of shock, as the heart is attempting to increase the cardiac output.

4 Correct answer—**D**

Shock is a complex clinical syndrome characterized by impaired cellular metabolism from decreased blood flow. It is a state in which there is an inadequate perfusion of body tissues. The major pathophysiologic problem occurs in the microcirculation at the capillary level. Inadequate tissue perfusion and decreased oxygen delivery result in a constellation of physiologic responses. As shock develops, a fall in cardiac output triggers compensatory mechanisms as pressoreceptors are stimulated to cause vasoconstriction. The net effect is an increase in mean arterial pressure and a restriction of peripheral blood flow. The available circulating volume is shunted to perfuse vital organs. As peripheral vasoconstriction progresses, a marked reduction in oxygen delivery to the cells forces a switch from aerobic to anaerobic metabolism. Increased lactic acid is produced, resulting in respiratory compensation; body-acid load is reduced by blowing off carbon dioxide. As a shock state continues, respiratory compensation fails and the progressive decline in pH from excessive lactate levels ensues. Metabolic acidosis causes impaired cellular function and impaired capillary permeability. Intravascular volume is further decreased as blood flows into capillary beds. The patient is now in the progressive state of shock as compensatory mechanisms fail to maintain an adequate cardiac output.

5 Correct answer—**D**

Respiratory alkalosis develops in the intitial phase of shock. A compensatory mechanism of tachypnea is initiated as a decrease in peripheral tissue perfusion occurs, resulting in hypoxia. In early shock, the patient hyperventilates to increase oxygenation, thus blowing off CO_2. During progressive stages, excessive and prolonged vasoconstriction causes lactic acid levels to increase within the body, producing the systemic acidosis.

6 Correct answer—**D**

During the compensatory stage of shock, the skin is cool, pale, and clammy as a result of peripheral vasoconstriction and increased sweat gland activity. If the cause of shock is not corrected and the compensatory mechanisms continue, the same physiologic events that were initiated to compensate for decreased cardiac output will lead to detrimental effects. Impaired cellular function leads to acidosis. The resultant decrease in cardiac contractility and loss of vasomotor tone will produce mottled skin. A decrease in capillary refill time occurs in shock.

7 Correct answer—**B**

Hypocalcemia is a potential problem during massive transfusions because citrate preservatives may bind ionized calcium. In fact, alkalosis may develop after multiple transfusions, as sodium citrate is converted to sodium bicarbonate. Patients who have these electrolyte and acid-base imbalances may demonstrate Chvostek's sign. This is a facial twitching that occurs when the side of the face is tapped. Brudzinski's sign indicates meningeal irritation; both the upper legs at the hips and the lower legs at the knees are flexed in response to the path of flexion of the head and the neck on the chest. Babinski's sign, which is the dorsiflexion of the big toe upon scratching the bottom of the foot, indicates upper motor neuron dysfunction. Cullen's sign, ecchymosis around the umbilicus, usually is seen in hemorrhagic pancreatitis.

8 Correct answer—**D**

The administration of vasopressors, such as dopamine (Intropin), would be least beneficial to the patient in hypovolemic shock. Natural vasoconstriction compensates for a hypovolemic state during the early shock phase. Giving a vasopressor in early shock increases vasoconstriction, possibly closing arterioles and further halting blood flow. Hypovolemia must be treated before dopamine can be given. For the patient in cardiogenic shock or septic shock (distributive shock), a vasopressor is appropriate because it increases myocardial contractility and raises cardiac output and systolic blood pressure.

9 Correct answer—**C**

The nurse should assess for manifestations of hypovolemic shock in the patient admitted with an intestinal obstruction. The obstruction could cause an alteration in fluid movement, which traps fluid in the interstitial space within the intestinal lumen and depletes the patient's intravascular volume (third-space fluid shift). Suspect neurogenic shock in the patient with drug overdose, septic shock in the postpartum patient with a fever, and cardiogenic shock in the patient with cardiac tamponade.

10 Correct answer—**C**

MAST is a single-unit suit with three compartments: an abdominal compartment and two individual lower-extremity compartments. It may achieve pressures ranging from 0 to 104 mm Hg. Each of the three compartments may be pressurized and deflated individually or in combination. Once a pressure of 104 mm Hg is achieved, automatic release, or pop-off, valves prevent further pressure increases.

11 Correct answer—**A**

The therapeutic effects produced by a MAST suit in the hypovolemic patient include augmentation of preload, thereby increasing blood return to the heart. This results in a greater cardiac output because of increased contractility and stroke volume. A MAST suit increases peripheral vascular resistance in the areas under pressure, decreases peripheral vascular resistance in the remainder of the body, and increases cerebral perfusion pressure. Although use of a MAST suit also decreases the patient's functional residual capacity and tidal volume, these effects are not considered therapeutic.

12 Correct answer—**D**

Indications for using a MAST suit include hypotension secondary to hypovolemia, as occurs in acute trauma; nontraumatic bleeding and nonhemorrhagic hypovolemia; hypotension secondary to volume maldistribution, as occurs in spinal shock, drug effects, and septic shock; and hypotension secondary to low cardiac output, as occurs in cardiac tamponade and cardiogenic shock. The MAST suit is beneficial in stabilizing patients with pelvic and lower-extremity fractures. Not only does the MAST suit support the fracture site and decrease unwanted movement, but it also decreases bleeding. It is useful in lower-extremity hemorrhage and intraabdominal bleeding. A MAST suit would not be indicated for the patient with bilateral hemothorax; it is contraindicated in shock secondary to hemorrhage above the diaphragm.

13 Correct answer—**C**

After a MAST suit is applied, the leg segments are inflated; the abdominal segment may then be inflated, if needed. The end point of pressurization is determined in all instances by the stabilization of the patient's blood pressure, which must be continuously monitored. When desired blood pressure is achieved and maintained, inflation stops. During inflation the patient's feet may turn a bluish color. The suit's maximum pressure, 104 mm Hg, usually is not sufficient to totally occlude perfusion; however, routine palpation of the dorsalis pedis pulses is mandatory. When deflation of the garment is indicated, the abdominal segment is depressurized first, then the leg segments. At no time should suit deflation continue if the patient's systolic blood pressure drops more than 5 mm Hg. Such a drop implies an inadequate circulating volume, and I.V. fluids should be administered until the patient's vital signs are stable.

14 Correct answer—**C**

The postoperative cardiac patient with acute pericarditis is least likely to develop cardiogenic shock. Cardiogenic shock is a vicious cycle that involves loss of myocardial contractility; resultant hemodynamic and metabolic reflex mechanisms cause further ischemia and the deterioration of contractility. Acute pericarditis, an inflammation of the pericardium, has a self-limiting, short-term clinical course when related to an acute MI or cardiac surgery. The cause is not irritation but, rather, an autoimmune response lasting 2 to 6 weeks. Pericardial effusion usually does not develop. Pain, the most characteristic symptom of acute pericarditis, usually can be alleviated by leaning forward. A pericardial friction rub is the most important physical finding. Most commonly, cardiogenic shock occurs as a complication of an MI, especially when at least 40% of the left ventricle is necrotic and ischemic. When the heart's ability to pump blood declines, the risk of cardiogenic shock increases. This occurs in conditions that produce deficient cardiac filling, such as cardiac tamponade and dysrhythmias in a compromised patient.

15 Correct answer—**D**

The clinical manifestations of cardiogenic shock are the result of the impaired contractility of the heart, which decreases cardiac output and elevates LVEDP. The reduced cardiac output impairs perfusion to the vital organs and peripheral tissues. Thus, the patient exhibits changes in sensorium, such as restlessness, anxiety, or confusion. The skin is cold and clammy due to peripheral vasoconstriction. As the cardiac output declines, the pulse pressure narrows; peripheral pulses are rapid and thready. Systemic arterial pressure drops and hypotension ensues. Urine output decreases as kidney perfusion declines. A rise in the LVEDP increases left atrial and pulmonary pressures, resulting in pulmonary congestion. Tachypnea, dyspnea, and pulmonary edema develop; an S_3 can be heard as the left ventricle fails and becomes overdistended during diastole. Increased pressure on the left side of the heart progresses back through the pulmonary venous system into the right side of the heart. This increase in pulmonary pressure decreases the right ventricular performance and may result in right ventricular failure, which in turn produces an elevated CVP and jugular vein distention with hepatomegaly.

16 Correct answer—**C**

The goals of therapy for the patient in cardiogenic shock are to improve myocardial contractility, increase cardiac output, and reduce the myocardial demand for oxygen. Improvement of cardiovascular function is primarily managed by pharmacologic therapies. Nitroprusside (Nipride) and nitroglycerin (Tridil) are commonly used to decrease both preload (ventricular end-diastolic pressure) and afterload (vascular resistance). These vasodilators reduce blood return to the heart and decrease systemic peripheral vascular resistance. Cardiac output is further increased by a decrease in cardiac work load and oxygen demand and complete emptying of the ventricles during systole. Vasodilator therapy is used with sympathomimetic drugs, such as dopamine (Intropin) and dobutamine (Dobutrex). These vasopressors have an inotropic effect that enhances myocardial contractility and increases cardiac output.

17 Correct answer—**A**

An early assessment finding that may indicate cardiogenic shock in the patient with an acute MI is presence of an S_3. The patient with an acute MI is at high risk of developing cardiogenic shock because of a decrease in the contractile function of the left ventricle. Early recognition of signs and symptoms of left ventricular failure, which may lead to shock, are vital. Initially, the failing ventricle causes a decrease in cardiac output. The body compensates by increasing sympathetic stimulation to increase the heart rate and to shunt blood to vital organs via peripheral vasoconstriction. The skin is cool and clammy. Tachycardia and an increased afterload from vasoconstriction increase the cardiac work load and oxygen consumption. A decrease in ventricular emptying during systole occurs, preload increases, and an S_3 may be heard. Pulmonary congestion then follows from the backward transmission of left-sided pressure, resulting in dyspnea, orthopnea, and bilateral crackles. As left ventricular failure progresses, pulmonary congestion increases and cardiogenic shock ensues.

18 Correct answer—**C**

In the context of shock, the kidneys are peripheral organs. Thus, their perfusion declines from the onset of shock. Renal vessels are initially among the most constricted. As renal perfusion declines, the kidneys respond by conserving water; concentrating urine causes an increase in the urine specific gravity. Also, when the blood supply to the kidneys is decreased, the tubules respond by reabsorbing sodium. This results in a decreased urine sodium level. An increase in BUN and serum creatinine levels occurs because of a decrease in the rate at which the kidneys clear metabolic end products such as urea and creatinine from plasma.

19 Correct answer—**B**

The beneficial effect of vasodilator therapy in the management of cardiogenic shock is the reduction of preload and afterload. Vasodilator therapy reduces venous tone and increases venous capacitance. This decreases blood return to the heart, thereby lowering the LVEDP. Vasodilator therapy also reduces arterial vascular tone, which results in decreased impedance to left ventricular ejection (afterload); cardiac work load is decreased, and cardiac output is increased.

20 Correct answer—**B**

Inotropic agents improve tissue perfusion in the patient with cardiogenic shock. They increase the force of myocardial contraction; cardiac output increases because of enhanced contractility. Dopamine (Intropin) is a sympathomimetic drug that has positive inotropic properties. Its vasopressor effects increase coronary blood flow, thereby improving tissue perfusion. The positive chronotropic effects of dopamine increase heart rate. This potential adverse effect limits its use because tachycardia increases myocardial oxygen consumption.

21 Correct answer—**D**

Initial nursing measures include positioning the patient with shoulder and head elevated to decrease pulmonary congestion. Administration of oxygen is vital to increase the myocardial oxygen supply. This will protect the myocardium from further damage. After interventions are taken to ensure improvement in airway and breathing, arterial pressure should be stabilized. Measures, such as infusion of I.V. fluids and infusion of vasopressor drips, should be implemented on physician's order. The rapid infusion of a hypotonic solution, such as 0.45% saline, may result in a sudden decrease in serum osmolarity. This can cause a shift of fluid into the cells, resulting in intravascular depletion and symptoms of increased intracranial pressure. Dextran, glucose, normal saline, and albumin solutions can be used in patients with cardiogenic shock.

22 Correct answer—**D**

The patient who severed two fingers while using garden machinery has a low risk for developing septic shock. Factors that increase a patient's risk include any invasive procedure or foreign body, such as I.V., indwelling catheter line, and pacemaker; diseases affecting the reticuloendothelial system (RES), such as leukemia; and any therapy that suppresses the RES, such as radiation therapy and cytotoxic or immunosuppressive drug therapy.

23 Correct answer—**A**

Obtaining an allergy history from your patient has the highest priority because antibiotics cause anaphylaxis more often than any other substance. Next, make sure to obtain all culture specimens before giving the first drug dose. Initiating antibiotics before collecting cultures is a serious error. It is important to identify accurately the infecting organism in order to provide optimal antibiotic treatment. A switch to a more appropriate therapy can help ensure patient survival.

24 Correct answer—**C**

As septic shock develops, the patient's earliest signs and symptoms are those of the warm (early or hyperdynamic) stage. These include warm, flushed, moist skin; tachycardia with full bounding pulses; tachypnea; confusion; normal or slightly increased urine output; and normal or slightly decreased blood pressure.

25 Correct answer—**C**

Hyperpnea is seen in early sepsis, sometimes to a point of respiratory alkalosis, and is caused by the respiratory response to lactic acidosis, as well as by stimulation of the medullary respiratory control center by the release of endotoxins. Advanced shock is characterized by pulmonary edema, which produces bilateral crackles. Additionally, adult respiratory distress syndrome (ARDS) has been associated with gram-negative sepsis.

26 Correct answer—**D**

There are several reasons for hypovolemia in septic shock. Fluid and electrolytes can leave the body through events associated with infection, such as sweating during fever, diarrhea, vomiting, and respiratory losses during tachypnea. Also, plasma fluid can be sequestered in the extravascular spaces because of a local or generalized increase in vessel permeability, secondary to the production of histamine, bradykinin, and other agents. Vessel permeability is increased in septic shock; thus there is an increased tendency for fluid leakage into tissues.

27 Correct answer—**D**

Septic shock is more common in men than women because of the greater number of urinary tract infections and genitourinary procedures occurring in men. Women are most vulnerable to septic shock after pregnancy. ED nurses must ascertain whether the patient has had a recent pelvic examination, appendectomy, or Foley catheter insertion, especially during childbirth. These procedures are frequent methods for induction of causative organisms. Indwelling urinary tubes, intrauterine devices, instrumented abortions, and peritonitis from a ruptured appendix are additional ways in which gram-negative bacilli may be introduced.

28 Correct answer—**A**

The use of steroids is still controversial, although studies have shown that, overall, pharmacologic doses of steroids appear to be efficacious in the treatment of septic shock. Multiple mechanisms of action have been proposed to explain these reported therapeutic effects. The most common explanations involve the intracellular action of steroids in stabilizing lysosomal membranes. Stabilization of lysosomal membranes will decrease release of vasoactive substances and interrupt the pathogenesis of the shock syndrome. Vasopressors, such as dopamine (Intropin), dobutamine (Dobutrex), and norepinephrine (Levophed) are also used during shock because of their ability to improve the patient's hemodynamic status. Salicylates are used to decrease body temperature. Beta-adrenergic blockers are used rarely in septic shock because they depress myocardial function.

29 Correct answer—**B**

Early in septic shock, the sensorium may change from "awake, alert, and oriented" to "confused, agitated, and restless." Factors responsible for this change in the patient's mental status include decreased cerebral perfusion caused by the low flow state from the endotoxin-induced vasodilation which increases pooling of blood within the venous system. Also, endotoxins act directly on the central nervous system to alter mental status and cause increased stimulation on the respiratory center. The resultant hyperventilation produces an alkalotic state. Cerebral vascular constriction, occurring in response to alkalosis, decreases cerebral blood flow and produces a change in mental status. Elevated BUN and creatinine levels seen in septic shock are not responsible for the change in mental status.

30 Correct answer—**C**

Anaphylaxis is most frequently precipitated by antibiotics, although a variety of agents have been reported to precipitate anaphylaxis. Essentially any compound capable of acting as an allergen may cause an anaphylactic reaction. Some are more common than others, however, and notable examples include the antibiotics, especially penicillin (300 fatal anaphylactic reactions to penicillin occur each year in the United States), medicines derived from animal sources, insect bites and stings, and iodinated radioactive contrast media.

31 Correct answer—**A**

After exposure to an allergen, the patient will develop symptoms of anaphylaxis within 2 to 20 minutes. These immediate reactions are life-threatening and display typical symptoms of anaphylaxis. A reaction that occurs 20 minutes to 48 hours after exposure is called an accelerated reaction and is rarely life-threatening, manifesting itself principally as urticaria and occasionally laryngeal edema. A delayed reaction may develop 3 or more days after drug administration is initiated and usually consists of a rash.

32 Correct answer—**D**

Angioneurotic edema is a cutaneous manifestation seen initially in anaphylaxis. The presence of stridor, hoarseness, and inspiratory wheezing indicate respiratory compromise. Airway obstruction and severe respiratory distress may follow quickly; therefore, these have the highest priority for intervention.

33 Correct answer—**D**

The classic manifestations of anaphylaxis include the triad of urticaria, laryngeal edema with bronchospasm, and hypotension. The intitial signs frequently are cutaneous and consist of diffuse erythema, pruritus, urticaria, or angioneurotic edema. These are frequently followed by pulmonary insufficiency of bronchospasm, laryngeal edema, or both. The patient will usually demonstrate stridor and wheezing. Airway obstruction may progress rapidly and lead to severe respiratory distress. Cardiovascular collapse may occur either before or after the cutaneous and pulmonary manifestations.

34 Correct answer—**A**

Corticosteroids have no place in the initial management of anaphylaxis. These drugs are to be used only in protracted cases and then only after I.V. fluids, epinephrine, and antihistamines have been administered. Epinephrine (Adrenalin) is generally regarded as the drug of choice; it can reverse all signs and symptoms of anaphylaxis. Its beta-adrenergic properties decrease histamine and bradykinin release and cause bronchodilation. Its alpha-adrenergic activity effects vasoconstriction, reversing hypotension.

35 Correct answer—**B**

During anaphylaxis, vasodilation, rather than a primary loss of myocardial contractility, is felt to be responsible for the hypotension. Thus, an agent with principally vasoconstrictive effects would be desirable. Dobutamine (Dobutrex) does not have enough vasoconstrictive effect to be useful in this situation. Norepinephrine (Levophed) does. I.V. aminophylline is indicated in instances of bronchospasm. Antihistamines are useful as adjunctive measures in relieving urticaria, and hydrocortisone, a steroid, decreases inflammation.

36 Correct answer—**D**

The most important principle that should be considered when caring for the patient with a history of allergies is to obtain an accurate and thorough drug history, identifying and describing previous drug reactions. All of the other choices are important, but the drug history has the highest priority.

37 Correct answer—**D**

In neurogenic shock, the major problem is altered blood vessel capacity. A neurologic insult disrupts transmission of sympathetic nerve impulses from the brain's vasomotor center. The unopposed parasympathetic stimulation causes a loss of vasomotor tone, resulting in massive vasodilation. The result is relative hypovolemia, decreased venous return, and decreased cardiac output.

38 Correct answer—**A**

Neurogenic shock may result from any condition that shuts down the entire vasomotor system. The following conditions may lead to neurogenic shock: deep general anesthesia, which may severely depress the brain's vasomotor center and lead to vasomotor collapse; spinal anesthesia, which is the most common cause of neurogenic shock; head trauma; and spinal trauma.

39 Correct answer—**C**

Assessment findings seen in neurogenic shock include warm, dry, and flushed skin; normal to low blood pressure; full regular pulse; profound bradycardia; and an increased respiratory rate. These are the result of blocked sympathetic vasomotor regulation.

40 Correct answer—**A**

The patient with neurogenic shock should be kept supine to prevent orthostatic hypotension. This occurs as a result of relative hypovolemia caused by increased vascular capacity. I.V. fluids are instituted to expand the intravascular volume. Fluids must be administered cautiously, as they may cause fluid overload when vasomotor tone is restored. A Foley catheter is inserted to permit frequent measurement of urine output. The catheter also helps prevent urinary retention if the patient has a spinal cord injury that has paralyzed the bladder.

Selected References

Barrows, J.J. "Shock Demands Drugs—But Which One's Best for Your Patient?" *Nursing82* 12:34-41, February 1982.

Berne, R.M., and Levy, M.N. *Cardiovascular Physiology*, 4th ed. St. Louis: C.V. Mosby Co., 1981.

Bordricks, K. *Patterns of Shock, Implications for Nursing Care*, 2nd ed. New York: MacMillan Publishing Co., 1980.

Budassi, S., and Barber, J. *Emergency Nursing Principles and Practice*. St. Louis: C.V. Mosby Co., 1981.

Burrell, L.O., and Burrell, Z.L. *Critical Care*. St. Louis: C.V. Mosby Co., 1982.

Cohen, S. "Nursing Care of Patients in Shock. Part 3: Evaluating the Patient," *American Journal of Nursing* 82:1723-1746, November 1982.

Crumlish, C.M. "Cardiogenic Shock: Catch It Early!" *Nursing81* 11:34-41, August 1981.

Elenbaas, R. "Anaphylactic Shock," *Critical Care Quarterly* 2:77-83, 1980.

Emergencies. Nurse's Reference Library Series. Springhouse, Pa. Springhouse Corp., 1984.

Eskridge, R. "Septic Shock," *Critical Care Quarterly* 2:55-76, 1980.

Hammond, C.B. "Cardiogenic Shock: A Review," *Journal of Emergency Nursing* 4:201-205, 1983.

Holloway, M.N., *Emergency Department Nurses Association Core Curriculum*. Philadelphia: W.B. Saunders Co., 1985.

Keely, B. "Septic Shock," *Critical Care Quarterly* 7:59-67, 1985.

Lamb, L.S. "Think You Know Septic Shock? Read This." *Nursing82* 12:34-43, January 1982.

Park, G.D. "Cardiogenic Shock," *Critical Care Quarterly* 2:43-53, 1980.

Chapter 3

Cardiovascular Emergencies Questions and Answers

You must begin with Question 1 of this chapter and progress in sequence. **Do not skip around.** Subsequent answers build on previous ones.

Laura Gasparis, RN, MA, CCRN, CEN
Linda Anne Laner, RN, MSN, CS, CCRN, CEN
Eva Scripps, RN, BSN, CCRN, CEN

SITUATION

A 68-year-old man presents to the emergency department (ED) with a chief complaint of frequent episodes of substernal chest pain that became increasingly severe this morning. He is alert and denies nausea, vomiting, or radiation of chest pain. The episodes began during the past month, occur at rest, last 10 to 15 minutes, and are relieved by three sublingual nitroglycerin pills. Cardiac monitoring is begun, and 500 ml of dextrose and water is administered intravenously at a keep-vein-open (KVO) rate. Oxygen 24% is given via a Venturi mask. An EKG demonstrates ST-segment elevation. After assessing the patient's vital signs, the nurse gives the following medications: 1" of nitroglycerin paste, 10 mg of propranolol (Inderal), and 10 mg of nifedipine (Procardia) P.O. Vital signs are as follows: blood pressure, 130/90 mm Hg; pulse, 110 beats/minute; and respirations, 24 breaths/minute.

Questions 1 to 6 refer to the above situation.

1 The patient's history and EKG findings are consistent with:

A. Stable angina
B. Preinfarction angina
C. Prinzmetal's angina
D. Angina decubitus

2 Which of the following changes commonly occurs before or during an attack of angina pectoris?

A. A decrease in blood pressure
B. A decrease in myocardial oxygen demand
C. An increase in ventricular compliance
D. An increase in heart rate

3 Which of the following EKG findings is consistent with typical angina pectoris?

A. ST-segment depression
B. ST-segment elevation
C. T-wave elevation
D. U-wave appearance

4 Possible precipitating factors related to the patient's angina include all of the following *except*:

A. Stress
B. Heavy meals
C. Bed rest
D. Smoking

5 Which of the following symptoms occurs during an angina attack?

A. Transient diastolic murmur
B. Transient abnormal point of maximal impulse
C. Pulsus paradoxus
D. Ventricular gallop (S_3)

6 Administration of propranolol to a patient with angina is contraindicated in all of the following *except*:

A. Heart block
B. Uncompensated congestive heart failure (CHF)
C. Tachycardia
D. Asthma

SITUATION

A 54-year-old man comes to triage complaining of severe, left-sided, pressurelike chest pain and left arm numbness. The pain began 2 hours ago and is unrelieved by rest. He has no significant medical history. He is anxious and diaphoretic when brought into the ED. Cardiac monitoring is begun, and oxygen is given at 2 liters/minute. An I.V. line of dextrose 5% in water (D_5W) is initiated to a KVO rate. His blood pressure is 120/60 mm Hg; pulse, 88 beats/minute and irregular; and respirations, 20 breaths/minute. The cardiac rhythm is normal sinus rhythm with occasional unifocal premature ventricular contractions (PVCs).

Questions 7 to 11 refer to the above situation.

7 The triage nurse should suspect that the patient is having a myocardial infaction (MI) because:

A. This type of pain has not occurred previously
B. The pain is severe and radiating
C. The pain has lasted for 2 hours
D. The pain is accompanied by PVCs

8 A 12-lead EKG shows ST-segment elevations in leads V_1, V_2, and V_3. These data indicate an acute MI in the:

A. Inferior wall
B. Anteroseptal wall
C. Lateral wall
D. Posterior wall

9 The patient's pain is unrelieved by the oxygen and sublingual nitroglycerin (1/150 grain every 5 minutes for three doses). I.V. morphine sulfate is ordered by the physician because:

A. It is a powerful analgesic and decreases myocardial work load
B. It dilates coronary arteries when used with nitroglycerin
C. It produces sedation
D. It is effective and nonaddicting when given in small doses

10 The patient's pain is relieved after 6 mg of morphine. The physician orders lidocaine (Xylocaine), 50 mg bolus every 5 minutes for two doses, followed by an infusion of 2 mg/minute. Lidocaine is indicated because it:

A. Lowers the fibrillation threshold
B. Decreases the heart's need for oxygen
C. Eliminates irritability within necrotic areas of the myocardium
D. Eradicates potentially dangerous PVCs

11 While awaiting transfer to the coronary care unit, the patient becomes tachycardic; his blood pressure remains stable. At this point, which of the following nursing actions receives the highest priority?

A. Giving additional morphine and reassuring the patient
B. Decreasing the lidocaine to 1 mg/minute and getting a stat lidocaine level
C. Auscultating the patient's lungs
D. Placing the patient in a low Fowler's position

12 Which of the following goals is primary when planning care for a patient with an acute MI?

A. Preventing dysrhythmias
B. Minimizing further cardiac damage
C. Decreasing the oxygen needs of the patient
D. Alleviating patient anxiety

13 Which of the following statements regarding MI is *false*?

A. Patients with an inferior wall MI in most cases develop life-threatening conduction disturbances
B. Dysrhythmias associated with atrioventricular (AV) block are usually transient and usually are not considered dangerous when they occur with an inferior wall MI
C. Severe nausea and vomiting are most prevalent with an inferior wall MI
D. Ventricular irritability, demonstrated by PVCs, is a danger regardless of the type of MI

14 When a crescendo-decrescendo systolic murmur suddenly develops in a patient experiencing an MI, the nurse should suspect:

A. Aortic insufficiency
B. Papillary muscle dysfunction
C. Ventricular aneurysm
D. Early pericarditis

15 Which of the following assessment data indicates a lateral wall MI?

A. Q waves in leads II, III, and aVF
B. Q waves in leads I, aVL, V_5, and V_6
C. Q waves in leads V_1 through V_3
D. Tall R waves in leads V_1 and V_2

16 Which of the following is *not* a predisposing factor for MI?

A. Diabetes
B. Hypertension
C. Hyperlipidemia
D. High estrogen levels

SITUATION

A 56-year-old woman is brought to the ED by emergency medical service for evaluation of increasing shortness of breath. The symptoms began 2 days ago and increased in severity this morning. She is pale and diaphoretic; her skin is warm. Respirations are 36 breaths/minute, with increasing use of supraclavicular and abdominal muscles. Bilateral crackles are present, and pedal edema is noted. She has a history of coronary artery disease and had an MI 2 years ago. After assisting the patient into a high Fowler's position, the nurse records the following vital signs: blood pressure, 90/60 mm Hg; pulse, 116 beats/minute and irregular.

Questions 17 to 33 refer to the above situation.

17 The patient's pulse pressure is:

A. 30 mm Hg
B. 50 mm Hg
C. 70 mm Hg
D. 75 mm Hg

18 The patient's vital signs and symptoms are consistent with:

A. Right ventricular failure
B. Left ventricular failure
C. Biventricular failure
D. Backward failure

19 Nursing assessment of physical findings in a patient with right ventricular failure includes:

A. Gallop rhythm and pulsus alternans
B. Elevated pulmonary artery (PA) diastolic pressure and pulmonary capillary wedge pressure (PCWP)
C. Hepatosplenomegaly, with or without pain
D. Cough, dyspnea, and crackles

20 Which of the following nursing interventions is *not* indicated for a patient in left ventricular failure?

A. Assess fluid intake and output and electrolyte balance
B. Restrict fluids
C. Maintain flow of normal saline solution
D. Maintain dietary sodium at 2 grams

21 The most common cause of right ventricular failure is:

A. Left ventricular failure
B. MI
C. Pulmonary hypertension
D. Cor pulmonale

22 A flow-directed, balloon-tipped catheter is introduced through the patient's right subclavian vein into the pulmonary artery to monitor all of the following *except*:

A. Ventricular pressures
B. Atrial pressures
C. Pulmonary pressures
D. Colloid osmotic pressures

23 During the insertion of the balloon-tipped catheter, which of the following should be available at the bedside?

A. Pacemaker wire and generator
B. Ambu bag and oxygen
C. Lidocaine and defibrillator
D. Heparin

24 The following pressures are recorded: right atrial pressure, 7 mm Hg; right ventricular pressure, 32/7 mm Hg; pulmonary artery, 32/22 mm Hg; and CWP, 22 mm Hg. The normal range of PCWP is:

A. 4 to 8 mm Hg
B. 5 to 12 mm Hg
C. 6 to 18 mm Hg
D. 8 to 14 mm Hg

25 Nursing interventions for a patient undergoing the insertion of a balloon-tipped catheter include all of the following *except*:

A. Supporting and observing the patient
B. Monitoring pressure tracing and EKG
C. Monitoring for thrombotic events
D. Monitoring vital signs

26 The most common complication associated with use of a balloon-tipped catheter is:

A. Infection
B. Thromboembolism
C. Pulmonary infarct
D. Knotting of the catheter

27 Appropriate medical management of the patient's CHF is:

A. Decreasing preload, increasing afterload, decreasing contractility
B. Decreasing preload, decreasing afterload, increasing contractility
C. Increasing preload, decreasing afterload, increasing contractility
D. Increasing preload, increasing afterload, decreasing contractility

28 Treatment-induced complications of CHF include which of the following?

A. Hypervolemia
B. Pulmonary hypertension
C. Digitalis toxicity
D. Cor pulmonale

29 The patient's CHF is being treated with digoxin (Lanoxin) and aminophylline (Aminophyllin). The pharmacologic effects of digoxin are:

A. Negative inotropy and positive chronotropy
B. Negative inotropy and negative chronotropy
C. Positive inotropy and negative chronotropy
D. Positive inotropy and positive chronotropy

30 EKG changes associated with digoxin toxicity include all of the following *except*:

A. Prolonged PR interval, shortened QT interval
B. ST-segment changes, decreased T-wave amplitude
C. Tachydysrhythmias, ventricular ectopy
D. Sinus tachycardia

31 Which of the following measures is appropriate in the treatment of digoxin toxicity?

A. Monitor patient for hyperkalemia
B. Administer quinidine for tachydysrhythmias
C. Administer phenytoin (Dilantin) for ventricular bigeminy
D. Administer calcium to desensitize the heart to digoxin

32 Which of the following effects does aminophylline (Aminophyllin) produce?

A. Bronchiole constriction
B. Decreased heart rate
C. Increased cardiac output
D. Decreased urinary output

33 After administration of aminophylline, the patient should be observed for which of the following signs of toxicity?

A. Bradycardia
B. Hypertension
C. Abdominal pain
D. Lethargy

34 Which of the following is likely to be seen on an EKG taken from a patient whose potassium level is 6 mEq/liter?

A. ST-segment depression
B. PVCs
C. Peaked T waves
D. Prominent U waves

35

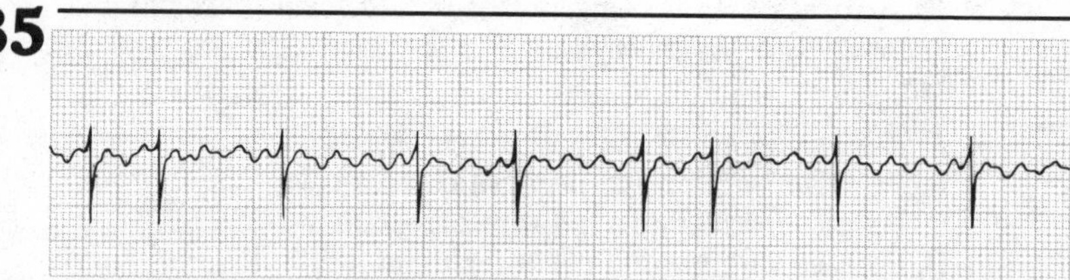

The above EKG strip represents:

A. Ventricular flutter
B. Atrial flutter
C. Atrial fibrillation
D. Paroxysmal atrial tachycardia (PAT) with block

36

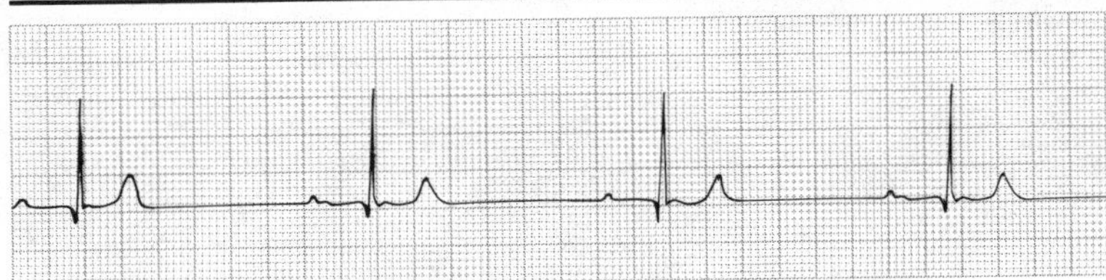

Commonly all of the following are associated with the above cardiac rhythm *except*:

A. The use of digoxin
B. Inferior wall MI
C. Hypokalemia
D. Organic heart disease

37

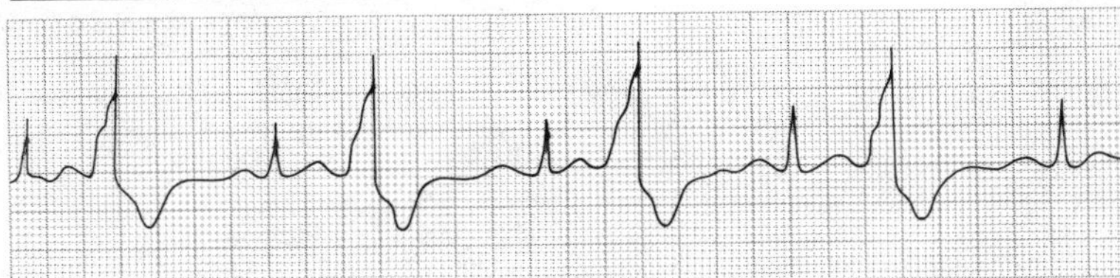

The above strip was taken from a patient having nausea. The patient's pulse indicates perfusion of all beats. This rhythm:

A. May be associated with digoxin toxicity
B. Should be treated with lidocaine
C. Represents ventricular trigeminy
D. Is caused by multiple ectopic foci in the ventricle

SITUATION

A patient is experiencing an acute MI. While speaking to the nurse, he suddenly becomes unresponsive and pulseless.

Questions 38 to 40 refer to the above situation.

38

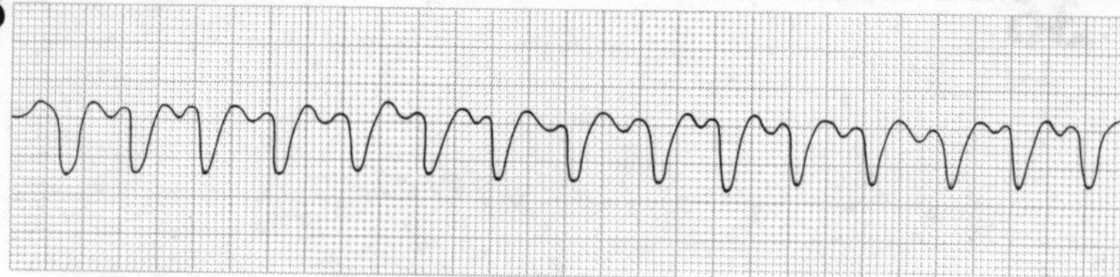

The above rhythm is seen on the monitor. A precordial thump is unsuccessful. The nurse's next action should be to call for help and:

A. Administer lidocaine 1 mg/kg bolus
B. Defibrillate using 200 joules
C. Perform synchronized cardioversion using 100 joules
D. Repeat the precordial thump

39

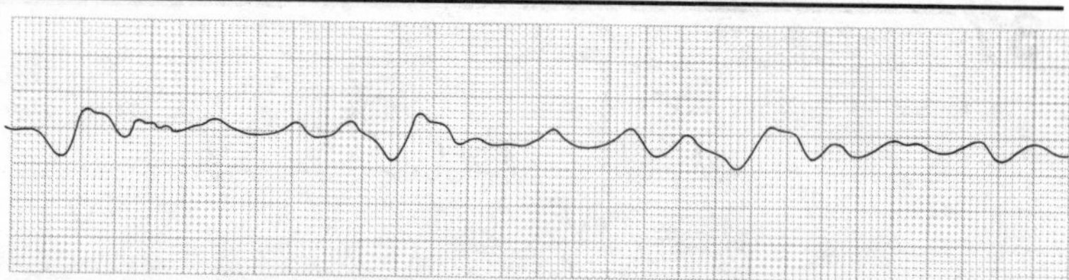

The patient's cardiac rhythm displays as shown above. Pulse remains undetectable. What should be done next?

A. Administer lidocaine 1 mg/kg bolus
B. Administer bretylium (Bretylol) 350 to 500 mg I.V. bolus
C. Defibrillate with 300 joules
D. Perform synchronized cardioversion with 300 joules

40 The patient's cardiac rhythm converts to sinus bradycardia with a rate of 30 beats/minute. Frequent PVCs are also noted. Which of the following is the treatment of initial choice in this situation?

A. Placement of temporary pacemaker
B. Bolus administration of an appropriate antiarrhythmic agent
C. I.V. bolus administration of atropine 0.5 mg
D. Infusion of isoproterenol (Isuprel)

41

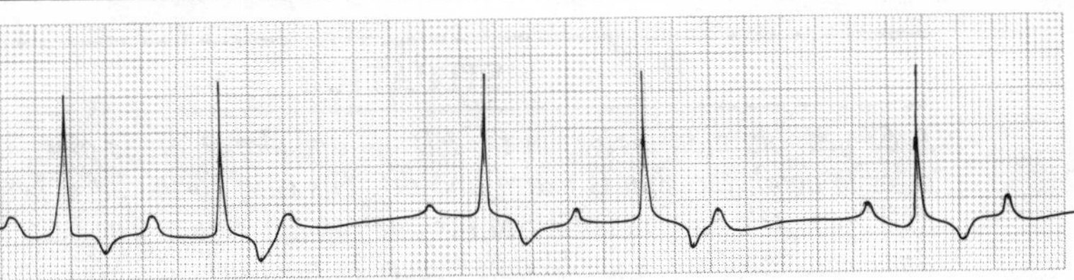

The above strip represents:

A. Wandering atrial pacemaker
B. Second-degree AV block, Mobitz I
C. Second-degree AV block, Mobitz II
D. Third-degree heart block

42

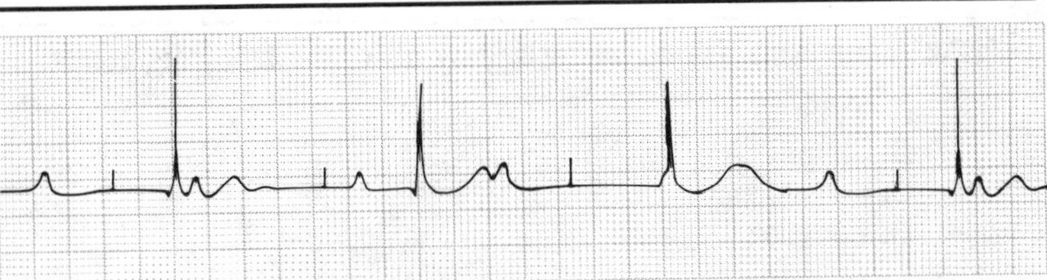

The above rhythm is noted in a patient with a temporary pacemaker. Which of the following actions would *not* be appropriate?

A. Turn the patient on his side
B. Increase the pacemaker rate
C. Check the pacemaker connections
D. Turn up the output (milliamperes) dial

43

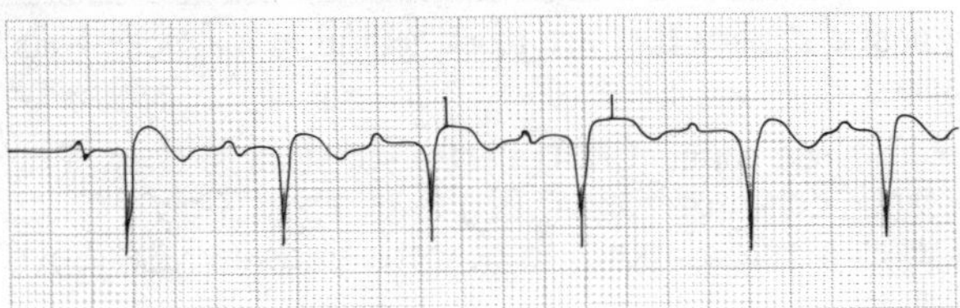

Which of the following problems does the above rhythm strip represent?

A. Runaway pacemaker
B. Loss of capture
C. Loss of sensing
D. Inadequate connection between the distal wire of the catheter and the negative terminal of the pulse generator

SITUATION

A 63-year-old man arrives in the ED via ambulance. He is alert, and his color is good; the skin is warm and dry. His chief complaint is persistent dull epigastric pain radiating to the intercapular region. The pain began 2 days ago. Vital signs are blood pressure in right arm, 120/60 mm Hg; in left arm, 220/100 mm Hg; right radial pulse, 2+; left radial pulse, 3+. Bilateral basilar crackles are present. A systolic cardiac murmur is noted at the second right intercostal space. The patient has a 33-year history of hypertension, which is treated with chlorthalidone (Hygroton), 50 mg daily, and methyldopa (Aldomet), 250 mg, three times a day.

Questions 44 to 48 refer to the above situation.

44 Aneurysms are characterized by all of the following *except*:

A. Type
B. Shape
C. Consistency
D. Location

45 The common manifestations of a proximal dissecting aortic aneurysm include:

A. Hypotension, tachycardia, radiating back pain
B. Hypotension, bradycardia, EKG changes
C. Anterior chest pain, disturbances of consciousness, paraparesis
D. Hypertension, vomiting, chest pain

46 The diagnostic studies that are most helpful in diagnosing aortic aneurysms are:

A. Complete blood count (CBC), electrolyte studies, chest X-ray
B. CBC, lactic dehydrogenase (LDH) level, chest X-ray
C. LDH level, serum glutamic oxaloacetic transaminase (SGOT) level, EKG
D. SGOT level, EKG, echocardiogram

47 The physician prescribes an antihypertensive agent for the patient. The main objective of therapy is to maintain the:

A. Systolic blood pressure at 100 to 120 mm Hg
B. Systolic blood pressure at 140 to 160 mm Hg
C. Diastolic blood pressure at 90 to 120 mm Hg
D. Diastolic blood pressure at 130 to 150 mm Hg

48 Aneurysms are most commonly found in which of the following?

A. Cerebral arteries
B. Aorta
C. Iliac arteries
D. Popliteal arteries

49 In a patient with suspected cardiac tamponade, the nurse should assess for which of the following signs?

A. Pulsus alternans
B. Wide pulse pressure
C. Large R wave in V leads on the EKG
D. Restlessness

50 Initially, the administration of I.V. fluid to patients with acute cardiac tamponade:

A. Is important to replace lost volume
B. Increases preload, thereby temporarily increasing cardiac output
C. Increases afterload, thereby temporarily increasing blood pressure
D. Is usually contraindicated because of accompanying pulmonary edema

51 In the treatment of cardiac tamponade, which of the following receives the highest priority?

A. Thoracotomy
B. Administration of I.V. fluids
C. Pericardiocentesis
D. Application of medical antishock trousers (MAST)

52 All of the following are common complications of pericardiocentesis *except*:

A. Ventricular perforation
B. Pneumothorax
C. Complete heart block
D. Ventricular fibrillation

53 A nursing responsibility during pericardiocentesis is to:

A. Prepare an infusion of isoproterenol
B. Monitor the patient's EKG tracings in a V lead
C. Place the patient flat, if possible
D. Encourage the patient to perform Valsalva's maneuver, if possible

54 The most common cause of acute cardiac tamponade is:

A. MI
B. Penetrating chest trauma
C. Blunt chest trauma
D. Cancer

SITUATION

A 50-year-old man comes to the ED complaining of headache, nausea, vomiting, and blurred vision. His blood pressure is 210/144 mm Hg. When asked if he takes any medications, the patient states that he has not taken clonidine (Catapres) in 2 days because he "ran out of pills."

Questions 55 and 56 refer to the above situation.

55 Which of the following assessment data is *least* important in alerting the nurse that the patient should be treated as quickly as possible?

A. Systolic blood pressure of 210 mm Hg
B. Diastolic blood pressure of 144 mm Hg
C. Headache and blurred vision
D. Nausea and vomiting

56 The nurse should suspect that the patient's hypertensive crisis is probably the result of:

A. Retention of sodium and water
B. Renal failure
C. Increased peripheral vascular resistance
D. Increased sympathetic stimulation from the brain

57 Sodium nitroprusside (Nipride) is frequently used in hypertensive emergencies. This medication:

A. Must be administered slowly, through microdrip tubing
B. Has a direct vasodilating action on smooth muscles of arteries and veins
C. Has an onset of action within 2 to 3 minutes
D. Stimulates alpha-adrenergic receptors, producing sympathetic inhibition of blood pressure

58 The most common cause of hypertension is:

A. Renal disease
B. Endocrine disorders
C. Poor dietary habits
D. Idiopathic

SITUATION

A patient arrives via ambulance stretcher with cardiopulmonary resuscitation (CPR) in progress. The cardiac monitor shows ventricular fibrillation. An endotracheal tube is in place; 100% oxygen is administered by Ambu bag. Dopamine (Intropin) is infused at 10 mg/kg/minute via right subclavian catheter; normal saline solution is infused at a KVO rate via right antecubital line. Defibrillation has been attempted three times without success.

Questions 59 and 60 refer to the above situation.

59 The drug of choice, after unsuccessful defibrillation, is:

A. Epinephrine (Adrenalin)
B. Calcium chloride
C. Bretylium
D. Lidocaine

60 Ventricular fibrillation continues. Arterial blood gases (ABGs) reveal: pH, 7.25; PCO_2, 35 mm Hg; PO_2, 60 mm Hg; and HCO_3^-, 15 mEq/liter. The drug of choice is:

A. Sodium bicarbonate
B. Calcium chloride
C. Bretylium
D. Lidocaine

61 After termination of ventricular fibrillation or ventricular tachycardia, which of the following medications should be infused?

A. Digoxin
B. Lidocaine
C. Verapamil (Isoptin)
D. Dopamine

62 If ventricular fibrillation is refractory to lidocaine, which of the following medications should be infused?

A. Verapamil
B. Calcium
C. Epinephrine
D. Bretylium

63 Which of the following drugs is indicated for the control of symptomatic complete heart block that is refractory to atropine?

A. Dopamine
B. Epinephrine
C. Isoproterenol
D. Propranolol

64 A therapeutic effect of propranolol (Inderal) administration is:

A. Increased myocardial contractility
B. Decrease in cardiac output
C. Decreased myocardial oxygen supply
D. Decreased AV conduction time

65 Which of the following drugs is most likely to be used in the treatment of severe hypotension?

A. Dopamine
B. Dobutamine (Dobutrex)
C. Isoproterenol
D. Epinephrine

66 Which of the following statements is true about dopamine (Intropin)?

A. It should be administered through a central line
B. The dose should be regulated through microdrip tubing
C. It is the preferred agent in the presence of uncontrolled dysrhythmia
D. In low doses, it may increase oxygen demand

67 The drug of choice to treat severe heart failure is:

A. Epinephrine
B. Dopamine
C. Dobutamine
D. Digoxin

68 A thrombolytic agent used in the first few hours of an MI is:

A. Heparin
B. Streptokinase (Streptase)
C. Thrombokinase
D. Warfarin (Coumadin)

69 Thrombolytic therapy is contraindicated in:

A. Deep vein thrombosis
B. Pulmonary emboli
C. Cerebrovascular accident (CVA)
D. Coronary occlusion

70 Thrombolytic therapy should be discontinued if which one of the following occurs?

A. Low-grade fever
B. Vomiting
C. Dyspnea
D. Relief of chest pain

71 The most serious adverse effect of I.V. nitroglycerin therapy is:

A. Hypotension
B. Bradycardia
C. CHF
D. Ventricular fibrillation

72 Rapid I.V. infusion of nitroprusside can cause:

A. Hypertension, bradycardia
B. Chest pain, muscle twitching
C. Dyspnea, dysrhythmia
D. Syncope, vomiting

SITUATION

A 32-year-old man is brought to the ED by ambulance after being in an automobile accident. He was the driver of the car. He is now complaining of chest pain and shortness of breath. Cardiac monitor shows sinus tachycardia with frequent PVCs.

Questions 73 to 77 refer to the above situation.

73 The nurse suspects this patient's symptoms indicate:

A. MI
B. Fractured ribs
C. Pericarditis
D. Cardiac contusion

74 The nurse understands that blunt chest trauma commonly results in damage to the:

A. Left ventricle
B. Right ventricle
C. Septum
D. Right atrium

75 Pharmocologic therapy for this condition would *not* include:

A. Nitroglycerin
B. Lidocaine
C. Morphine sulfate
D. Oxygen

76 The ED nurse should monitor this patient for the development of which one of the following complications?

A. Adult respiratory distress syndrome (ARDS)
B. Pulmonary embolism
C. CHF
D. Cardiomyopathy

77 Which of the following medications is contraindicated in this situation?

A. Heparin
B. Digoxin
C. Dopamine
D. Bretylium

SITUATION

A 56-year-old man is seen in the ED with complaints of chest pain and shortness of breath. He underwent open-heart surgery 1 month ago and, until today, had "felt fine." A diagnosis of pericarditis is made.

Questions 78 to 81 refer to the above situation.

78 During the initial nursing assessment, it is imperative to observe for:

A. An increase in temperature
B. A pericardial friction rub
C. Pulsus paradoxus
D. Kussmaul's sign

79 When pericarditis is present, the patient will probably exhibit:

A. Further chest pain when sitting upright
B. Immediate relief of discomfort during deep inspiration
C. Bradycardia with ST-segment depression
D. Dyspnea and tachypnea

80 This patient's condition may best be relieved by which of the following pharmacologic measures?

A. Indomethacin (Indocin)
B. Penicillin
C. Acetaminophen (Tylenol)
D. Digoxin

81 All of the following medical histories predispose patients to pericarditis *except*:

A. Rheumatic fever
B. Postmyocardial infarction
C. Chronic obstructive pulmonary disease
D. Kidney disease

SITUATION

A 26-year-old man with a long history of I.V. drug abuse enters the ED complaining of fever, shaking, chills, and severe night sweats. He is diagnosed as having endocarditis.

Questions 82 to 84 refer to the above situation.

82 Which of the following nursing assessment parameters holds the *lowest* priority for the patient with endocarditis?

A. Auscultate for an S_3
B. Monitor for PVCs
C. Monitor patient's temperature
D. Auscultate for crackles

83 The nurse should evaluate the patient's laboratory studies to show:

A. Leukocytopenia
B. Elevated erythrocyte sedimentation rate
C. Polycythemia vera
D. Thrombocytosis

84 The nurse would consider which of the following laboratory studies as a prime diagnostic tool for endocarditis?

A. Blood cultures
B. CBC with differential
C. Electrolyte studies
D. Clotting profile

SITUATION

A 42-year-old woman is admitted to the ED complaining of a sudden onset of severe pain in the right leg. After a thorough assessment, a diagnosis of acute arterial occlusion of the right leg is made.

Questions 85 to 88 refer to the above situation.

85 Which of the following medical histories would *not* be typical for an acute arterial occlusion?

A. Atrial fibrillation
B. Postpartum
C. Prosthetic cardiac valve
D. MI

86 Which of the following symptoms would the nurse expect to see in a patient with acute arterial occlusion?

A. Swelling of affected extremity and trophic changes
B. Positive Homans' sign with nonpalpable pulses
C. Tenderness to deep pressure and pale extremity
D. Paresthesias

87 An appropriate action for the ED nurse to take during the care of a patient with an arterial occlusion is to:

A. Apply hot compresses to extremity
B. Elevate the ischemic extremity
C. Administer heparin infusion, as ordered
D. Measure calf width

88 The nurse could anticipate the need to prepare this patient for all of the following procedures *except*:

A. Arteriovenous shunt
B. Embolectomy
C. Thrombolytic infusion
D. Balloon-tipped catheter extraction of emboli

Answer Sheet

	A	B	C	D		A	B	C	D		A	B	C	D
1	○	○	○	○	31	○	○	○	○	61	○	○	○	○
2	○	○	○	○	32	○	○	○	○	62	○	○	○	○
3	○	○	○	○	33	○	○	○	○	63	○	○	○	○
4	○	○	○	○	34	○	○	○	○	64	○	○	○	○
5	○	○	○	○	35	○	○	○	○	65	○	○	○	○
6	○	○	○	○	36	○	○	○	○	66	○	○	○	○
7	○	○	○	○	37	○	○	○	○	67	○	○	○	○
8	○	○	○	○	38	○	○	○	○	68	○	○	○	○
9	○	○	○	○	39	○	○	○	○	69	○	○	○	○
10	○	○	○	○	40	○	○	○	○	70	○	○	○	○
11	○	○	○	○	41	○	○	○	○	71	○	○	○	○
12	○	○	○	○	42	○	○	○	○	72	○	○	○	○
13	○	○	○	○	43	○	○	○	○	73	○	○	○	○
14	○	○	○	○	44	○	○	○	○	74	○	○	○	○
15	○	○	○	○	45	○	○	○	○	75	○	○	○	○
16	○	○	○	○	46	○	○	○	○	76	○	○	○	○
17	○	○	○	○	47	○	○	○	○	77	○	○	○	○
18	○	○	○	○	48	○	○	○	○	78	○	○	○	○
19	○	○	○	○	49	○	○	○	○	79	○	○	○	○
20	○	○	○	○	50	○	○	○	○	80	○	○	○	○
21	○	○	○	○	51	○	○	○	○	81	○	○	○	○
22	○	○	○	○	52	○	○	○	○	82	○	○	○	○
23	○	○	○	○	53	○	○	○	○	83	○	○	○	○
24	○	○	○	○	54	○	○	○	○	84	○	○	○	○
25	○	○	○	○	55	○	○	○	○	85	○	○	○	○
26	○	○	○	○	56	○	○	○	○	86	○	○	○	○
27	○	○	○	○	57	○	○	○	○	87	○	○	○	○
28	○	○	○	○	58	○	○	○	○	88	○	○	○	○
29	○	○	○	○	59	○	○	○	○					
30	○	○	○	○	60	○	○	○	○					

Answer Sheet

	A	B	C	D		A	B	C	D		A	B	C	D
1	○	○	○	○	31	○	○	○	○	61	○	○	○	○
2	○	○	○	○	32	○	○	○	○	62	○	○	○	○
3	○	○	○	○	33	○	○	○	○	63	○	○	○	○
4	○	○	○	○	34	○	○	○	○	64	○	○	○	○
5	○	○	○	○	35	○	○	○	○	65	○	○	○	○
6	○	○	○	○	36	○	○	○	○	66	○	○	○	○
7	○	○	○	○	37	○	○	○	○	67	○	○	○	○
8	○	○	○	○	38	○	○	○	○	68	○	○	○	○
9	○	○	○	○	39	○	○	○	○	69	○	○	○	○
10	○	○	○	○	40	○	○	○	○	70	○	○	○	○
11	○	○	○	○	41	○	○	○	○	71	○	○	○	○
12	○	○	○	○	42	○	○	○	○	72	○	○	○	○
13	○	○	○	○	43	○	○	○	○	73	○	○	○	○
14	○	○	○	○	44	○	○	○	○	74	○	○	○	○
15	○	○	○	○	45	○	○	○	○	75	○	○	○	○
16	○	○	○	○	46	○	○	○	○	76	○	○	○	○
17	○	○	○	○	47	○	○	○	○	77	○	○	○	○
18	○	○	○	○	48	○	○	○	○	78	○	○	○	○
19	○	○	○	○	49	○	○	○	○	79	○	○	○	○
20	○	○	○	○	50	○	○	○	○	80	○	○	○	○
21	○	○	○	○	51	○	○	○	○	81	○	○	○	○
22	○	○	○	○	52	○	○	○	○	82	○	○	○	○
23	○	○	○	○	53	○	○	○	○	83	○	○	○	○
24	○	○	○	○	54	○	○	○	○	84	○	○	○	○
25	○	○	○	○	55	○	○	○	○	85	○	○	○	○
26	○	○	○	○	56	○	○	○	○	86	○	○	○	○
27	○	○	○	○	57	○	○	○	○	87	○	○	○	○
28	○	○	○	○	58	○	○	○	○	88	○	○	○	○
29	○	○	○	○	59	○	○	○	○					
30	○	○	○	○	60	○	○	○	○					

1 Correct answer—**C**

Prinzmetal's angina is severe, non–effort-induced pain that occurs when the person is at rest. It has a cyclic pattern and may occur at the same time each day. The pain may be of greater duration than other types of angina. It is frequently seen in women under age 50 and is attributed to spasms of a large coronary artery. The pain associated with stable angina is chronic in nature, not changing in duration, intensity, or frequency for at least 2 months. The pain can be debilitating or mild. Preinfarction angina is a term for unstable angina that increases in frequency, duration, and severity of pain. Preinfarction angina or unstable angina usually develops into an MI. Angina decubitus is diagnosed when pain occurs upon assuming a recumbent position.

2 Correct answer—**D**

During the ischemic event, angina pectoris is associated with the hemodynamic pattern characterized by a mild increase in blood pressure and heart rate before the pain episode. Typically, angina is precipitated by activities that increase myocardial oxygen demand, such as exercise. Oxygen demand in excess of oxygen supply results in localized ischemia. Transient ischemia causes reversible changes at both the tissue and cellular levels, impairing left ventricular function (compliance) and decreasing myocardial contractility. Ideally, a critical balance exists between oxygen supply and demand. Whenever myocardial oxygen demand increases, oxygen supply must increase concurrently. The oxygen requirements of the heart are greater than those of most other body tissues and are affected by the cardiac work load.

3 Correct answer—**A**

Ischemia produces ST-segment depression or T-wave inversion. Angina pectoris is chest pain or discomfort resulting from transient myocardial ischemia. An EKG may record transient ischemic changes during anginal episodes. Prinzmetal's angina produces ST-segment elevation during anginal episodes. A U wave develops with hypokalemia.

4 Correct answer—**C**

The underlying cause of angina pectoris is a disequilibrium between myocardial oxygen supply and demand. Stress and heavy meals increase oxygen demands, whereas smoking decreases blood supply through vasoconstriction. Thus, all three factors cause an imbalance between myocardial oxygen supply and demand. Bed rest decreases myocardial oxygen demand.

5 Correct answer—**B**

During an anginal attack, the following symptoms may be manifested: anxiety, diaphoresis, pain or discomfort, cold and clammy skin, dyspnea, increased heart rate, pulsus alternans, transient abnormal displaced point of maximal impulse (PMI), atrial gallop (S_4), and a rare transient systolic murmur. Transient ischemia will produce reversible cellular changes. The myocardium will shift from aerobic to anaerobic metabolism, resulting in lactic acid accumulation. Calcium release from the endoplasmic reticulum may be reduced, impairing myocardial function and hemodynamic stability. The aftermath may lead to a decrease in cardiac output, with increasing left ventricular end-diastolic volume. This increase in preload further taxes the ischemic myocardium.

6 Correct answer—**C**

Reflex tachycardia is induced by the use of nitrates, which is compensated by the bradycardic effects of beta blockade. Beta blockers, such as propranolol, are usually administered until relief is obtained or adverse effects occur. Common contraindications of beta blockers include heart block, uncompensated CHF, and asthma. Myocardial contractility, blood pressure, and heart rate decrease with beta blockade. After abrupt cessation of propranolol, exacerbation of angina occurs, possibly inducing an acute MI.

7 Correct answer—**C**

Chest pain that lasts longer than 30 to 45 minutes is most likely caused by an MI. Chest pain associated with angina rarely lasts longer than 30 minutes and may also be severe and radiating, but it is usually relieved by rest. PVCs can occur as a result of myocardial ischemia and may be present during an anginal episode.

8 Correct answer—**B**

In this setting, ST-segment elevations are indicative of acute myocardial injury. Leads V_1, V_2, and V_3 represent the anterior septal wall of the left ventricle. Leads II, III, and aVF represent the inferior wall, and leads I, V_5, and V_6 represent the lateral wall. ST-segment elevations are not characteristic of posterior wall MI; mirror images, that is, ST-segment depression, would be present in leads V_1, V_2, and V_3.

9 Correct answer—**A**

Morphine is a powerful analgesic. It reduces preload by causing peripheral vasodilation and reduces sympathetic activity, thereby decreasing myocardial work load. It has no direct effect on coronary arteries. Although morphine may produce sedation and is nonaddictive in small doses, it is not administered for these reasons.

10 Correct answer—**D**

PVCs are a result of myocardial irritability and are dangerous in the setting of an acute MI because they are precursors to life-threatening ventricular dysrhythmias. The ischemic area surrounding the area of infarction is the source of irritability. Necrotic tissue can neither generate nor transmit impulses. Lidocaine is an antiarrhythmic that raises the fibrillation threshold and has little effect on myocardial oxygen needs.

11 Correct answer—**C**

Auscultating the patient's lungs has the highest priority. Before action can be taken, the cause of the tachycardia should be found. Tachycardia is frequently often the first sign of heart failure in the patient with an MI. It is a compensatory mechanism for low stroke volume. Tachycardia may also be caused by anxiety and chest pain, but it is not a symptom of lidocaine toxicity. If heart failure is the cause of the tachycardia, a high Fowler's position would be the most comfortable for the patient. Morphine administration is not warranted initially for tachycardia.

12 Correct answer—**C**

Decreasing the patient's oxygen needs is primary. In MI, there is an imbalance between myocardial oxygen supply and demand. Measures that reduce the body's need for oxygen, such as giving supplemental oxygen, promoting rest, and reducing the patient's anxiety, can decrease the occurrence of complications, such as dysrhythmias, and prevent further myocardial damage.

13 Correct answer—**A**

A patient with an anterior wall MI is more likely to develop life-threatening conduction disturbances because the left anterior descending coronary artery supplies the His bundle and bundle branches, as well as the anterior wall of the left ventricle. These patients should be closely monitored because second-degree heart block, especially Mobitz II, is more likely to progress to complete heart block and cardiac arrest. First-degree AV and second-degree AV, Mobitz I (Wenckebach) blocks are common in patients with an inferior wall MI. They are caused by vagus nerve stimulation and AV node ischemia and edema. In 90% of the population, the right coronary artery supplies the AV node as well as the inferior wall of the left ventricle. In this setting, progression to more serious blocks is rare.

14 Correct answer—**B**

This murmur is characteristic of a papillary muscle dysfunction, namely mitral valve insufficiency. When a papillary muscle infarcts, improper valve closure results in regurgitation of blood from the left ventricle into the left atrium. Aortic insufficiency produces a diastolic murmur, and pericarditis produces a friction rub. Various murmurs can accompany ventricular aneurysm, depending on the aneurysm's location. Alone, none of these is diagnostic.

15 Correct answer—**B**

Q waves are indicative of myocardial necrosis. Leads I, aVL, V_5, and V_6 represent the lateral wall of the left ventricle. Leads II, III, and aVF represent the inferior wall, and leads V_1, V_2, and V_3, the anterior wall. Tall R waves in leads V_1 and V_2 are characteristic of a posterior infarction, reflecting the mirror image of Q waves.

16 Correct answer—**D**

Estrogen is thought to decrease lipoprotein levels and help the coronary arteries resist atherosclerosis. For this reason, MI is a rare occurrence in women of childbearing age. When a woman reaches menopause, her chance of developing coronary artery disease approaches that of men. Diabetes and hyperlipidemia are considered predisposing factors for the development of an MI.

17 Correct answer—**A**

Pulse pressure is the difference between the systolic and diastolic blood pressure, and a blood pressure of 90/60 mm Hg corresponds to a pulse pressure of 30 mm Hg. If arterial pressure falls and sympathetic compensatory vasoconstriction occurs, the pulse pressure is narrowed. The pulse pressure is influenced by stroke volume and peripheral resistance. A narrow pulse pressure indicates a low stroke volume (lowering systolic pressure) or high peripheral resistance (raising diastolic pressure).

18 Correct answer—**B**

A falling blood pressure and narrowing pulse pressure are ominous signs of left ventricular failure, or forward failure. CHF can be described as right-sided or left-sided, although failure of both sides may be present at the same time, or one may progress to the other. In left-sided heart failure, fluid accumulates in the pulmonary bed, whereas in right-sided heart failure, fluid accumulates in the systemic circulation. CHF can also be described according to the direction of the main force of blood flow. Cardiac output is decreased in forward failure. Backward failure occurs when blood accumulates in one or both ventricles and the venous system, thus decreasing cardiac output.

19 Correct answer—**C**

Hepatosplenomegaly is a common finding in patients who exhibit signs of right ventricular failure. The signs of right-sided heart failure are a result of venous congestion. With systemic vascular engorgement, the pressure in the capillaries of the abdominal organs will rise, resulting in edema. The edema produces a sense of fullness in the abdomen and may cause anorexia, nausea, and vomiting. Liver congestion causes tenderness over the hepatic area. The liver should be palpated for tenderness and engorgement. (Normally, the liver cannot be palpated.) Gallop rhythm, pulsus alternans, elevated PA diastolic pressure and PCWP, dyspnea, and crackles are seen in left ventricular failure.

20 Correct answer—**C**

Nursing intervention for the patient in CHF includes maintaining blood pressure, thereby maintaining warm, dry skin; adequate diuresis; and normal mental status. Sodium and fluid intake also must be monitored closely. Although the serum sodium concentration level may be low, dilution from excessive fluid retention masks the underlying problem of sodium excess. Fluid restriction is necessary to allow the sodium concentration to reach a normal level. The administration of saline solution worsens CHF. Sodium intake should also be limited to decrease the patient's thirst and water intake.

21 Correct answer—**A**

Right ventricular failure is frequently a sequel of left ventricular failure with its high pulmonary venous and arterial pressures. Right ventricular failure also may be caused by intrinsic lung disease, valvular disease, right ventricular infarction, or pulmonary hypertension. Cor pulmonale is right ventricular failure that occurs from prolonged pulmonary hypertension.

22 Correct answer—**D**

Colloid osmotic pressure (COP) is a reflection of edema production. COP represents the ability of plasma proteins to keep fluid in the vascular space. The normal range of COP is 30 to 35 mm Hg. When colloid osmotic pressure falls below hydrostatic pressure, transudation of fluids from capillary membranes to the interstitium occurs. The introduction of a balloon-tipped catheter via a central vein permits the following: measurement of pulmonary artery diastolic and wedge pressures, continuous monitoring of pulmonary artery systolic and mean pressures, sampling of mixed venous blood, and evaluation of cardiac output. These measurements give information on myocardial and hemodynamic function.

23 Correct answer—**C**

The catheter tip may irritate the right ventricle as it is being passed and may produce PVCs. The physician may elect to withdraw the catheter or order the administration of I.V. lidocaine.

24 Correct answer—**B**

Normal pressures are as follows: PCWP, 5 to 12 mm Hg; right atrial pressure, 0 to 5 mm Hg; right ventricular pressure, 25/0 to 5 mm Hg; and pulmonary artery pressure, 25/5 to 12 mm Hg. The PCWP is recorded when the tip of the balloon catheter wedges into a smaller branch of the pulmonary artery. Deflation of the balloon results in a pulmonary artery pressure reading. Lung changes shown on X-ray are closely related to changes depicted in PCWP.

25 Correct answer—**C**

Nursing responsibilities during the insertion of a balloon-tipped catheter include monitoring and recording pressure tracings and pressures, monitoring vital signs, providing emotional support and direction, and maintaining sterile technique. Monitoring for thrombotic events would not be required during insertion of a balloon-tipped catheter, thrombi being relegated to a long-term complication from this procedure.

26 Correct answer—**A**

The insertion of a flow-directed, balloon-tipped catheter is an invasive procedure, having a complication rate of 2%. The most common complication is infection, resulting from either catheter-associated infections or poor sterile technique during insertion. Other complications include damage to the lung parenchyma, pulmonary infarct, cardiac dysrhythmias, balloon rupture, and knotting of the catheter.

27 Correct answer—**B**

The aim of therapy for CHF is to decrease left ventricular demands and increase myocardial oxygen supply. This is accomplished by decreasing preload and afterload along with increasing contractility. These three parameters are the primary determinants of the stroke volume.

28 Correct answer—**C**

Complications occurring from the treatment of CHF include hypovolemia, hypokalemia, digitalis toxicity, cardiac dysrhythmia, and emboli formation. Hypovolemia and hypokalemia may occur from excessive use of diuretic therapy, resulting in sodium, potassium, and water loss. Hypokalemia may lead to cardiac dysrhythmias. Digitalis toxicity can occur with digoxin overmedication, hypokalemia, or renal dysfunction. Dysrhythmias may occur in response to electrolyte imbalances, sympathomimetic drugs, or digoxin. Emboli formation can be caused by bed rest or excessive diuretic therapy, resulting in an elevated hematocrit hemoconcentration. Cor pulmonale is the dilation and hypertrophy of the right ventricle resulting from lung disease. The prerequisite for the development of cor pulmonale is pulmonary hypertension.

29 Correct answer—**C**

Digoxin is widely used to treat CHF and supraventricular dysrhythmias, especially atrial fibrillation. Digoxin exerts a positive inotropic action, increasing contractility in normal and failing hearts. In the failing heart, digitalis decreases ventricular size and reduces wall tension. Antiarrhythmic action of the drug prolongs conduction time and the refractory features of the AV node. As a negative chronotropic agent, digitalis produces vagotonia, resulting in a slow heart rate.

30 Correct answer—**D**

The PR interval, QT interval, and QRS complex, as well as the atrial and ventricular rates, should be monitored in a patient taking digoxin. The cardiac rhythm should also be noted. The enhanced automaticity and facilitation of reentry produced by the drug can result in atrial, junctional, or ventricular tachydysrhythmias. Sinus tachycardia, however, is not produced. Other manifestations of digoxin toxicity are PAT with block, AV blocks, atrial ectopic beats, atrial fibrillation, sinus arrest, and sinoatrial block. However, the hallmark dysrhythmia in digoxin toxicity is ventricular bigeminy. In diseased hearts, digoxin toxicity is more likely to result in tachydysrhythmias; in normal hearts, AV blocks result.

31 Correct answer—**C**

Dilantin is the antiarrhythmic drug of choice in digoxin toxicity. The patient should be monitored for hypokalemia because a low potassium level enhances digoxin toxicity. Hypercalcemia may sensitize the heart to the drug's effects, precipitating digoxin-induced dysrhythmias. Quinidine administration potentiates and may precipitate digoxin toxicity.

32 Correct answer—**C**

Aminophylline is a useful agent to treat CHF because it increases myocardial contractility and cardiac output, resulting in diuresis. It also acts directly on peripheral arteries and veins, producing vasodilation. The drug relieves bronchospasm associated with lung disease, pulmonary edema, and asthma. An undesirable adverse effect of aminophylline administration is tachycardia.

33 Correct answer—**C**

Adverse effects related to aminophylline administration and toxicity include nausea, vomiting, abdominal pain, tachycardia, hypotension, and convulsions. If any of these occur, the drug should be discontinued.

34 Correct answer—**C**

A potassium level greater than 5 mEq/liter causes hyperkalemia, peaked T waves, as well as prolonged PR interval and widened QRS complex. Hypokalemia, a potassium level less than 3 mEq/liter, causes the appearance of a prominent U wave, flattened T waves, ST-segment depression, and PVCs.

35 Correct answer—**B**

The interpretation of this strip is atrial flutter, which is characterized by an atrial rate of 300 beats/minute, sawtooth pattern of flutter waves, and normal QRS complexes. In the given strip, varying degrees of block are represented. PAT with block is characterized by an atrial rate of 150 to 250 beats/minute. P waves precede each QRS complex, but when block occurs, they are not conducted. The P waves may be buried in the preceding T wave and are often different in configuration because they arise from an ectopic focus. Atrial fibrillation is characterized by an atrial rate of 350 to 600 beats/minute, so fast that P waves cannot be distinguished. QRS complexes are normal in configuration and occur in an irregular rhythm.

36 Correct answer—**C**

The interpretation of this strip is first-degree AV block. The PR interval is greater than 0.20 seconds. Prolongation of the PR interval may be associated with hyperkalemia. First-degree AV block is a common finding in inferior wall MI because of AV-node ischemia. The effects of digoxin and organic heart disease can cause delayed conduction through the AV node, thus prolonging the PR interval.

37 Correct answer—**A**

The interpretation of this strip is ventricular bigeminy, one of several dysrhythmias associated with digitalis toxicity. A PVC occurs after every other beat. Phenytoin is the ventricular antiarrhythmic most useful in treating this condition. In this particular situation, lidocaine would not be given because these PVCs perfuse. Eliminating the PVCs would decrease the heart rate by 50%, severely diminishing cardiac output. The PVCs are unifocal and therefore arise from the same ectopic focus. The patient had nausea, a well established symptom of digitalis toxicity. Other symptoms include anorexia, visual disturbances, and fatigue.

38 Correct answer—**B**

The interpretation of this strip is ventricular tachycardia, and the treatment of choice is defibrillation. If the patient had a pulse, synchronized cardioversion would be indicated. The defibrillator would then be synchronized with the cardiac monitor so that the electrical impulse is discharged on the QRS complex (depolarization) and not on the T wave, which can cause the rhythm to deteriorate. A precordial thump is not warranted because it was previously unsuccessful. Lidocaine may be administered *after* defibrillation.

39 Correct answer—**C**

The interpretation of this strip is ventricular fibrillation. Immediate defibrillation is the treatment of choice. Lidocaine or bretylium may be administered after defibrillation. The rhythm is totally chaotic, without evidence of P waves or QRS complexes.

40 Correct answer—**C**

Atropine is the treatment of choice initially for symptomatic bradycardia, as well as bradycardia associated with PVCs. It may be repeated every 5 minutes to a maximum dose of 2 mg, if necessary. A temporary pacemaker may then be inserted. PVCs may be a symptom of hypoxia caused by the bradycardia. If this is the case, increasing the heart rate would eliminate the PVCs; hence, they should not be treated with an antiarrythmic. Isoproterenol is used to treat symptomatic heart block that does not respond to atropine. It is used only until a pacemaker can be inserted. Isoproterenol increases myocardial oxygen consumption and predisposes the heart to dysrhythmias, which is detrimental in the face of an MI.

41 Correct answer—**B**

The interpretation of this strip is second-degree AV block, Mobitz I (Wenckebach). This dysrhythmia is characterized by a PR interval that becomes progressively wider until a QRS complex is dropped. Then the sequence begins again. Second-degree AV block, Mobitz II, is characterized by a constant PR interval and unpredictable dropping of QRS complexes. Wandering atrial pacemaker is characterized by P waves that vary in size and configuration. The PR interval also varies, depending on the distance of the pacemaker to the AV node. In third-degree heart block, no relationship exists between the P waves and QRS complexes. The atria and ventricles beat independently; the atrial rate may be 60 to 100 beats/minute, with regularly occurring P waves. The ventricular rate can be anywhere from 20 to 60 beats/minute, depending on whether the impulse originates in the AV node or the ventricles. The rate will be slowest if the beat arises from the ventricle.

42 Correct answer—**B**

The interpretation of this strip is loss of capture. The pacemaker is sensing the patient's slow rate and firing appropriately. However, the pacing spikes are not followed by QRS complexes. Increasing the pacemaker rate will not solve the problem—it will just produce more spikes. Possible causes of capture loss include an inadequate amount of energy (measured in milliamperes [MA]) and displacement of the catheter tip. Turning up the output (MA) dial will increase the amount of electrical energy delivered by the pacemaker to the myocardium. Turning the patient on either side may cause the catheter to move back toward the endocardium. Another possible cause of loss of capture is when the negative terminal of the pulse generator becomes disconnected from the distal wire of the pacing catheter. The distal electrode delivers the energy that paces the heart.

43 Correct answer—**C**

The interpretation of this strip is failure to sense the cardiac rhythm. The pacemaker continues to fire at the preset rate even though the patient's own heart rate is higher. Pacemaker spikes should never be seen when the patient's own rate is consistently higher than the one set for the demand pacemaker. When this occurs, the patient's own pacemaker and the temporary pacemaker compete for control of the heart. Some pacemaker spikes will be followed by a QRS complex; others will not. This can be a dangerous situation if a pacemaker spike occurs on a T wave, which represents the repolarization or vulnerable phase of the cardiac cycle. Ventricular fibrillation can result. Runaway pacemaker, which may be seen in battery depletion, results in the pacemaker firing at a rate faster than the pacemaker setting. The absence of pacemaker spikes will occur if an inadequate connection between pacemaker wire and generator exists.

44 Correct answer—**C**

Aneurysms are usually described according to shape and identified according to type and location. Their shape is either fusiform or saccular. A fusiform aneurysm is a uniform, round arterial dilation. A saccular aneurysm is a vascular outpouching with a small neck attaching to the arterial wall. A true aneurysm results from dilation enclosed by an intact arterial wall. Whenever there is an extravascular accumulation of blood from a disruption of all three layers of the arterial wall, a false aneurysm exists. A dissecting aneurysm results from a separation of arterial layers; blood accumulates in the middle layer secondary to a tear in the inner lining.

45 Correct answer—**C**

A common finding in a patient with a proximal aortic dissection is anterior central chest pain, which rarely radiates to the back. The patient frequently experiences neurologic deficits, including cerebral apoplexy, paraparesis, peripheral neuropathy, and changes in mental status. Another common finding is blood pressure variations between the arms and pulse deficits. Hypertension is a major manifestation in a patient with a distal dissection.

46 Correct answer—**B**

The most frequent findings of dissection are an elevated LDH level, leukocytosis, and a widened aorta. An important EKG finding is left ventricular hypertrophy. Angiography is the most definitive diagnostic procedure to determine the location and extent of dissection. The status of the renal, mesenteric, and iliac circulations is also evaluated by contrast angiography. Emergency anteroposterior and lateral lumbosacral spinal X-ray studies or ultrasonography should be done. If the aneurysm is small and the patient is symptomatic, ultrasound studies should be performed approximately every 6 months to monitor size and determine need for surgery.

47 Correct answer—**A**

The initial therapy and treatment of choice for all types of dissecting aneurysms is drug therapy, the primary objective of which is to decrease the systolic pressure to 100 to 120 mm Hg for 24 to 48 hours. Agents such as reserpine (Serpasil), trimethaphan (Arfonad), nitroprusside (Nipride), and propranolol may be administered to control blood pressure. Cardiac contractility also must be decreased. Diuretics may be given concurrently. Drug therapy hastens the fibrotic phase of the healing process, reduces edema, and reduces bleeding in the subsequent surgery. Once pain is relieved and blood pressure controlled, aortography is performed to select the appropriate, definitive therapy. If the aortogram indicates a type I or type II dissection, immediate surgery is warranted. Types I and II aortic aneurysms involve the ascending aorta. Type I progresses beyond the aortic arch; type II ends before the aortic arch. Type II involves most or all of the descending aorta. Types I and II are more often associated with cardiac tamponade and severe aortic regurgitation. In these types, aortic valve replacement may accompany aneurysm repair. If the dissection is type III and no contraindications to medical therapy exist, antihypertensive therapy can be initiated as planned.

48 Correct answer—**B**

Aneurysms are most commonly found in the aorta, although they also occur in the left ventricle after an acute MI, in the cerebral arteries, and in other central and peripheral arteries. Aortic aneurysms are categorized according to location, such as thoracic-ascending, transverse, descending, thoracoabdominal, and abdominal. Ascending thoracic aneurysms are located in the area of the aorta that is closest to the heart. Aneurysms of the transverse arch include the carotid, subclavian, and upper vertebral arteries. Aneurysms of the descending thoracic aorta are found in the proximal part of the descending aorta. Abdominal aneurysms are found below the arteries of the kidney and above the bifurcation of the iliac arteries. Thoracoabdominal aneurysms extend from immediately above the diaphragm to the area immediately below it and are typically associated with decreased blood supply to the celiac, superior mesenteric, and renal arteries. Dissecting aneurysms occur when there is progressive horizontal tearing of the middle layer from the inner layer, or intima.

49 Correct answer—**D**

Restlessness is a sign of cardiac tamponade, a result of hypoxia caused by a decreased cardiac output. Other signs are narrow pulse pressure, pulsus paradoxus, and decreased amplitude of QRS complexes. Pulse pressure narrows because of a decrease in systolic pressure caused by the drop in cardiac output; diastolic pressure rises because of peripheral vasoconstriction. Pulsus paradoxus refers to an exaggerated decrease in the systolic pressure during inspiration. To check for pulsus paradoxus, inflate the blood pressure cuff and slowly deflate. If pulsus paradoxus is present, the sounds will be absent during inspiration for a period greater than 10 mm Hg during cuff deflation. The amplitude of the QRS complexes may decrease as fluid accumulation increases the distance of the heart from the chest wall, thereby interfering with EKG recording.

50 Correct answer—**B**

Preload refers to the stretching force of the ventricle immediately before contraction. According to Starling's law, an increase in the left ventricular volume can increase the volume pumped out during systole. Beyond a certain point, however, this mechanism no longer works. Therefore, increasing the patient's circulating volume can temporarily support a failing cardiac output until measures can be instituted to relieve the pressure of the tamponade. Large amounts of blood are seldom lost when tamponade occurs quickly. As little as 100 ml of blood in the pericardial space is enough to cause a severe decrease in cardiac output. Patients with cardiac tamponade usually do not have pulmonary edema. They will usually have normal chest X-rays, although a widened cardiac silhouette may be apparent. Afterload refers to the force against which the left ventricle must pump (peripheral vascular resistance).

51 Correct answer—**C**

During pericardiocentesis, a 16- or 18-gauge intracardiac needle is inserted into the pericardial sac to withdraw blood or fluid. When blood in the pericardial space causes myocardial compression and decreased cardiac output, immediate aspiration is the priority. Removing as little as 20 ml of blood may save the patient's life. After hemodynamic stability is restored, the patient may be taken for a thoracotomy, if indicated. Administration of I.V. fluids and the application of a MAST suit do not hold the highest priority as they only temporarily increase the cardiac output.

52 Correct answer—**C**

Heart block is not a complication of pericardiocentesis. Ventricular perforation can occur if the needle is advanced too quickly, and ventricular fibrillation can result from the needle making contact with the myocardium. Pneumothorax can occur if the needle is accidently introduced into the pleural space.

53 Correct answer—**B**

A precordial (V lead) EKG lead should be attached to the hub of the intracardiac needle. During pericardiocentesis, the EKG machine should be recording in V lead. If the needle makes contact with the myocardium, a current of injury pattern, ST-segment elevation, will be recorded. During the procedure, a high Fowler's position will provide maximum comfort for the awake patient. Isoproterenol and Valsalva's maueuver are not indicated in the treatment of pericardial tamponade.

54 Correct answer—**B**

Penetrating chest trauma is the most common cause of acute cardiac tamponade. Blunt trauma is the second next frequent cause. Tamponade is also an infrequent and serious complication following a transmural MI. Chronic fluid accumulation in the pericardial sac can result from various disorders, such as cancer, autoimmune disease, and uremia. Because these effusions occur chronically, the pericardium has a chance to stretch to accommodate as much as 1,500 ml of fluid. In this situation, the onset of symptoms is much more gradual and less immediately life-threatening.

55 Correct answer—**A**

Hypertensive crisis is characterized by a diastolic pressure greater than 130 mm Hg. When symptoms such as headache, visual disturbances, nausea, and vomiting accompany a critically elevated diastolic pressure, hypertensive encephalopathy should be suspected. Hypertensive encephalopathy is a medical emergency and occurs when arterial spasm and cerebral edema produce neurologic symptoms. Other symptoms of this syndrome include papilledema, transient hemiparesis, disorientation, and convulsions. If untreated, hypertensive encephalopathy can lead to death.

56 Correct answer—**D**

Clonidine lowers blood pressure by acting directly on alpha-adrenergic receptors in the central nervous system, thereby causing a decrease in sympathetic outflow from the brain. Abrupt discontinuation of this drug can cause a withdrawal reaction leading to severe rebound hypertension. This may occur within 12 to 48 hours. Clonidine does not have any effect on sodium and water balance and is not known to have any direct effect on the peripheral vasculature. Nothing in the patient's history warrants suspicion of renal failure.

57 Correct answer—**B**

Nitroprusside has a powerful vasodilating effect and acts directly on peripheral vascular smooth muscle. The onset of action is 30 to 60 seconds. This medication should always be administered through an infusion pump. Profound hypotension can occur quickly in response to this medication; therefore, the patient's blood pressure must be closely monitored, preferably with the use of an arterial line.

58 Correct answer—**D**

Although various factors predispose an individual to hypertension, the majority of patients have no known medical problems directly causing hypertension. Predisposing factors include old age, elevated cholesterol levels, heredity, obesity, and sedentary life-style. A minority of patients have secondary hypertension in which there is an identifiable cause. These include the use of substances such as tobacco, alcohol, caffeine, and certain drugs; cardiovascular disorders, such as coarctation of the aorta; endocrine disorders, such as pheochromocytoma and disorders of the adrenal cortex; neurologic disorders, such as increased intracranial pressure; kidney disorders, such as renal artery stenosis, acute or chronic renal failure, and renin-secreting tumors; and pregnancy.

59 Correct answer—**A**

Epinephrine is an endogenous catecholamine with both alpha- and beta-adrenergic actions. During resuscitation, epinephrine elevates perfusion pressure generated during chest compression, improves myocardial contractility, and increases the vigor of ventricular fibrillation. It is also used in ventricular standstill in an attempt to generate electrical and mechanical activity. Recommended dose of epinephrine is 0.5 to 1 mg of a 1:10,000 solution. If an I.V. line is unavailable, 1 mg may be given endotracheally. Because of its short duration of action, it may be necessary to repeat the dose at 5-minute intervals. Epinephrine should not be added to an alkaline solution because that may result in inactivation. Lidocaine and/or bretylium are indicated medications after epinephrine administration. Calcium chloride is no longer recommended as advanced life-support medication because research studies have shown no therapeutic effects from its use.

60 Correct answer—**A**

Sodium bicarbonate is an extracellular buffer responsible for controlling acid-base balance. During cardiac resuscitation, the body is in a state of ventilatory failure, which leads to respiratory acidosis and circulatory failure. Metabolic acidosis is the result of these events. Efficient ventilation of the lungs is essential for the elimination of carbon dioxide, as well as the provision of oxygenation. The need for therapy must be guided by evaluation of ABGs and is appropriate only if metabolic acidosis exists. Sodium bicarbonate is administered at a dose of 1 mEq/kg.

61 Correct answer—**B**

Lidocaine is the drug of choice after termination of ventricular fibrillation or tachycardia, especially when defibrillation has been used. The use of lidocaine may terminate reentrant activity responsible for ventricular dysrhythmias in ischemic zones. A common therapeutic dose is 1 mg/kg as a bolus, followed by a continuous infusion of 2 to 4 mg/minute via an infusion pump. Blood levels of lidocaine should be maintained in the effective suppressive range of 1.5 to 6 mcg/ml. Blood levels of lidocaine above 9 mcg/ml may produce toxic effects. Lidocaine is degraded by the liver; the dosage should be reduced in patients with impaired liver function. Digoxin, verapamil, and dopamine are indicated to treat ventricular dysrhythmia.

62 Correct answer—**D**

Bretylium possesses antiarrhythmic effects, adrenergic-blocking properties, and positive inotropic action. Bretylium is beneficial in terminating ventricular fibrillation and tachycardia refractory to lidocaine. In ventricular fibrillation, 5 mg/kg of undiluted bretylium should be administered intravenously. If unsuccessful, the dose can be increased to 10 mk/kg and repeated as needed. The onset of action of bretylium seems to be within a few minutes; however, in ventricular tachycardia, it may be delayed up to 20 minutes or more. In the awake patient, the bolus should be diluted and infused over 10 minutes. Bretylium is contraindicated in the treatment of ventricular tachycardia caused by digitalis toxicity. The most common adverse effects of bretylium are postural hypotension, nausea, and vomiting.

63 Correct answer—**C**

The principal use for isoproterenol is in the immediate control of hemodynamically significant, atropine-refractory complete heart block until a pacemaker is made available. Isoproterenol is a pure beta-adrenergic agent possessing positive inotropic and chronotropic properties. It increases cardiac output and heart rate. The recommended infusion rate is 2 to 10 mcg/minute titrated to maintain a heart rate of 60 beats/minute. Because of its cardiac-stimulating properties, isoproterenol is contraindicated when tachydysrhythmias are present. Extreme caution must be exercised when the drug is used to treat MI because isoproterenol may cause the areas of ischemia and infarction to enlarge.

64 Correct answer—**D**

An effect of propranolol administration is decreased AV conduction time. Propranolol is used for beta-adrenergic blockade in the treatment of angina pectoris, cardiac dysrhythmias, and hypertension. Beta-blockade action is useful in controlling the ventricular response to atrial flutter or fibrillation and to prevent recurrences of paroxysmal supraventricular tachycardia, as it decreases AV conduction. Propranolol also decreases myocardial contractility, which results in decreased myocardial oxygen demand. A decrease in cardiac output would not be a therapeutic effect.

65 Correct answer—**A**

Dopamine, an endogenous catecholamine, is an important agent to treat various types of shock because it directly increases cardiac output and renal blood flow. The hemodynamic effects depend on the dosage. At dosages less than 7 mcg/kg/minute, increases in cardiac output, myocardial contractility, and renal blood flow predominate; little or no vasoconstriction occurs. At dosages higher than 7 mcg/kg/minute, alpha-adrenergic effects predominate, leading to peripheral vasoconstriction and an increase in mean arterial pressure.

66 Correct answer—**A**

Dopamine should be infused into a central line by an infusion pump. Dopamine is contraindicated in the presence of uncontrolled dysrhythmia, pheochromocytoma, and use of monoamine oxidase (MAO) inhibitors. The most serious effect of dopamine is the onset or exacerbation of cardiac dysrhythmia. At high doses, dopamine increases myocardial oxygen demand and may cause ischemia to extend in the presence of coronary artery disease.

67 Correct answer—**C**

Dobutamine is the preferred agent to treat severe heart failure. It produces a greater increase in cardiac output, a lessened increase in heart rate and peripheral vascular resistance, and fewer cardiac dysrhythmias than equivalent doses of dopamine. Adverse effects of dobutamine include nausea, headache, dyspnea, and angina. Digoxin and epinephrine increase myocardial oxygen consumption.

68 Correct answer—**B**

Streptokinase is a nonenzymatic protein thrombolytic agent excreted by group C beta-hemolytic streptococci. Thrombolytic therapy is effective in treating massive pulmonary emboli, extensive deep vein thrombosis, and lysis of a thrombus-occluded arteriovenous cannula. Substantial evidence supports the use of streptokinase in treating acute MI in its early stages. Heparin and wararin are anticoagulant agents. Thrombokinase is nonexistent.

69 Correct answer—**C**

The use of streptokinase is contraindicated in surgical procedures performed within the past 10 days (including paracentesis, thoracentesis, and invasive biopsy), active gastrointestinal bleeding, coagulation disorders, recent CVA, cardiac trauma or massage, intracranial neoplasia, severe hypertension, mitral valve disease with atrial fibrillation, subacute bacterial endocarditis, and acute or chronic renal or hepatic failure. To avoid complication, a detailed history, a physical examination, and laboratory studies should be obtained before starting therapy. Anticoagulant or antiplatelet agents should not be given concurrently. The prothrombin time, partial thromboplastin time, thrombin time, and total platelet count should be measured before streptokinase therapy is begun and monitored frequently during therapy.

70 Correct answer—**C**

Thrombolytic therapy should be discontinued immediately if dyspnea occurs, as it may indicate a severe allergic reaction. Adverse reactions to streptokinase therapy include hemorrhagic complications with bleeding at I.V. sites, incision sites, and wounds. These can be treated with pressure and discontinuation of therapy. In severe hemorrhage, fresh frozen plasma can be administered and aminocaproic acid (Amicar) may be needed. Allergic reactions include urticaria, pruritus, headache, musculoskeletal pain, bronchospasm, edema, hypertension, and fever. Febrile reactions and mild allergic symptoms can be treated with acetaminophen, antihistamines, and steroids. Severe allergic reactions warrant discontinuation of the infusion. Rare adverse reactions include gastrointestinal upset, hepatitis symptoms, depression, delirium, and tachycardia.

71 Correct answer—**A**

Adverse effects from the use of I.V. nitroglycerin include headache, methemoglobinemia, bradycardia, and hypotension. Hypotension is the most serious effect and can result in ischemia to organs that are dependent on perfusion pressure, such as the heart, kidneys, and brain. Hypotension can be treated with fluid administration. Bradycardia can be corrected with the use of atropine; continuous infusion is initiated at 10 to 20 mcg/minute and increased by 5 to 10 mcg/minute until desired hemodynamic or clinical results are achieved. Congestive heart failure and ventricular fibrillation are not adverse effects of I.V. nitroglycerin therapy.

72 Correct answer—**B**

Nitroprusside is a potent vasodilator, decreasing preload and afterload. Rapid infusion of I.V. nitroprusside results in hypotension, apprehension, restlessness, muscle twitching, palpitations, and chest and abdominal pain. Treatment consists of lowering or discontinuing the infusion rate. The dose of nitroprusside should be regulated by an infusion pump because of its potency and rapid onset of action. Thiocyanate levels should be monitored if high doses of nitroprusside are infused for longer than 48 hours.

73 Correct answer—**D**

Cardiac contusion occurs following blunt chest trauma, such as steering wheel injuries. Myocardial edema and hemorrhage result in myocardial ischemia and necrosis. The signs and symptoms of cardiac contusion are similar to those of an MI: chest pain, shortness of breath, EKG changes (ST-segment elevation, T-wave inversion, and Q-wave formation), and cardiac enzyme elevation. The precipitating event is of traumatic rather than coronary artery origin.

74 Correct answer—**B**

The right ventricle is the most common area of damage after a cardiac contusion because it is situated directly behind the sternum.

75 Correct answer—**A**

Nitroglycerin is not indicated in the treatment of cardiac contusion because the pain is not of coronary artery origin, and dilation of the coronary arteries would not relieve it. Morphine sulfate is the analgesic of choice for the pain associated with cardiac contusion. Oxygen should be given to improve the oxygen supply to the damaged myocardium. Lidocaine is indicated in the treatment of ventricular dysrhythmias associated with cardiac contusion.

76 Correct answer—**C**

The complications of cardiac contusion are a result of damage to the myocardium from edema and microscopic hemorrhage. These complications include ventricular dysrhythmias, pericarditis, CHF, cardiac tamponade, and cardiogenic shock.

77 Correct answer—**A**

Anticoagulants are contraindicated in cardiac contusion because of the microscopic hemorrhage that occurs after the trauma. Hemopericardium, or bleeding into the pericardium, may result if heparin is administered. Digoxin and dopamine may be indicated if CHF develops. Bretylium or procainamide (Pronestyl) may be indicated if the ventricular dysrhythmias are not suppressed by lidocaine.

78 Correct answer—**C**

Of paramount importance during the initial assessment of the patient with pericarditis is observing for pulsus paradoxus, an exaggeration of the normal physiologic response to inspiration. Normally, upon inspiration, there is a fall of less than 10 mm Hg in arterial systolic pressure. With pulsus paradoxus, arterial pressure drops, upon inspiration, exceeding 10 mm Hg. During further assessment, a pericardial friction rub is present but is of no help in evaluating the severity of the condition. Fever is not a constant finding. Kussmaul's sign, which is paradoxic inspiratory neck vein filling, is rarely seen in the acute setting. Pericarditis, or inflammation of the pericardial sac, may occur alone or with an inflammatory process of the myocardium.

79 Correct answer—**D**

When pericarditis is present, the patient will probably exhibit dyspnea and tachypnea. Those factors that increase pain include deep inspiration, rotation of the trunk, or lying flat. Palliative measures include sitting upright or leaning forward. Pericarditis usually is evidenced by a severe pleuritic substernal chest pain with widespread ST-segment elevation on the EKG.

80 Correct answer—**A**

The treatment of pericarditis requires the relief of pain and resolution of the acute inflammatory process. Treatment with anti-inflammatory drugs, such as aspirin, indomethacin, or steroids, is usually employed. If pericarditis is the result of an infectious process, antibiotics would also be used. In this instance, the patient is postcardiotomy; thus, the developing pericarditis is an autoimmune reaction to pericardial injury.

81 Correct answer—**C**

The causes of pericarditis are multiple. Medical histories include viral infections, inflammatory processes, such as systemic lupus erythematosus, rheumatic fever, and scleroderma; and hypersensitivity or autoimmune responses that include postcardiotomy and postmyocardial infarction (Dressler's syndrome). Some metabolic disturbances, such as uremia or myxedema, may cause pericarditis as well as blunt or penetrating trauma. Chronic obstructive pulmonary disease is not associated with pericarditis.

82 Correct answer—**B**

The patient with endocarditis presents with sudden fever, which is the most essential feature of this disease, along with septicemia, and CHF. Therefore, priority nursing assessments include monitoring for the symptoms of CHF, which includes auscultation for S_3 and crackles. The patient should be placed on a cardiac monitor for assessment of heart rate, because the tachycardia is frequently out of proportion to the patient's temperature. PVCs are seldom associated with infective endocarditis.

83 Correct answer—**B**

Laboratory studies usually reflect leukocytosis (increased white blood cell count), anemia, and an elevated erythrocyte sedimentation rate, which is present in virtually all cases.

84 Correct answer—**A**

Blood cultures are of prime diagnostic, as well as therapeutic, importance. Culture specimens from several sites should be obtained as the fever is climbing. Culture media and techniques for identifying fungi and anaerobic bacteria should be used, as should the standard techniques for aerobic strains. Although a nonspecific test, measurement of the erythrocyte sedimentation rate is useful in a negative sense; that is, if the rate is not elevated, a diagnosis of bacterial endocarditis becomes most unlikely.

85 Correct answer—**B**

Patients who develop acute arterial occlusion commonly have a medical history that predisposes them to mural thrombi formation. This may occur in rheumatic valvular disease, atrial fibrillation, MI, and previous cardiac surgery, such as prosthetic valve replacement. A postpartum patient may be predisposed to a venous occlusion.

86 Correct answer—**D**

Physical examination of the involved extremity would reveal a pale or cyanotic extremity that is cold to touch; nonpalpable pulses distal to the occlusion; paresthesias; and trophic changes, such as thin, shiny, hairless skin. Swelling and tenderness in the affected extremity and a positive Homans' sign are symptoms of a venous occlusion.

87 Correct answer—**C**

Appropriate nursing interventions for a patient with acute arterial occlusion include providing warm environmental temperature to relieve arterial spasms (heat is never applied to the extremity); elevation of the head of the bed or stretcher on 8- to 10-inch (20- to 25-cm) blocks so that gravity will augment flow of blood to the ischemic extremity (the affected extremity should never be elevated); and heparin administration, as ordered.

88 Correct answer—**A**

The nurse would anticipate that this patient would possibly undergo the following therapeutic procedures: balloon-tipped catheter extraction of an emboli, embolectomy, thrombolytic infusion, or a bypass graft.

Selected References

Andreoli, K., and Wallace, A. *Comprehensive Cardiac Care*. St. Louis: C. V. Mosby Co., 1983.

Ballenger, J. "More Field Drugs: Mechanisms of Action," *Emergency Medicine*, January 1985.

Chatterjee, K. "Acute Management of Unstable Angina," *Emergency Medicine*, August 1983.

Conley, K., and Small, R.E. "Administering IV Nitroglycerin: Nursing Implications," *DCCN* (Dimensions in Critical Care Nursing), January/February 1983.

Conti, R. "Sorting Out Chest Pain," *Emergency Medicine*, February 1984.

Cosgriff, J.A., and Anderson, D. L. "A Man with Abdominal and Back Pain," *Journal of Emergency Nursing* 12:109-110, March/April 1986.

Cowley, R.A., and Dunham, C.M. *Shock Trauma/Critical Care Manual*. Baltimore: University Park Press, 1982.

Eisenhaur, L.A., and Gerald, M.C. *The Nurse's 1984-85 Guide to Drug Therapy*. Englewood Cliffs, N.J.: Prentice Hall, 1984.

Hedges, R. "Preload and Afterload Revisited," *Journal of Emergency Nursing* 9:262-267, September/October 1983.

Holloway, N.M. *Emergency Department Nurses Association Core Curriculum*. Philadelphia: W. B. Saunders Co., 1985.

Huang, S., et al. *Coronary Care Nursing*. Philadelphia: W. B. Saunders Co., 1983.

Kransover, T. "A Conceptual Approach to the Electrocardiogram," *Critical Care Nurse* 2:66-76, March/April 1982.

Lamb, H. "The Angina that Can Kill: Variant Angina that Results from Coronary Artery Spasm," *RN* 48:28-34, August 1985.

May, H.L. *Emergency Medicine*. New York: John Wiley & Sons, 1984.

McCauley, C.M., et al. *McGoon's Cardiac Surgery: An Interprofessional Approach to Patient Care*. Philadelphia: F. A. Davis Co., 1985.

O'Boyle, C., et al. *Emergency Care: The First 24 Hours*. East Norwalk, Conn.: Appleton-Century-Crofts, 1985.

Parker, J.G. *Emergency Nursing, A Guide to Comprehensive Care*. New York: John Wiley & Sons, 1984.

Patrizzi, J.O., and Tackett, M.K. *Emergency Nursing: A Case Study Approach*. Bowie, Md.: Robert J. Brady Co., 1984.

Price, S., et al. *Pathophysiology: Clinical Concepts of Disease Processes*. New York: McGraw-Hill Book Co., 1984.

Sanderson, R., et al. *The Cardiac Patient: A Comprehensive Approach*. Philadelphia: W. B. Saunders Co., 1983.

Sheehy, S.B., and Barber, J. *Emergency Nursing: Principles and Practice*. St. Louis: C. V. Mosby Co., 1985.

"Standards for Cardiopulmonary Resuscitation (CPR) and Emergency Cardiac Care (ECC)," Supplement to *Journal of the American Medical Association*, June 6, 1986.

Underhill, S.L., et al. *Cardiac Nursing*. Philadelphia: J. B. Lippincott Co., 1982.

Vaughan, P., and Rice, V. "Complications of Myocardial Infarction," *Critical Care Nurse* 2:51-55, May/June 1982.

Zullo, M., and Scheidt, S. "Treatment of Arrhyt[illegible]ias in Acute Myocardial Infarction," *Clinical Cardiology in Practice*, March/April 1984.

Chapter 4

Respiratory Emergencies Questions and Answers

You must begin with Question 1 of this chapter and progress in sequence. **Do not skip around.** Subsequent answers build on previous ones.

Mary Blum, RN, MSN
Deborah Gough, RN, MSN, CCRN, CEN
Marilyn McDonald, RN, MA
Janet A. Neff, RN, MN, CCRN, CEN

1 Atelectasis is indicated when bronchial breath sounds are heard over the:

A. Carina
B. Right middle lobe
C. Right main stem bronchus
D. Left main stem bronchus

2 During percussion, consolidated dense areas will produce:

A. Tympany
B. Flatness or dullness
C. Hollowness
D. Hyperresonance

3 During auscultation, bronchovesicular sounds are heard over the:

A. Large bronchi
B. Lung periphery
C. Entire lung surface area
D. Trachea

4 Vesicular breath sounds are decreased or absent in:

A. Pulmonary fibrosis
B. Pleural effusion
C. Chronic obstructive pulmonary disease (COPD)
D. All of the above

5 Which of the following techniques is used to determine the degree of respiratory excursion?

A. Cardiothoracic ratio on chest X-ray
B. Percussion
C. Palpation
D. Auscultation

6 The most frequent cause of upper airway obstruction in the unconscious adult is:

A. Food
B. Dentures
C. Bronchospasm
D. Relaxed tongue

7 Symptoms of complete upper airway obstruction include:

A. Hoarseness
B. Inability to speak
C. Forceful cough
D. Wheezing

8 In a conscious adult with complete upper airway obstruction by a foreign body, initial management consists of:

A. Four quick back blows with the heel of the hand between the victim's shoulder blades
B. Six to ten abdominal thrusts (Heimlich maneuver)
C. Endotracheal intubation
D. Emergency tracheotomy

SITUATION

A 50-year-old man is admitted to the emergency department (ED) with a diagnosis of suspected pulmonary embolus. He is dyspneic and anxious. The physician plans to start heparin therapy.

Questions 9 to 12 refer to the above situation.

9 Which of the following sets of laboratory test results is consistent with a diagnosis of pulmonary embolus?

A. Elevated lactic dehydrogenase (LDH) level and PaO_2 of 70 mm Hg
B. Normal LDH level and a PaO_2 of 70 mm Hg
C. White blood cell (WBC) count of 10,000/mm^3 and a PaO_2 of 85 mm Hg
D. WBC count of 20,000/mm^3 and a PaO_2 of 85 mm Hg

10 The patient complains of calf pain upon dorsiflexion of the foot. This is termed a positive:

A. Trousseau's sign
B. Homans' sign
C. Kehr's sign
D. Babinski's reflex

11 The most frequent electrocardiograph (EKG) finding in patients with pulmonary embolus is:

A. Sinus tachycardia
B. Increased R waves in V_1
C. First-degree atrioventricular (AV) block
D. Right axis deviation

12 Which of the following statements concerning heparin therapy for pulmonary embolus is *true*?

A. Heparin will assist in dissolving the existing clot
B. Heparin reduces the risk of secondary thrombi formation
C. The dosage of heparin is based on the prothrombin time (PT)
D. Bolus administration is preferred for the high-risk patient

13 For a patient in respiratory arrest, the first action that should be taken is:

A. Auscultate for breath sounds
B. Feel for a carotid pulse
C. Insert an oropharyngeal airway
D. Open the airway

14 Which of the following statements concerning endotracheal intubation for respiratory arrest is *true*?

A. It is always necessary for adequate ventilation
B. It should be performed as the initial step in airway management
C. It should be preceded by oxygenation of the lungs through other methods
D. It should be performed in 1 to 2 minutes

15 Which of the following statements concerning the esophageal obturator airway is *true*?

A. It presents some potential for damage to the trachea
B. It requires visualization of the airway for insertion
C. It should be removed before endotracheal intubation is performed
D. Its removal is frequently followed by immediate regurgitation

16 Which of the following statements is *false* regarding respiratory arrest?

A. It can precede cardiac arrest
B. It always follows cardiac arrest
C. It can be a result of adult respiratory failure
D. It may be reversed by opening the airway

17 Early signs of respiratory failure include all of the following *except*:

A. Restlessness
B. Tachycardia
C. Cyanosis
D. Tachypnea

18 Acute respiratory failure caused by a ventilation impairment *initially* produces:

A. Hypoxia
B. Hypocapnia
C. Hypercapnia
D. Hypoventilation

19 In patients with essentially normal lung tissue, acute respiratory failure is usually indicated by:

A. Shortness of breath, $Pa{O_2}$ of 80 mm Hg, and $Pa{CO_2}$ of 40 mm Hg
B. Diaphoresis, chest pain, and shortness of breath
C. $Pa{CO_2}$ above 50 mm Hg and $Pa{O_2}$ below 50 mm Hg
D. $Pa{CO_2}$ below 40 mm Hg and $Pa{O_2}$ above 50 mm Hg

20 The initial emergency treatment for patients in acute respiratory failure secondary to COPD includes:

A. 24% oxygen via Venturi mask and bronchodilator therapy
B. 50% oxygen via humidity mask and bronchodilator therapy
C. 100% oxygen via mask and morphine sulfate 2 mg I.V. push to decrease anxiety
D. Endotracheal intubation and positive pressure ventilation

SITUATION

A 56 year-old man comes to the ED with dyspnea and anxiety. His symptoms became progressively worse while he and his family were at the movies. The patient is an accountant. He has been smoking for more than 35 years and has been told that he has chronic bronchitis. This is his worst episode.

Questions 21 to 32 refer to the above situation.

21 In this patient's history, the *most* important factor contributing to this situation is:

A. Anxiety
B. Smoking habits
C. Occupation
D. Activity level

22 The patient questions why this episode has been so severe, particularly because he has smoked for so many years and only had a "cigarette cough." The best response is:

A. "Disease is not evident symptomatically for 20 to 30 years"
B. "You've been asking for a health problem since the day you started smoking"
C. "There is no point in stopping. The disease is too far gone"
D. "Just be grateful that you don't have cancer. That's worse"

23 The patient also wonders whether it is too late to quit smoking. He should be told that if he stops smoking now:

A. "Your symptoms will disappear and you will be healed"
B. "Your cough and sputum will decrease and your pulmonary function tests will improve"
C. "The damage has been done by this time, so enjoy what is left"
D. "It will be too stressful for you to try quitting while you are ill"

24 Before this admission, this patient had been treated for chronic bronchitis, which became increasingly severe with each successive attack. Which of the following describes patients who have this medical history and who demonstrate alveolar destruction?

A. "Pink puffers"
B. "Blue bloaters"
C. Hyperreactive airway
D. Twitchy lung disease

25 Cor pulmonale is a complication of COPD secondary to:

A. Atrophy of the right ventricle caused by heart failure
B. Stimulation of erythropoiesis, which decreases blood viscosity
C. Decreased intravascular blood volume with arterial congestion
D. Pulmonary hypertension caused by vasoconstriction in response to hypoxia

26 The pathophysiology of obstruction of the small airways is usually *irreversible* in:

A. Asthma
B. Atelectasis
C. Pneumonia
D. Emphysema

27 Effective measures by which this patient will maintain health and prevent illness include:

A. Annual chest X-rays and spirometry
B. Weight control and vitamin supplements
C. Flu and pneumonia vaccines
D. Living in a warm, dry climate with air conditioning

28 Patients with emphysema characteristically develop barrel chest, which is a result of:

A. Hyperinflation and overdistention of the alveoli
B. Distention and destruction of the primary lobules
C. Hyperventilation in response to hypoxemia and hypocapnia
D. Hypoventilation in response to hypoxemia and hypercapnia

29 Chronic bronchitis is classified as COPD because of which pathogenic occurrence(s)?

A. Increase in goblet cells and disappearance of cilia
B. Hyperplasia of mucus-secreting glands in the bronchi
C. Hyperplasia, inflammatory swelling, and thick mucus production
D. Increased production and stimulation of neutrophils and macrophages

30 Which of the following is a collaborative measure between nursing and respiratory therapy staff that is useful early in the management of patients with dyspnea with COPD?

A. Inspiratory muscle training
B. Intermittent positive-pressure breathing (IPPB)
C. Pursed-lip breathing exercises
D. Diaphragmatic breathing exercises

31 Chronic cough is a common symptom of COPD; therefore, the patient should be told to avoid:

A. Hydration and aerosol humidification
B. Spicy foods
C. Cough suppressants and self-medication with antihistamines
D. Chest physiotherapy and postural drainage

32 The most difficult task for the COPD patient is:

A. Developing good nutritional habits
B. Mastering coping skills
C. Recognizing signs and symptoms of respiratory infection
D. Learning drug and oxygen therapies

SITUATION

At 3 a.m., a 13-year-old girl is brought to the ED because of coughing and severe dyspnea. Her medical history includes allergic rhinitis and eczema since childhood. A diagnosis of acute asthmatic attack is made.

The patient is wheezing and talking with effort. When questioned about precipitating factors, her mother states that she was using makeup for the first time. She also wore a new acrylic sweater and new down jacket.

Questions 33 to 39 refer to the above situation.

33 With known allergies as the causative agents, this type of asthma is categorized as:

A. Intrinsic
B. Extrinsic
C. Mixed
D. Idiopathic

34 The most likely precipitating factor of this asthma attack is the:

A. Season of the year
B. Makeup
C. Acrylic sweater
D. Down jacket

35 The patient is dyspneic and complains of tightness in her chest. These symptoms are the result of:

A. Bronchospasm and inflammation of the airways
B. Mucus production in response to mucosal edema
C. Constriction of the bronchioles during expiration
D. Constriction of the alveoli during respiration

36 The characteristic symptoms of an asthma attack include:

A. Wheezing with labored inspiratory breathing
B. Coughing and pursed-lip breathing
C. Prolonged wheezing expiration with nonproductive cough
D. Shallow wheezing inspiration with productive cough

37 Which of the following early treatments is likely to produce a dramatic improvement in the patient's condition?

A. Prednisone (Deltasone) P.O. and epinephrine (Adrenaline) S.C.
B. Cromolyn sodium (Intal) by inhalation and terbutaline (Brethine) S.C.
C. Metaproterenol (Alupent) by inhalation and aminophylline (Phyllocontin) I.V.
D. Oxygen via Venturi mask and lactated Ringer's solution I.V.

38 A primary goal for the management of this asthmatic patient is to teach her the importance of:

A. Getting prompt treatment for upper respiratory tract infections
B. Attending aerobic exercise programs on a regular basis
C. Participating in outdoor activities to improve respiratory aeration
D. Eliminating any exercise regimen to prevent undue exertion

39 Which of the following interventions should be implemented throughout the asthma attack?

A. Maintain a calm, reassuring attitude while with the patient
B. Teach the patient about preventive measures
C. Administer fluids P.O. and I.V. for adequate hydration
D. Provide diversional therapy to avoid panic or anxiety

SITUATION

A 21-year-old man is seen in the ED. His temperature is 103.6° F. (39.8° C.) rectally; pulse, 88 beats/minute; and respiratory rate, 28 breaths/minute. He complains of chills and productive cough with rust-colored sputum. A diagnosis of bacterial pneumonia is made.

Questions 40 and 41 refer to the above situation.

40 The most common type of bacterial pneumonia is caused by:

A. *Staphylococcus aureus*
B. *Streptococcus pneumoniae*
C. *Streptococcus pyogenes*
D. *Bacillus anthracis*

41 Which of the following diagnostic studies will be helpful in the assessment of this patient?

A. Bronchoscopy and electrolyte studies
B. Pulmonary function tests and arterial blood gas (ABG) measurements
C. Chest X-rays and Gram stain of sputum
D. Lung scan and cultures of sputum

SITUATION

A 4-year-old child is brought to the ED because of dysphagia, excessive salivation, mild respiratory distress, orthopnea, and fever. The child's father reports an abrupt onset of symptoms, with the child refusing to lie down for a nap. A diagnosis of epiglottitis is made, and the child is admitted to the pediatric unit.

Questions 42 to 46 refer to the above situation.

42 Which of the following assessment findings are associated with epiglottitis?

A. Cherry-red, edematous epiglottis; muffled voice sounds
B. Cyanotic, edematous epiglottis; muffled voice sounds
C. Greyish, edematous epiglottis; muffled voice sounds
D. Pink, edematous epiglottis; aphonia

43 When a child in the acute stage of epiglottitis begins to exhibit airway obstruction, the nursing priority is to:

A. Request the parents to leave the room
B. Secure intubation and tracheotomy equipment
C. Obtain consent for a tracheotomy
D. Administer oxygen via a face mask

44 Which of the following should be considered when planning for the child's care?

A. Agitation and combative behavior from the child
B. Bacteremia in almost all cases of epiglottitis
C. A productive cough and vomiting
D. Laryngospasm upon attempted visualization of the epiglottis

45 What is the *primary* reason for administering chloral hydrate (Noctec) to an intubated child with epiglottitis?

A. To produce mild sedation without respiratory depression
B. To produce sedation and decrease respiratory secretions
C. To sedate the child to prevent removal of the endotracheal tube
D. To reduce epiglottal edema and promote rest

46 When a tracheotomy is performed during an episode of epiglottitis, which of the following findings has the highest priority to be included in the nurses' notes?

A. Clear lung sounds bilaterally
B. Scant secretions from the tracheotomy site
C. Agitation and anxiety
D. Oxygen concentration delivered

SITUATION

A 19-month-old boy with respiratory distress is seen in the ED. His mother reports he has a temperature of 101° F. (38.3° C.), fatigue, and hoarseness for 2 days before examination. The hoarseness and fatigue have progressively increased, and the patient developed a "barking" cough during the night. A diagnosis of laryngotracheobronchitis croup is made.

Questions 47 to 51 refer to the above situation.

47 Early signs of hypoxemia include:

A. Use of accessory respiratory muscles and a resonant cough
B. Expiratory stridor and cyanosis
C. Lethargy and tachypnea
D. Restlessness and rapidly increasing heart rate

48 The management of children with croup is primarily directed toward:

A. Airway maintenance and adequate respiratory exchange
B. Respiratory acid-base balance
C. Increased humidification of inspired air
D. Liquefied respiratory secretions

49 The parents must be told that during the child's illness, the following medications, including sedatives, should *not* be administered:

A. Antitussives
B. Acetaminophen
C. Acetylsalicylic acid
D. Decongestants

50 Which of the following nursing actions is *most* effective in aiding adequate respiratory exchange for a child with croup?

A. Placing the child in a semi-Fowler's position with the neck slightly extended
B. Placing the child in a semi-Fowler's position with the neck slightly flexed
C. Placing the child in a supine position
D. Placing the child in a prone position

51 The nurse initiates I.V. therapy as directed. The patient's hydration status should be monitored by measurement of:

A. Weight, fluid intake and output, and urine specific gravity
B. Weight, fluid intake and output, and fontanel tension
C. Skin turgor, fluid intake and output, and fontanel tension
D. Skin turgor, fluid intake and output, and urine specific gravity

52 Innervation of the diaphragm occurs at which level of the spinal cord?

A. C2
B. C4
C. T1
D. T8

53 Naloxone (Narcan) is *not* effective in reversing depressant effects associated with an overdose of:

A. Methadone (Dolophine) and oxycodone (Percodan)
B. Diazepam (Valium)
C. Morphine and meperidine (Demerol)
D. Chloral hydrate

54 Aspiration of gastric contents:

A. Is a minimal risk to unconscious patients because they do not regurgitate
B. Occurs more commonly in adults than children
C. Can cause adult respiratory distress syndrome (ARDS) because of the high pH
D. Often results from ventilatory attempts in an obstructed airway

55 Which of the following factors is most important in the prevention of aspiration?

A. Level of consciousness
B. Body position
C. Degree of gastric distention
D. Cardiac sphincter integrity

56 A 34-year-old woman is found unconscious in the waiting room. She is diaphoretic and apneic, with a slightly irregular pulse of 88 beats/minute. She is ventilated effectively with oxygen. Administration of which of the following drugs has *highest* priority?

A. Lidocaine (Xylocaine)
B. Naloxone
C. Epinephrine
D. Glucose

57 Which of the following statements regarding airway management is correct?

A. Nasotracheal intubation is a logical choice in a patient with maxillofacial injury
B. Cricothyroidotomy is the formation of an opening for an artificial airway above the vocal cords
C. Tracheotomy is a less hazardous procedure than cricothyroidotomy
D. The carina is the landmark by which proper depth of endotracheal intubation can be measured

58 Which is the most common cause of altered gas exchange after blunt chest trauma?

A. Apnea or hypopnea
B. Flail chest
C. Pulmonary contusion
D. Phrenic nerve paralysis

59 Fracture of the scapula or first or second rib indicates serious force of injury and a high probability of underlying tissue damage. In the emergent phase of care, pulmonary contusion is best documented by:

A. Auscultation
B. ABG analysis
C. Radiographic studies
D. Symptoms of dyspnea

60 Which of the following findings is indicative of hypoxia?

A. Deterioration in level of consciousness
B. Change in respiratory rate or depth
C. Peripheral vasoconstriction
D. Delayed capillary refill

61 An increase in negative pressure inside the pleural space will result in:

A. Lung collapse
B. Tension pneumothorax
C. Normal inspiration
D. Normal expiration

62 In a patient who sustains a stab wound to the left upper abdominal quadrant, dyspnea is most likely caused by:

A. Pain and anxiety
B. Peritoneal irritation
C. Gastric rupture
D. Associated chest injury

63 Development of sudden subcutaneous emphysema and a crunching or crackling sound associated with auscultation of apical heart rate is indicative of:

A. Empyema
B. Mediastinal air leak
C. Pericarditis
D. Fat embolism

SITUATION

A 64-year-old man with emphysema is admitted with sudden onset of dyspnea. No breath sounds are present on the right side. The diagnosis is spontaneous pneumothorax. A chest tube is inserted.

Questions 64 and 65 refer to the above situation.

64 The patient's chest tube is ordered to be on suction, at 20 cm of water pressure (cmH_2O). When checking the chest tube drainage system at the start of the shift, the nurse notices continuous bubbling in the suction chamber. This indicates which of the following?

A. There is a leak in the tubing or system
B. Bronchial disruption has developed
C. An esophageal fistula has developed
D. The system is functioning normally

65 The lung is well expanded, and the chest tube is placed to water-seal drainage without suction. The water-seal level will:

A. No longer be needed
B. Rise upon spontaneous inspiration
C. Rise with positive-pressure ventilation
D. Fall during forceful coughing

66 Upon discharge from the ED after treatment of rib contusion and a minor rib fracture, a patient should be instructed to report fever, dyspnea on exertion, sputum production, or chest pain. These signs and symptoms occur in association with which of the following?

A. Pneumonia or costochondritis
B. Empyema
C. Pulmonary hypertension
D. Pneumothorax

SITUATION

A 26-year-old man diagnosed with spontaneous pneumothorax is being monitored in the holding room overnight. He had limited symptoms and lung involvement; therefore, decompression of the pleural cavity was not initiated.

Questions 67 and 68 refer to the above situation.

67 What assessment is most important to report to the physician?

A. Pain on deep inspiration
B. Expanding hyperresonance on percussion of the lung
C. Respiratory rate of 20 breaths/minute, moderate depth, easy arousal
D. Heart rate of 64 beats/minute

68 The next morning, an expiratory upright chest X-ray shows full expansion of the lung. The patient is instructed to report to a physician findings indicative of recurrence. Which of the following is least significant?

A. Activity intolerance
B. Fever and chills
C. Sudden, sharp chest pain
D. Diaphoresis and dyspnea

69 What size French chest tube should be prepared for a suspected hemothorax in an adult?

A. 20
B. 28
C. 36
D. 44

70 Autotransfusion is indicated for patients with which of the following conditions?

A. Left-sided hemothorax with hypotension
B. Hypotension secondary to spinal cord injury
C. Avulsion amputation of the left thigh
D. Hepatic hemorrhage secondary to a gunshot wound

71 A patient with a history of coronary artery disease complains of chest pain and then collapses in full cardiac arrest. Bystanders initiate basic life support measures. Emergency medical technicians facilitate adequate airway control and ventilation; an automatic chest compressor (Thumper) also is utilized. The patient is not responding. Which of the following contributing factors would be of least concern?

A. Pericardial tamponade
B. Hypocapnia
C. Tension pneumothorax
D. Volume deficit

SITUATION

A paramedic radios data to the base station regarding a 64-year-old man who has been in a motor vehicle accident and who has signs and symptoms of an acute tension pneumothorax. A needle thoracotomy is ordered by the mobile intensive care nurse.

Questions 72 to 75 refer to the above situation.

72 The paramedic will insert the needle:

A. Under the fourth rib at the anterior axillary line
B. Over the third rib at the midclavicular line
C. On the side toward which the trachea is deviated
D. On the right side to avoid puncture of the heart

73 Signs and symptoms of tension pneumothorax include:

A. Cyanosis, chest pain, vasodilation
B. Tachycardia, subcutaneous emphysema, dullness to percussion
C. Paradoxical chest movement, bradycardia, high cardiac output
D. Dyspnea, jugular venous distention, hypotension, tracheal deviation

74 After thoracotomy, the patient's condition does not improve despite assisted ventilation with 100% oxygen and rapid infusion of crystalloids. Which other condition causes similar symptoms?

A. Large diaphragmatic hernia
B. Cardiac contusion
C. Chronic airway obstruction
D. 10% hemothorax

75 When the patient arrives in the ED, a chest tube is inserted. The tube is connected to a water-seal bottle that has a moderate air and fluid leak seen on expiration. When the patient is taken to the radiology department, the bottle is accidently broken. Which of the following actions should be taken?

A. Remove the chest tube immediately to prevent aspiration of glass particles
B. Apply a clamp to the chest tube near the insertion site and instruct the patient to exhale deeply
C. Pinch the chest tube, place the end in a bottle of sterile saline or cup of water, and encourage the patient to cough and deep breathe
D. Use the phone in radiology to order a new bottle, and do not manipulate the chest tube

76 A 25-year-old man fell off a roof and landed on his right side on a cement abutment. He drove himself to the ED but is complaining of dyspnea and significant chest pain. All of the following actions ensure proper ventilation and perfusion in this patient *except*:

A. High-flow oxygen
B. Insertion of large-bore venous access devices
C. Positioning the patient on his right side
D. Positioning the patient on his left side

77 What specific anatomic injuries constitute a flail chest?

A. Single fractures of the fourth, fifth, sixth, and seventh left lateral ribs
B. Single fracture of seventh and eighth left and right anterior ribs
C. Fractured xiphoid process
D. Fractured sternum

78 Flail chest is easiest to assess:

A. When the thoracic fracture occurs posteriorly
B. When the thoracic fracture occurs anteriorly
C. In a conscious patient with well-developed musculature
D. Immediately after the injury

79 A massive flail chest is detected. Criteria for ventilatory support include all of the following *except*:

A. Age and actual-versus-ideal weight
B. Progressive fatigue
C. Hypercapnia, hypoxia, and dyspnea
D. Imminent abdominal surgery

80 After multiple rib fracture, appropriate interventions to alleviate pain and encourage optimal ventilation include:

A. High-dose I.V. morphine sulfate and binding of the chest wall
B. Low-dose narcotics and intercostal nerve block
C. Postural drainage and incentive spirometry
D. Forceful coughing after chest percussion

Answer Sheet

	A	B	C	D		A	B	C	D		A	B	C	D
1	○	○	○	○	**31**	○	○	○	○	**61**	○	○	○	○
2	○	○	○	○	**32**	○	○	○	○	**62**	○	○	○	○
3	○	○	○	○	**33**	○	○	○	○	**63**	○	○	○	○
4	○	○	○	○	**34**	○	○	○	○	**64**	○	○	○	○
5	○	○	○	○	**35**	○	○	○	○	**65**	○	○	○	○
6	○	○	○	○	**36**	○	○	○	○	**66**	○	○	○	○
7	○	○	○	○	**37**	○	○	○	○	**67**	○	○	○	○
8	○	○	○	○	**38**	○	○	○	○	**68**	○	○	○	○
9	○	○	○	○	**39**	○	○	○	○	**69**	○	○	○	○
10	○	○	○	○	**40**	○	○	○	○	**70**	○	○	○	○
11	○	○	○	○	**41**	○	○	○	○	**71**	○	○	○	○
12	○	○	○	○	**42**	○	○	○	○	**72**	○	○	○	○
13	○	○	○	○	**43**	○	○	○	○	**73**	○	○	○	○
14	○	○	○	○	**44**	○	○	○	○	**74**	○	○	○	○
15	○	○	○	○	**45**	○	○	○	○	**75**	○	○	○	○
16	○	○	○	○	**46**	○	○	○	○	**76**	○	○	○	○
17	○	○	○	○	**47**	○	○	○	○	**77**	○	○	○	○
18	○	○	○	○	**48**	○	○	○	○	**78**	○	○	○	○
19	○	○	○	○	**49**	○	○	○	○	**79**	○	○	○	○
20	○	○	○	○	**50**	○	○	○	○	**80**	○	○	○	○
21	○	○	○	○	**51**	○	○	○	○					
22	○	○	○	○	**52**	○	○	○	○					
23	○	○	○	○	**53**	○	○	○	○					
24	○	○	○	○	**54**	○	○	○	○					
25	○	○	○	○	**55**	○	○	○	○					
26	○	○	○	○	**56**	○	○	○	○					
27	○	○	○	○	**57**	○	○	○	○					
28	○	○	○	○	**58**	○	○	○	○					
29	○	○	○	○	**59**	○	○	○	○					
30	○	○	○	○	**60**	○	○	○	○					

Answer Sheet

	A	B	C	D		A	B	C	D		A	B	C	D
1	○	○	○	○	31	○	○	○	○	61	○	○	○	○
2	○	○	○	○	32	○	○	○	○	62	○	○	○	○
3	○	○	○	○	33	○	○	○	○	63	○	○	○	○
4	○	○	○	○	34	○	○	○	○	64	○	○	○	○
5	○	○	○	○	35	○	○	○	○	65	○	○	○	○
6	○	○	○	○	36	○	○	○	○	66	○	○	○	○
7	○	○	○	○	37	○	○	○	○	67	○	○	○	○
8	○	○	○	○	38	○	○	○	○	68	○	○	○	○
9	○	○	○	○	39	○	○	○	○	69	○	○	○	○
10	○	○	○	○	40	○	○	○	○	70	○	○	○	○
11	○	○	○	○	41	○	○	○	○	71	○	○	○	○
12	○	○	○	○	42	○	○	○	○	72	○	○	○	○
13	○	○	○	○	43	○	○	○	○	73	○	○	○	○
14	○	○	○	○	44	○	○	○	○	74	○	○	○	○
15	○	○	○	○	45	○	○	○	○	75	○	○	○	○
16	○	○	○	○	46	○	○	○	○	76	○	○	○	○
17	○	○	○	○	47	○	○	○	○	77	○	○	○	○
18	○	○	○	○	48	○	○	○	○	78	○	○	○	○
19	○	○	○	○	49	○	○	○	○	79	○	○	○	○
20	○	○	○	○	50	○	○	○	○	80	○	○	○	○
21	○	○	○	○	51	○	○	○	○					
22	○	○	○	○	52	○	○	○	○					
23	○	○	○	○	53	○	○	○	○					
24	○	○	○	○	54	○	○	○	○					
25	○	○	○	○	55	○	○	○	○					
26	○	○	○	○	56	○	○	○	○					
27	○	○	○	○	57	○	○	○	○					
28	○	○	○	○	58	○	○	○	○					
29	○	○	○	○	59	○	○	○	○					
30	○	○	○	○	60	○	○	○	○					

1 Correct answer—**B**

Atelactasis is indicated when bronchial breath sounds are heard over the right middle lobe. Bronchial sounds are normally heard only over the manubrium of the sternum and along the sternal borders. They are characteristically high pitched, loud, and harsh in quality, with a pause between the inspiratory and expiratory phases. The appearance of bronchial breath sounds over the periphery of the lung may indicate abnormal sound transmission because of consolidated lung tissue, as in atelectasis.

2 Correct answer—**B**

When percussion is performed over an area of pneumonic consolidation, the resulting sound will be dull because of the increased mass. Percussion over the normal lung produces a resonant or hollow sound that is of low pitch and intensity. An overinflated lung, such as in emphysema, will produce a sustained hyperresonant sound. Tympanic sounds are high pitched and are produced by air-containing organs, such as the stomach.

3 Correct answer—**A**

Bronchovesicular lung sounds are best heard over the large bronchi, below the clavicles and between the scapulae. These sounds are of moderate amplitude, medium to high in pitch, and represent a mixture of bronchial and vesicular sounds. In other parts of the lung, bronchovesicular sounds may indicate consolidation or other abnormalities. Bronchial sounds are loud, high pitched, and heard over the trachea.

4 Correct answer—**D**

Any pathologic condition that produces disruption of alveolar function, consolidation, or compression will decrease or cause an absence of vesicular sounds. Vesicular sounds are produced by the alveoli opening on inspiration and a glottic hiss (air movement through the larynx) during expiration. They are of low amplitude, medium to low pitch, and may be described as swishing or rustling.

5 Correct answer—**C**

Palpation has four uses in respiratory assessment: to identify areas of tenderness, to assess any observed abnormality, to elicit fremitus, and to assess respiratory excursion. To assess respiratory excursion, determine if each lung expands to the same degree at different chest locations. Place the hands, with thumbs together and fingers spread, over the center of the chest. As the patient takes a deep breath, note if the fingers and thumbs move apart to an equal degree. Each lobe of the lung, or its equivalent area, should be assessed in this manner.

Unequal excursion may be caused by conditions such as atelectasis or pneumothorax.

6 Correct answer—**D**

A relaxed tongue is the most common cause of upper airway obstruction in the unconscious adult. Without sufficient muscle tone, the relaxed tongue will fall over the back of the throat, obstructing the pharynx and the larynx. Because the tongue is attached to the lower jaw, moving the lower jaw forward (as in the head-tilt-chin-lift maneuver) will lift the tongue away from the back of the throat and open the airway. Performing this maneuver may restore spontaneous respirations in the apneic patient.

7 Correct answer—**B**

When the airway is completely obstructed, there will be no air movement, coughing will be absent, and the victim will be unable to speak. A partial airway obstruction may produce good or poor air exchange. If the air exchange is good, a forceful cough is evident, although wheezing between coughs may be present. A poor air exchange produces an ineffective, weak cough, inspiratory stridor, and cyanosis.

8 Correct answer—**B**

The American Heart Association recommends the abdominal thrust, or Heimlich maneuver, as the initial management measure for relieving foreign-body airway obstruction. A subdiaphragmatic abdominal thrust, by elevating the diaphragm, can force air from the lungs in sufficient quantity to create an artificial cough, intended to move and expel an obstructing foreign body in the airway. The foreign body obstruction must be relieved before intubation or tracheotomy can be performed, if necessary. The efficacy of back blows in relieving airway obstruction is not well documented.

9 Correct answer—**A**

A decreased oxygen tension or room air (PaO_2 below 80 mm Hg) and elevated LDH levels are the most frequent laboratory findings with a pulmonary embolus. If the PaO_2 is above 80 mm Hg on room air, pulmonary embolus is unlikely. LDH elevations are seen in many diseases, and this finding is not specifically diagnostic for pulmonary embolus. The WBC count may be elevated or normal.

10 Correct answer—**B**

Calf pain on dorsiflexion of the foot is termed a positive Homans' sign and is indicative of deep vein thrombosis. Trousseau's sign is a carpal spasm elicited by compressing the upper arm, causing ischemia of the distal nerves, and is indicative of tetany. Babinski's reflex is dorsiflexion of the great toe and fanning of the smaller toes in response to a strong stimulus on the sole of the foot. Kehr's sign is radiating shoulder pain that occurs when the diaphragm is irritated from blood loss in the peritoneum, and is usually seen in a ruptured spleen.

11 Correct answer—**A**

Pulmonary emboli rarely cause specific EKG changes. However, sinus tachycardia caused by apprehension, pain, and a decreased PO_2 is the most frequent EKG finding. Some EKG findings that may suggest a pulmonary embolus include enlarged P waves, depressed ST segment, inverted T waves, and atrial fibrillation. If a massive pulmonary embolus has occurred, the EKG may show right axis deviation, indicating right ventricular failure.

12 Correct answer—**B**

Heparin impedes clotting by preventing thrombi formation. It does not act on existing clots. Adequate anticoagulation is documented by the partial thromboplastin time (PTT), and the dosage is adjusted to achieve a PTT range from 55 to 85 seconds. Continuous I.V. heparin administration is preferred for the high-risk patient because it maintains a steady therapeutic blood level. Heparin bolus administration produces peak levels for a short time, but subtherapeutic levels are evident before the next dose is due.

13 Correct answer—**D**

In an emergency, the ABCs (A = airway, B = breathing, C = circulation) of assessment and intervention always apply. Before other assessments are made, the airway should be opened by the head-tilt-chin-lift or the jaw-thrust maneuver. This action may allow the victim to resume spontaneous respirations without further intervention.

14 Correct answer—**C**

Endotracheal intubation should never be used as the initial procedure for ventilation in respiratory arrest. Intubation requires the skill of a trained individual who can efficiently complete the procedure in 20 to 30 seconds. Adequate ventilation can be provided with the use of a bag-valve-mask device, and the lungs should be well oxygenated before any intubation attempt.

15 Correct answer—**D**

With the use of an esophageal obturator airway, regurgitation of stomach contents must be expected and suction must be available. The patient who does not have an endotracheal tube in place should be turned on the left side before the removal of an esophageal obturator airway to prevent aspiration of stomach contents. The esophageal obturator airway is a tube approximately 14½″ (37 cm) long that is open at the top and has a blind end at the bottom. The blind end is inserted into the esophagus; the airway is not visualized. An inflatable cuff is located just above the blind end, and several side holes located near the upper end allow passage of air from the interior of the tube into the pharynx. Possible hazards associated with the use of the esophageal obturator airway include laceration and rupture of the esophagus. It is possible to perform endotracheal intubation with the esophageal obturator airway in place.

16 Correct answer—**B**

Respiratory arrest can precede cardiac arrest for a few seconds or even a few minutes. The heart may continue to beat because of its inherent automaticity and rhythmicity. In a respiratory arrest without cardiac arrest, ventilations must be provided at the rate of 1 breath every 5 seconds or 12 breaths/minute. Respiratory arrest ensues after untreated respiratory failure. Spontaneous breathing may return after opening the airway.

17 Correct answer—**C**

Restlessness, tachycardia, and tachypnea are early signs of hypoxia and hypoxemia. Cyanosis occurs secondary to unoxygenated hemoglobin in the capillaries and is not perceptible until there are 5 grams of reduced (unoxygenated) hemoglobin per 100 ml of blood. Therefore, cyanosis is a later sign of respiratory failure. Cyanosis may not be present in a patient with a decreased hematocrit.

18 Correct answer—**C**

Conditions impairing ventilation initially produce hypercapnia because oxygen does not reach the alveoli, and so the gas exchange does not take place. Such conditions may include asthma, atelectasis, or emphysema. Conditions impairing oxygenation will initially produce hypoxia because although oxygen does reach the alveoli, it is not absorbed or utilized. Hypoxia may be instigated by lung tumors, near-drowning, aspiration, pulmonary edema, or toxic chemical inhalation. When the body senses hypercapnia, hypoxia, or both, it responds with an increased respiratory depth and rate, resulting in hyperventilation.

19 Correct answer—**C**

In patients without underlying lung disease, respiratory failure is said to be present when the PaO_2 level falls below 50 mm Hg (oxygen saturation below 85%) or when the $PaCO_2$ level rises above 50 mm Hg. Respiratory failure is defined as any condition in which blood oxygen content is not sufficient to fulfill tissue demands for oxygen, secondary to decreased lung function. Patients who have obstructive disorders, such as COPD, will function with abnormal blood gas levels. The diagnosis of respiratory failure must be made based on history, clinical appearance, and changes in serial arterial blood gas (ABG) studies.

20 Correct answer—**A**

The initial emergency treatment for patients in acute respiratory failure, secondary to COPD, includes 24% oxygen administered by Venturi mask, and bronchodilator therapy. Unless the patient with COPD has severe acidosis or is obtunded, a conservative approach to treatment is initially recommended. Most patients with COPD are dependent on the hypoxic drive to maintain adequate ventilation. Uncontrolled or high-flow oxygen therapy may precipitate severe carbon dioxide narcosis and respiratory arrest. Precise oxygen therapy delivered by a Venturi mask may allow time for use of other therapeutic measures, such as bronchodilators, and thereby avoid the need for mechanical ventilation. The respiratory depressant effects of morphine sulfate render it inappropriate for this situation.

21 Correct answer—**B**

Cigarette smoking appears to be the single most important factor leading to chronic airway obstruction. Cigarette smoking also interacts with virtually every other contributing factor. Anxiety does affect breathing patterns. In certain occupational groups, such as auto mechanics and miners, the incidence of COPD is high. An increased activity level by the patient with existing lung disease may exacerbate it.

22 Correct answer—**A**

Chronic bronchitis and emphysema have an insidious onset. By the time the patient's symptoms develop, pulmonary function is usually irreversibly impaired. Emphasis should be placed on controlling the symptoms and increasing self-esteem and a sense of mastery and well-being.

23 Correct answer—**B**

In the early stages, cessation of cigarette smoking is probably the most significant factor in halting the progression of the disease. After discontinuation of cigarette smoking, the accelerated decline in pulmonary function slows and pulmonary function returns to the more normal level of nonsmokers. Thus, the sooner smoking is stopped, the less there is loss of pulmonary function along with a decrease in cough and sputum production.

24 Correct answer—**B**

People with severe bronchial abnormalities and little emphysema are often labeled "blue bloaters." In this condition, hypoventilation leads to hypoxemia and hypercapnia. People with severe emphysema and little bronchitis are often labeled "pink puffers." In this condition, hyperventilation assists in adequate oxygenation; thus, cyanosis is absent. Asthmatic symptoms are caused by a hyperreactive airway.

25 Correct answer—**D**

In COPD, pulmonary hypertension is caused primarily by constriction of the pulmonary vessels in response to alveolar hypoxia; acidosis further potentiates the vasoconstriction. Chronic alveolar hypoxia causes ventricular hypertrophy and stimulates erythropoiesis, which increases the blood viscosity. Clinical manifestations are related to dilation and failure of the right ventricle, with subsequent intravascular volume expansion and systemic venous congestion.

26 Correct answer—**D**

The usually reversible chronic obstructive airway disease is asthma, while emphysema and chronic bronchitis are usually irreversible. Pneumonia is an inflammatory process of the lung substance and not of the small airways. Atelectasis can be reversed by improving ventilation.

27 Correct answer—**C**

The patient should be encouraged to receive influenza vaccine at the prescribed times and to seek medical advice about receiving vaccine against streptococcal pneumonia. Individuals with COPD are more prone to respiratory infections, which subsequently intensify the pathologic destruction of lung tissue and the progression of COPD. The most common causative organisms are *Hemophilus influenzae* and *Streptococcus pneumoniae*. Retained secretions provide a good medium for the proliferation of these organisms. Chest X-rays are not recommended annually. Vitamin supplements are not encouraged unless the patient also has a vitamin deficiency. Dry climates could be harmful for expectorating sputum that is not liquefied.

28 Correct answer—**A**

In emphysema there is destruction of elastin and collagen, which are the supporting structures of the lung. Because there is no traction or pull on the walls of the bronchioles, they tend to collapse, and the air is trapped in the distal alveoli, resulting in hyperinflation and overdistention of the alveoli. This trapped air gives the patient a barrel chested appearance.

29 Correct answer—**C**

Hyperplasia, inflammatory swelling, and excess thick mucus cause narrowing of the airway lumens and result in diminished airflow, which chronically spans 20 to 35 years. The constant irritation of the bronchioles leads to hypertrophy of mucus-secreting glands, goblet cell hyperplasia, and increased mucus production, leading to bronchial plugging and narrowing.

30 Correct answer—**C**

Pursed-lip breathing slows expiration and prevents collapse of lung units. It also helps the patient to control the rate and depth of respirations and to relax, which decreases dyspnea and feelings of panic. The use of IPPB in patients with COPD is controversial. It is used only in patients who have end-stage disease and poor respiratory muscle function. Use of inspiratory muscle training devices must be judiciously monitored by a health care professional. Indiscriminate use can produce inspiratory muscle exhaustion and acute ventilatory failure. Diaphragmatic breathing is also a later adjunct to prolong expiration.

31 Correct answer—**C**

The use of expectorants is not uniformly recommended for patients with COPD, but cough suppressants must be avoided. Antihistamines cause drying of the respiratory mucosa, which can result in thickening of the mucus, leading to airway obstruction. Hydration, aerosol humidification, chest physiotherapy, and postural drainage loosen and remove thick secretions. The patient with COPD does not need to avoid spicy foods.

32 Correct answer—**B**

Healthy psychological coping is often the most difficult task to master. People with COPD frequently have to deal with many life-style changes. A vicious cycle of emotional entrapment can occur. Honest communication with supportive family and friends and avoidance of anxiety-producing situations may need to be learned. These skills are much more difficult to learn than factual matters concerning nutrition, infection, and therapies.

33 Correct answer—**B**

Extrinsic asthma is caused by a known allergen or allergies. Individuals with extrinsic asthma usually have a family history of allergies and a medical history of infantile eczema or allergic rhinitis. Intrinsic asthma is exacerbated by cold air, air pollution, and primary infection. Mixed asthma is associated with some allergic tendencies, and idiopathic asthma has unknown causative factors.

34 Correct answer—**D**

Extrinsic asthma attacks are precipitated by exposure to certain allergens, such as pollen, dander, feathers (as in a down jacket), mold, dust, and some foods. The other answer choices are not likely to be allergens.

35 Correct answer—**C**

Normally, the bronchioles constrict during expiration. However, expiration becomes more difficult when the bronchioles are constricted, edematous, and filled with mucus. Bronchospasm and mucus production are present during asthma attacks, but inflammation is not present at this time. The alveoli are not constricted.

36 Correct answer—**C**

The characteristic clinical manifestations of asthma are wheezing, coughing, dyspnea, and chest tightness after exposure to the causative allergen or precipitating factor. Expiration is more difficult than inspiration. Prolonged wheezing expirations are characteristic. The cough may be nonproductive, possibly indicating widespread bronchiolar plugging. Production of thick, tenacious, white, gelatinous mucus also may occur, usually only after treatment has begun.

37 Correct answer—**C**

Metaproterenol and aminophylline will produce the most dramatic improvement. To relieve bronchospasm, treatment is aimed toward decreasing mucosal edema and facilitating secretion removal. Beta-adrenergic agents and bronchodilators, such as aminophylline, epinephrine, and terbutaline, administered by inhalation or direct I.V. therapy, offer the most rapid relief. Corticosteroids are usually effective 6 to 9 hours after administration. Cromolyn sodium is used prophylactically but should not be used for an acute attack. Oxygen and I.V. fluids will not reverse bronchospasm.

38 Correct answer—**A**

Prompt diagnosis and treatment of upper respiratory tract infection may prevent exacerbations. Physical exercise within the patient's limit of toleration is beneficial. Staying indoors when there is a high degree of air pollution is helpful.

39 Correct answer—**A**

An important nursing goal during an acute asthma attack is to decrease the patient's sense of panic. However, diversional therapy is not the best approach. A calm, quiet, reassuring attitude helps the patient to relax. Staying with the patient and being available provides additional comfort. The physician will prescribe fluids needed for hydration. Teaching is most effective after the attack subsides.

40 Correct answer—**B**

The most common type of pneumonia is pneumococcal, caused by *Streptococcus pneumoniae*. Staphylococcal pneumonia occurs more commonly in hospitalized patients than in people in the community. *Bacillus* pneumonia is associated with agricultural or industrial exposure to *Bacillus* microorganisms. Pneumonia caused by *Streptococcus pyogenes* is known to occur in military populations after influenza epidemics.

41 Correct answer—**C**

A Gram stain of sputum provides the information on which the initial therapy is based. Immediate identification of the infecting organism permits the institution of appropriate antimicrobial therapy. Sputum and blood cultures take 24 to 72 hours. Chest X-rays frequently show a pattern characteristic of the infecting organisms; lung scans do not show this. Bronchoscopy may be necessary if the patient cannot voluntarily produce a sputum specimen. ABG measurements and an SMA-6 are helpful but are not critical, unless the patient is tachypneic and diaphoretic.

42 Correct answer—**A**

Epiglottitis is associated with a large, cherry-red, edematous epiglottis; muffled voice sounds or aphonia; dysphagia; drooling; and a croaking or froglike sound on inspiration. There is a rapid onset of symptoms, and the child may complain of a sore throat. The child seldom struggles to breathe, but rather prefers to remain still for better air exchange. Frequently the child assumes an upright position and leans forward with the chin thrust forward (tripod position). Additionally, younger children may protrude their tongues. The temperature may range from 100° to 105° F. (37.8° to 40.5° C.). Epiglottitis usually occurs between ages 3 and 7.

43 Correct answer—**B**

Intubation or tracheotomy equipment must be available when epiglottitis is suspected, because complete airway obstruction can occur suddenly. Suction equipment and humidified oxygen should also be accessible. Epiglottitis requires immediate intervention, and the child should be admitted to the pediatric intensive care unit. The child should never be left unattended. Separation from the parents may increase the anxiety and agitation of the child, thus increasing the oxygen need. The need for a tracheotomy consent will vary according to locale and institution. Usually, the physician obtains the informed consent for surgical procedures or medical care. Oxygen may not be needed once an airway is established.

44 Correct answer—**D**

Attempts to directly visualize the epiglottis with a tongue depressor can precipitate sudden laryngospasm and result in complete airway obstruction. A nurse should never attempt to visualize the epiglottis. Such visualization should occur within the operating room, with intubation or tracheotomy equipment available. An I.V. infusion should be started before the procedure. To prevent trauma, the endotracheal tube should be smaller than that normally used. To prevent laryngospasm, a culture of the epiglottis should be obtained after the airway is established. *Hemophilus influenzae* is the most common bacterial agent in epiglottitis. Bacteremia is present in 50% of cases; thus, blood cultures should be obtained. The WBC is generally elevated above 15,000/mm³. Children with epiglottitis are usually quiet because they have better air exchange with little activity. There is no cough or vomiting with epiglottitis, although occasionally a child may have some retching.

45 Correct answer—**A**

Chloral hydrate produces mild sedation without respiratory depression or drying of secretions. Restlessness, agitation, or anxiety can increase the respiratory rate and oxygen demand. Sedation may be required to prevent the child from removing the artificial airway, as restraints usually increase the child's agitation. Steroids may be administered to reduce epiglottal edema.

46 Correct answer—**C**

Restlessness, anxiety, or agitation can increase the respiratory rate and oxygen demand. The artificial airway equipment and the inability to talk are frequently sources of fear for the child, and thus an explanation of all procedures is important. Because of the abruptness and severity of epiglottitis, parents are encouraged to stay with the child without restrictions. Epiglottitis is seldom recurrent, which may reassure the child and parents. Clear lung sounds bilaterally, scant secretions from the tracheotomy, and the oxygen concentration are also important parts of the nursing report.

47 Correct answer—**D**

The earliest signs of hypoxemia in children are restlessness, tachypnea, and a rapidly increasing heart rate. Use of accessory respiratory muscles, retractions, and nasal flaring are advanced signs of hypoxemia. Cyanosis and lethargy are late signs and require immediate intervention. The cough is brassy or barking and resonant. Inspiratory stridor is caused by partial upper airway obstruction. The normal respiratory rate for a 19-month-old child is 24 to 40 breaths/minute. In children, an increase in metabolism will increase oxygen consumption and thus increase the respiratory rate. A fever can increase the respiratory rate by 4 breaths/minute for each Fahrenheit degree rise in temperature above normal.

48 Correct answer—**A**

Airway maintenance and adequate respiratory exchange are of prime importance and are more difficult to achieve in children than adults. A child's airway is smaller than an adult's and contains more soft tissue; thus, it is more susceptible to obstruction from edema or secretions. The child's respiratory mucous membranes are more susceptible to irritation, causing edema or coughing. The larynx of an infant is located two to three cervical vertebrae higher than in an adult. That location allows for greater proximity of the esophagus and trachea, resulting in a great risk of aspiration. Also, the tongue is proportionately larger, increasing the possibility of airway obstruction. Because of excessive carbon dioxide release, respiratory alkalosis is possible with tachypnea. Treatment for croup consists of high humidity with cold mist; this decreases mucosal edema and prevents drying of secretions. Oxygen and intubation are warranted for anoxia and obstruction.

49 Correct answer—**C**

Acetylsalicylic acid (aspirin) should not be administered to the child who has croup. Acetylsalicylic acid has been correlated with Reye's syndrome, which can cause fatal encephalopathy. Reye's syndrome frequently follows acute upper respiratory tract viral infections. Laryngotracheobronchitis, the most common form of croup, results from a viral infection and usually occurs in the fall and winter. It is more prevalent in males between ages 3 months and 3 years. Sedatives should also not be administered to children with potential respiratory distress because restlessness, an early indicator of hypoxemia, would be masked.

50 Correct answer—**A**

A semi-Fowler's position will aid in lung expansion, and slight extension of the neck will open the narrow airway of a child. A prone position helps to compress distended lungs during expiration, but this is not a problem in croup. During auscultation, the child should be placed in a sitting position to facilitate an accurate assessment. Additionally, auscultation of the entire chest is necessary; because the chest is small, breath sounds frequently are referred to other aspects of the chest.

51 Correct answer—**D**

Skin turgor, fluid intake and output, and urinary specific gravity are the most important measures of hydration status. Hydration is particularly important in infants and young children because their total water body composition differs from that of adults. At approximately age 2, the composition is similar to an adult's. The weight of an infant under age 2 is an important parameter for hydration assessment. However, if the child is older than age 2, other parameters are of greater importance. The skin turgor is poor with dehydration of a child. Intravenous fluid replacement may be necessary to decrease physical exertion and the possibility of aspiration, with an increased respiratory rate. Fluid intake and output measurements are essential to monitor the hydration status, especially to prevent overhydration with I.V. therapy. The posterior fontanel is usually closed by age 2 or 3 months, and the anterior fontanel closes by age 12 or 18 months; hence, it is not an appropriate indicator in this patient. Urine specific gravity is an excellent indicator of hydration, because the renal ability to concentrate and dilute urine increases with age. Because infants' kidneys are immature, specific gravity is not a good indicator of renal function.

52 Correct answer—**B**

Innervation of the diaphragm, which is responsible for inspiration, occurs at the C3 to C5 level. The diaphragm is the main muscle of respiration and is frequently the only muscle active in quiet inspiration. The intercostal muscles, innervated at the T1 to T11 level, are external muscles used during inspiration. The abdominal muscles, innervated at the T6 to L1 level, are used for active expiration and coughing. Accessory muscles of inspiration are the scalene and sternocleidomastoid muscles.

53 Correct answer—**D**

Chloral hydrate is a sedative-hypnotic drug with no known response to naloxone in people. Naloxone is a pure opioid antagonist. Methadone, oxycodone, morphine, and meperidine are opioid analgesics. The antagonistic effects of naloxone will increase respiratory rate within 1 to 2 minutes of administration and will reverse sedative effects and depressed blood pressure. Antagonism of some depressant effects of diazepam has been shown in people, and animal studies are demonstrating additional drug antagonism by naloxone.

54 Correct answer—**D**

Excessive pressure used for inflation of a partially or completely occluded airway results in gastric distention. The air follows the path of least resistance and travels down the esophagus to the stomach, creating a high risk of distention, regurgitation, and aspiration. The new Basic Life Support (BLS) guidelines have changed the speed of airflow delivery during mouth-to-mouth or mouth-to-mask respiration to reduce the chance of gastric distention. Children have a greater tendency for aerophagia (air swallowing) when crying and frightened; this increases the risk of gastric distention and aspiration. The low pH of gastric contents can lead to ARDS after aspiration.

55 Correct answer—**A**

Level of consciousness is a significant factor in determining the risk of aspiration. An alert, cooperative patient with intact cerebral, brain stem, and spinal input will be able to swallow with concurrent glottic closure, while maintaining a cough and gag reflex. A sedated or unconscious patient will have reduced protective reflex mechanisms. Nursing interventions include positioning (including alert patients who are immobilized for spinal precautions), providing access to suction, and monitoring gastric distention and the patency of nasogastric tubes. The cardiac sphincter is the lower esophageal sphincter near the opening of the stomach.

56 Correct answer—**D**

Administration of glucose takes the highest priority among drugs, although ensuring a patent airway is always first priority. The patient's symptoms and history suggest severe hypoglycemia. Neurons are dependent on glucose, and irreversible damage can occur if it is not available. To prevent further damage, I.V. dextrose should be administered and the patient assessed for response. It is preferable to draw a blood sample first to document the serum glucose level. In practice, both naloxone and glucose are given I.V. push early in therapy. Naloxone is given to reverse possible respiratory depression from a drug overdose. Lidocaine and epinephrine are not indicated because the patient has no lethal dysrhythmias.

57 Correct answer—**D**

Placement of the tip of the endotracheal tube too near or below the carina can result in right main stem bronchus intubation or atelectasis of the left lung. Placement too far above the carina risks damage to the vocal cords or inadvertent extubation. Nasotracheal intubation is safer than endotracheal intubation for suspected spinal cord injury because it requires less extension and manipulation of the neck. Despite the association of spinal cord injury with facial injury, the risk of nasal fracture and frontal skull and cribriform plate damage make nasotracheal intubation hazardous, possibly resulting in sinus or intracranial infection. Cricothyroidotomy is an emergency procedure performed to create an opening in the cricothyroid membrane, which is located below the thyroid cartilage (Adam's apple) and above the cricoid cartilage. The vocal cords are above these landmarks.

58 Correct answer—**C**

Pulmonary contusion is a frequent consequence of blunt thoracic trauma. Blunt or penetrating trauma to the lung characteristically causes an accumulation of blood and fluid in the involved interstitial tissue, alveoli, and small bronchi. The reduced vital capacity and pulmonary compliance, together with increased secretions from the injured lung, cause an increasing atelectasis. This combination of atelectasis, disrupted tissue, and extravasated blood results in an altered gas exchange. Flail chest is a type of penetrating chest trauma. Apnea, hypopnea, and phrenic nerve paralysis may occur after spinal cord injury.

59 Correct answer—**C**

Radiographic studies would document pulmonary contusion best. Pulmonary contusion is a bruise of the lung, which causes interstitial edema and hemorrhage. The chest X-ray initially may show patchy infiltrates but progresses to consolidation. Pulmonary contusion may evolve into ARDS. Auscultation may not initially reveal abnormalities unless other injuries are present. Hypoxemia may be delayed, and, therefore, dyspnea will not be prominent. ABG test results will be serially checked but may not demonstrate intrapulmonary shunting in the emergent phase. Signs and symptoms depend on the severity of contusion and associated injuries.

60 Correct answer—**A**

Changes in level of consciousness, such as restlessness, confusion, irritability, and decreased responsiveness, indicate serious hypoxia. Changes in respiratory rate or depth may result from many factors, such as pain or fear, but must be frequently assessed. Peripheral vasoconstriction and delayed capillary refill are related mainly to reduction in vascular volume and inadequate perfusion.

61 Correct answer—**C**

Airflow into the lungs is guided by the principle of flow from an area of higher pressure to an area of lower pressure. As the diaphragm contracts, the thorax enlarges and the visceral and parietal pleura move with it. Healthy lungs will recoil and pull away from the chest wall, which pulls the parietal pleural layer, creating negative (subatmospheric) pressure within the intrapleural space. The more the thorax enlarges, the more the lung stretches and tries to recoil, creating more and more negative pressure. Outside air at atmospheric pressure flows into the lungs during this inspiratory process. Positive pleural pressure will collapse the lung, resulting in a pneumothorax.

62 Correct answer—**D**

Dyspnea in this situation is most likely caused by an associated chest injury. The lungs extend to the sixth rib anteriorly to the eighth rib laterally and may descend to the twelfth rib posteriorly on deep inspiration. The downward stroke of the diaphragm can be 3¼″ (8.3 cm). A chest injury should be suspected in any blunt or penetrating injury to the upper abdomen or with gunshot wounds.

63 Correct answer—**B**

Subcutaneous emphysema is seen in conditions such as pneumothorax as well as with a sudden intrathoracic pressure increase, causing alveolar rupture. Air dissects to the loose mediastinal tissues and gravitates up to the neck, face, and supraclavicular area where it may be first detected. Mediastinal air can be heard as it is compressed by the contraction of the heart with each beat, creating a sign known as Hamman's sign. The air may arise from the esophagus or pulmonary anatomy.

64 Correct answer—**D**

The suction chamber should be bubbling constantly if connected to suction. When a patient has a significant air leak caused by bronchial damage or there is a leak in the chest tube connection or from the drainage holes in the end of the tube extending outside the chest wall, there usually is continuous bubbling in the water-seal chamber. This is where fluctuation with respiration and air leaks on expiration will be seen. Gastric drainage in the chest drainage system may indicate an esophageal fistula.

65 Correct answer—**B**

During spontaneous respiration, the intrapleural pressure becomes more negative (or subatmospheric), which will pull fluid in the water-seal chamber toward the patient. The opposite would be expected to occur if the patient is manually or mechanically ventilated with positive pressure or forcefully coughed. Gastric drainage in the chest drainage system may indicate an esophageal fistula.

66 Correct answer—**A**

Pneumonia and costochondritis are associated with these signs and symptoms. Pneumothorax is a rare occurrence after these injuries, but it is usually not associated with fever or sputum production. Empyema may develop after penetrating chest trauma. Pulmonary hypertension will not develop after rib fractures.

67 Correct answer—**B**

Extension of the pneumothorax rather than the desired reabsorption would be detected by auscultation of diminished breath sounds and a larger area of hyperresonance to percussion over the affected lung. Percussion creates vibration in the lung and chest wall; when it is performed over the air-filled intrapleural space, a tympanic sound results because of an increase in the normal resonance of the lung. The patient will have constant pain, tachypnea, and tachycardia.

68 Correct answer—**B**

Fever and chills may indicate atelectasis, but with full lung expansion and short duration of pulmonary abnormality, it is not likely. It is more apt to be caused by a viral infection. The other symptoms listed are typical of a pneumothorax and imply a more significant risk to the patient.

69 Correct answer—**C**

A large chest tube, with or without a trocar, is used to evacuate blood from the chest cavity to prevent obstruction from clots. The typical size used is 36 French or 40 French for hemothorax, 28 French for pneumothorax.

70 Correct answer—**A**

Hemothorax is the most frequent reason for autotransfusion in the emergency setting. Most basic autotransfusion devices are attached to the chest tube, which evacuates accumulated blood. Blood from other sites, such as the liver or thigh, holds the risk of bacterial contamination, has a higher likelihood of clotting and particulate matter, and would not be advantageous unless the patient were exsanguinating and blood products were not available. Hypotension from a spinal cord injury does not result from hemorrhage; hence, a transfusion is not required.

71 Correct answer—**B**

Hypocapnia may result from aggressive ventilation creating a mild respiratory alkalosis, which is offset by metabolic acidosis. Ventilatory efforts will prevent hypoxia. The other contributing factors, such as pericardial tamponade or pneumothorax, will seriously hinder resuscitation and can be rapidly corrected.

72 Correct answer—**B**

The needle should be inserted over the third rib because the intercostal artery and vein are located under the rib. Placement at the superior border should avoid vascular trauma. The procedure may be done at the second intercostal space midclavicular line or the fourth or fifth intercostal space midaxillary line. Tension pneumothorax is caused by excessive pressure on the injured side. This will eventually shift the mediastinal contents to the uninjured side, affecting vascular flow and ventilation. Treatment should be aimed at the side of origin of injury, the side opposite the tracheal deviation. Needle thoracotomy can be performed correctly on the left side of the chest without inducing cardiac injury.

73 Correct answer—**D**

Signs and symptoms of a tension pneumothorax include dyspnea, jugular venous distention, hypotension, and trachael deviation. In tension pneumothorax, the injured lung is collapsed and the contralateral lung is partially collapsed. This creates severe dyspnea from ineffective gas exchange. The mediastinal contents (large vessels, trachea, and heart) are shifted or deviated and compressed depending on the pressure created. This results in ineffective cardiac contraction and reduced venous return, resulting in jugular venous distention and low cardiac output. Tachycardia is a compensatory mechanism and hypotension would be present.

74 Correct answer—**A**

A large diaphragmatic hernia caused by a rupture or laceration of the diaphragm allows abdominal contents to enter the thoracic cavity. Pressure within the abdominal cavity is higher than intrathoracic pressure. Diaphragmatic hernias occur most often on the left side because the right side is better protected by the liver. Excursion of the bowel and other abdominal structures into the thorax creates excessive pressure that can also compress and shift the thoracic structures. A 10% hemothorax and COPD will not cause such severe symptoms. Cardiac contusion does not produce respiratory symptoms.

75 Correct answer—**C**

The best action is to pinch the tubing to prevent atmospheric air from entering the pleural space until a temporary water seal can be obtained. Be creative in seeking a new form of water seal and enlist the help of other personnel in the immediate area. Use of a clean urinal filled with water would be better than sustained clamping. Pinching is suggested, rather than clamping, because one then cannot forget to release the tube. This patient required a needle thoracotomy to relieve a tension pneumothorax. The current chest tube, if clamped, is ineffective in allowing escape of intrapleural air or fluid. It should not be removed or the tension will recur.

76 Correct answer—**C**

Turning the patient onto the injured side would cause great pain and might cause further internal injury. The opposite side would be optimal for positioning. This allows insertion of chest tubes as necessary, while providing the best ventilation and perfusion to the uninjured lung. Pulmonary blood flow follows gravity, and ventilation, per unit of lung volume, is greater in the dependent area of the lung. Positioning the patient on his left side would also assist in draining secretions from his affected side.

77 Correct answer—**D**

Flail chest is defined as two or more ribs fractured in two or more places, or with one fracture plus costochondral separation, or a fractured sternum. A flail segment or free-floating piece of thoracic cage must be present. This piece causes the chest wall to move paradoxically because of the defect in thoracic skeletal structure. The chest wall is pulled toward the negative intrapleural pressure during inspiration and pushed away from positive intrapleural pressure on expiration. Changes in ventilation and perfusion are most closely linked with underlying pulmonary damage rather than the paradoxical motion.

78 Correct answer—**B**

Fractured thoracic segments will be difficult to visualize in muscular individuals or if they are splinted by muscle contraction as the posterior chest is. To relieve pain, an alert patient will splint the area so the flail will be less evident until the victim becomes fatigued. Splinting is not present if the patient is unconscious and does not react to the discomfort. Anterior thoracic structures are least supported by muscle and are easier to see. Lateral flail segments are intermediate.

79 Correct answer—**A**

A victim of flail chest may need assisted ventilation if breathing fatigue is increasing and if signs and symptoms of inadequate oxygen and carbon dioxide exchange are evident. All trauma victims are intubated and ventilated during surgery. When associated injuries are present, assisted ventilation may be provided on a temporary basis to ensure proper oxygenation. Although advanced age and obesity can contribute to reduced ventilatory reserve, they are not finite criteria.

80 Correct answer—**B**

In the early stages of injury, patients will not tolerate chest percussion or postural drainage because of pain and unstable condition. High-dose morphine may alleviate the pain but will also depress respiratory rate or depth, leading to atelectasis. Chest binding and taping also limit chest excursion and air exchange. The most effective method of pain control is through physician-initiated intercostal nerve blocks or thoracic epidural analgesia. These allow for optimal chest wall movement and ventilation; then incentive spirometry may be used.

Selected References

American College of Surgeons Committee on Trauma. *Advanced Trauma Life Support Course Instructor Manual.* Chicago: American College of Surgeons, 1985.

Brunner, L., and Suddarth, D. *Textbook of Medical-Surgical Nursing,* 5th ed. Philadelphia: J.B. Lippincott Co., 1984.

Budassi, S.A. "Chest Trauma," *Journal of Emergency Nursing* 9:356-360, November/December 1983.

Cosgriff, J.H., and Anderson, D.L. *The Practice of Emergency Care,* 2nd ed. Philadelphia: J.B. Lippincott Co., 1984.

Elpren, W.H. "Asthma Update: Pathophysiology and Treatment," *Heart and Lung* 9:665-670, July/August 1980.

Harmon, A.L., ed. *Nursing Care of the Adult Trauma Patient.* New York: John Wiley & Sons, 1985.

Hudak, C., and Gallo, B. *Critical Care Nursing: A Holistic Approach,* 4th ed. Philadelphia: J.B. Lippincott Co., 1985.

Knezevich, B. *Trauma Nursing: Principles and Practice.* East Norwalk, Conn.: Appleton and Lange, 1986.

Langfitt, D. *Critical Care: Certification Preparation and Review.* East Norwalk, Conn.: Appleton and Lange, 1984.

Lehrer, S. *Understanding Lung Sounds.* Philadelphia: W.B. Saunders Co., 1984.

Lewis, S., and Collier, I. *Medical-Surgical Nursing: Assessment and Management of Clinical Problems,* 2nd ed. New York: McGraw-Hill Book Co., 1987.

Lundberg, G., ed. "Standards and Guidelines for Cardiopulmonary Resuscitation and Emergency Cardiac Care," *Journal of the American Medical Association* 225:2905-2989, June 1986.

May, H. *Emergency Medicine.* New York: John Wiley & Sons, 1984.

McFadden, E.R., and Dusten, E.F. "Asthma," in *Harrison's Principles of Internal Medicine,* 10th ed. Edited by Isselbacker, K., et al. New York: McGraw-Hill Book Co., 1983.

McGraw, J.P. "Triage of a Patient Exhibiting Hamman's Crunch After a Fall," *Journal of Emergency Nursing* 13:64-65, January/February 1987.

O'Boyle, C., et al. *Emergency Care: The First 24 Hours.* East Norwalk, Conn.: Appleton and Lange, 1985.

Respiratory Emergencies. Nursing Now Series. Springhouse, Pa.: Springhouse Corporation, 1984.

Shaffer, M.A., and Walraven, G., eds. "Pulmonary Trauma," *Trauma Quarterly* 2:1-79, 1986.

Sheehy, S., and Barber, J. *Emergency Nursing: Principles and Practice,* 2nd ed. St. Louis: C.V. Mosby Co., 1985.

Summer, W.R. "Status Asthmaticus," *Chest* 87:875-945 (Suppl. 1), January 1985.

Tammelin, B.R. "Respiratory Management of the Trauma Patient," *Topics in Emergency Medicine* 25-34, April 1984.

Traver, G.A. *Respiratory Nursing: The Science and the Art.* New York: John Wiley & Sons, 1982.

West, J.B. *Respiratory Physiology: The Essentials,* 3rd ed. Baltimore: Williams & Wilkins Co., 1985.

Chapter 5

Neurologic Emergencies Questions and Answers

You must begin with Question 1 of this chapter and progress in sequence. **Do not skip around.** Subsequent answers build on previous ones.

Kathy Daly, RN, CCRN, CEN
Laura Gasparis, RN, MA, CCRN, CEN
Maureen Sheehy, RN, CCRN, CEN

SITUATION

A 45-year-old man with a history of seizure disorders comes to the emergency department (ED) via ambulance. His family states he had a seizure 30 minutes before arrival. He takes phenytoin (Dilantin) and phenobarbital daily. Vital signs are blood pressure (BP) 120/60 mm Hg; pulse, 110 beats/minute; and respiratory rate, 12 breaths/minute. His pupils are equal and reactive to light. At present, he grimaces only in response to tactile stimuli.

Questions 1 to 6 refer to the above situation.

1 Which statement accurately describes the mechanism of epilepsy?

A. The abnormal excessive firing of brain cells causes the clinical signs and symptoms of a seizure
B. The entire brain is involved in a seizure
C. The metabolism of the involved cells is greatly decreased during a seizure
D. The abnormal firing of the neurons, once initiated, is perpetuated indefinitely until therapy is instituted

2 Which nursing action has the highest priority for a patient in a postictal state?

A. Obtain a complete history from the family
B. Institute an I.V. administration of 0.9% saline solution
C. Place the patient on his side and administer an I.V. solution
D. Call the physician and obtain a suction apparatus at the bedside

3 Which factor would not be considered initially to precipitate seizure activity?

A. Head trauma
B. Ingestion of toxic substances
C. Discontinuation of anticonvulsant medication by the patient
D. Cerebral edema

4 When administering phenytoin intravenously, it is essential to:

A. Place the patient on a cardiac monitor
B. Obtain serum phenytoin levels immediately after administration
C. Administer the drug in a dextrose solution
D. Administer the drug at a rate no faster than 500 mg/minute

5 Which life-threatening situation can be expected if I.V. phenytoin is administered by a rapid bolus?

A. Ventricular tachycardia
B. Supraventricular tachycardia
C. Third-degree heart block
D. Electromechanical dissociation

6 Discharge teaching regarding phenytoin should include what information?

A. Alcohol may cause phenytoin toxicity
B. Phenytoin must be taken even in the absence of seizures
C. Missed doses should not be made up
D. Aspirin, rather than acetaminophen, should be taken for headaches

SITUATION

A 21-year-old woman is admitted to the ED in a coma. She is accompanied by her husband, who states that she had a seizure. The patient is 1½ weeks postpartum. Vital signs are BP, 180/128 mm Hg; pulse 120 beats/minute; respiratory rate, 12 breaths/minute.

Questions 7 and 8 refer to the above situation.

7 After initial management, the most appropriate medication is:

A. Phenobarbital (Luminal)
B. Diazepam (Valium)
C. Magnesium sulfate
D. Phenytoin (Dilantin)

8 Which statement accurately describes the clinical manifestations of eclampsia?

A. Signs and symptoms occur most frequently during the third trimester and can occur up to 2 months postpartum
B. Signs and symptoms include hypertension, proteinuria, oliguria, and seizures
C. Eclampsia most commonly occurs in women who are multigravida
D. Eclampsia is idiopathic and not associated with any preexisting diseases

SITUATION

A middle-aged man who was found unconscious on the street is brought to the ED by paramedics. No identification or further information is available. Vital signs are BP, 160/90 mm Hg; pulse 120 beats/minute; and respiratory rate, 16 breaths/minute. Upon arrival, the patient begins to have sustained grand mal seizures and requires intubation. An I.V. access is established.

Questions 9 and 10 refer to the above situation.

9 The drug of choice to control status epilepticus is:

A. Phenytoin (Dilantin) 18 mg/kg I.V.
B. Diazepam (Valium) 5 mg/minute I.V. every 5 to 10 minutes
C. Phenobarbital (Luminal) 10 to 20 mg/kg I.V.
D. Lorazepam (Ativan) 4 mg I.V. over 2 minutes

10 After controlling this patient's seizure activity, which drug would *not* be given routinely?

A. 50% dextrose 50 ml
B. Phenobarbital (Luminal) 10 to 20 mg/kg I.V.
C. Thiamine 100 mg I.V.
D. Naloxone (Narcan) 2 mg I.V.

11 The drug of choice in the treatment of seizures caused by traumatic head injury is:

A. Diazepam (Valium)
B. Dexamethasone (Decadron)
C. Phenytoin (Dilantin)
D. Phenobarbital (Luminal)

SITUATION

A 60-year-old man with a history of seizures is brought to the ED because of recurrent seizure activity. While in the ED, he develops tonic-clonic movements of the right arm and leg.

Questions 12 and 13 refer to the above situation.

12 This type of seizure activity is called:

A. Grand mal
B. Petit mal
C. Jacksonian
D. Psychomotor

13 In this patient, the ED nurse should expect to observe which postictal problem?

A. Paralysis of the right side
B. Loss of consciousness
C. Incontinence
D. Seizure activity of the left side

14 While caring for a patient with head trauma, the nurse would assess for signs of uncal herniation. Which factor is an early indication of the condition?

A. Absent doll's eye reflex
B. Ipsilateral dilated pupil
C. Ataxic breathing
D. Impairment of motor function

15 Manifestations indicative of increased intracranial pressure (ICP) include:

A. Narrowing pulse pressure, rising systolic blood pressure, bradycardia
B. Narrowing pulse pressure, rising systolic blood pressure, tachycardia
C. Widening pulse pressure, rising diastolic blood pressure, bradycardia
D. Widening pulse pressure, rising systolic blood pressure, bradycardia

16 Which statement concerning epidural and subdural hematomas is correct?

A. Epidural bleeding occurs below the dura mater and above the arachnoid layer
B. Signs and symptoms of epidural bleeding develop more slowly than do those of subdural bleeding
C. Epidural hematomas are usually caused by arterial bleeding, and subdural hematomas are usually caused by injury to a vein
D. Temporal bone fractures are associated with subdural hematomas

17 Conditions that further increase ICP include:

A. Hypoxemia, hypercapnia, alkalosis
B. Hypoxemia, hypercapnia, acidosis
C. Hypoxemia, hypocapnia, alkalosis
D. Hypoxemia, hypocapnia, acidosis

18 In the treatment of increased ICP, the use of mannitol is supported by which rationale?

A. It induces diuresis by raising the osmotic pressure of glomerular filtrate
B. It increases the rate of electrolyte excretion, particularly of sodium, chloride, and potassium
C. It increases plasma osmolality, thus inducing diffusion of water from cerebrospinal fluid (CSF) back into the plasma and extravascular space
D. It results in a shifting of intracellular fluid into the interstitial space, thus decreasing cellular edema

19 Factors that contribute to the elevation of ICP include:

A. Valsalva's maneuver
B. Coughing or sneezing
C. Isometric muscle contraction or hip flexion
D. All of the above

20 Which method of determining ICP in a patient with a head injury is *unsafe*?

A. Lumbar puncture
B. Epidural monitoring
C. Intraventricular catheter
D. Subarachnoid screw

SITUATION

A 25-year-old man, disoriented to time and place, is admitted to the ED. His co-worker states that 2 hours ago the patient was hit on the head with a beam. That caused momentary unconsciousness. The patient was fine until a half hour ago, when he became tired and "wasn't making any sense." Physical examination reveals a dilated nonreactive left pupil. Blood pressure is 160/80 mm Hg; pulse, 80 beats/minute; respiratory rate, 16 breaths/minute.

Questions 21 to 23 refer to the above situation.

21 Which diagnostic test is indicated initially?

A. Lumbar puncture
B. Computed tomography (CT) scan
C. Cervical spine and skull X-rays
D. Cerebral angiography

22 Diagnostic studies reveal a temporal fracture with a pineal shift. This finding frequently is associated with:

A. Subdural hematoma
B. Epidural hematoma
C. Subarachnoid hemorrhage
D. Intracerebral bleeding

23 The ED nurse would anticipate the treatment for this patient to be:

A. Direct ICP monitoring in the intensive care unit (ICU)
B. Pharmacologic management
C. Lumbar puncture
D. Surgical evacuation of clot

24 The primary objective in caring for a patient with a traumatic head injury is:

A. Decreasing ICP
B. Maintaining ventilation
C. Maintaining body alignment
D. Hyperventilating the patient

25 Increased ICP is *best* relieved by which of the following nursing interventions?

A. Elevating the head of the bed 30 degrees
B. Administering oxygen
C. Administering diuretics
D. Hyperventilating the patient

26 Which observation is the first indication of increased ICP?

A. Elevation of systolic blood pressure
B. Elevation of body temperature
C. Change in respiratory patterns
D. Change in level of consciousness

27 Which symptom is *not* likely to be exhibited by a patient who sustains a cerebral concussion?

A. Loss of consciousness
B. Loss of memory
C. Visual disturbances
D. Bleeding from the nose and ears

28 At the time of discharge, the patient who sustains a cerebral concussion should be instructed that all neurologic symptoms should subside within:

A. 2 to 4 hours
B. 4 to 8 hours
C. 8 to 12 hours
D. 24 to 48 hours

29 In a patient who has a head injury that has damaged the sixth cranial nerve, which condition will be observed by the nurse?

A. Absent gag reflex
B. Fixed and dilated pupils
C. Nystagmus
D. Inward deviation of the eyes

30 A man is brought to the ED by ambulance after hitting his head when he dove into a 4-foot-deep swimming pool. After determining the patient's level of consciousness and checking his vital signs, the most important diagnostic test is:

A. CT scan of the head
B. X-ray of the cervical spine
C. Arterial blood gas (ABG) studies
D. Routine laboratory work

31 An accurate method by which the ED nurse can determine a patient's level of consciousness is:

A. Assessment of pupillary reaction
B. Measurement of vital signs
C. Assessment of muscle strength in the extremities
D. Glasgow Coma Scale

32 Consciousness is determined by:

A. Reticular activating system (RAS)
B. Spinothalamic tract
C. Extrapyramidal tracts
D. Hypothalamus

33 The Glasgow Coma Scale measures:

A. Pupillary reaction, motor response, verbal response
B. Eye movement, motor response, verbal response
C. Eye movement, vital signs, verbal response
D. Pupillary reaction, motor response, vital signs

34 A comatose patient brought to the ED is exhibiting decerebrate posturing. Which areas of the brain have been injured?

A. Cerebrum and cerebellum
B. Cerebrum and brain stem
C. Hypothalamus and brain stem
D. Cerebellum and hypothalamus

35 The physiologic event that precipitates most neurologic emergencies is:

A. Head trauma
B. Cerebrovascular accident (CVA)
C. Intracerebral hemorrhage
D. Increased ICP

36 In assessing consciousness, the ED nurse begins by using:

A. Auditory stimulation
B. Tactile stimulation
C. Light pain
D. Deep pain

37 The single most reliable index of a patient's neurologic condition is:

A. Level of consciousness
B. Pupillary responses
C. Vital signs
D. Motor function

38 Which breathing pattern is demonstrated by a patient who has a lesion at the lower midbrain level?

A. Hyperventilation
B. Hypoventilation
C. Apneustic breathing
D. Cluster breathing

SITUATION

A patient admitted to the ED after a motor vehicle accident is found to have a basal skull fracture with middle meningeal artery damage.

Questions 39 to 44 refer to the above situation.

39 This patient is likely to develop which condition?

A. Subdural hemorrhage
B. Subarachnoid hemorrhage
C. Epidural hematoma
D. Aneurysm

40 This patient should be assessed for the presence of Battle's sign, which is:

A. A postconcussion syndrome
B. An ecchymosis over the mastoid bone
C. Black-and-blue discoloration around the eyes
D. A superficial hematoma on the skull

41 This patient may also suffer injury to the:

A. Oculomotor nerve
B. Olfactory nerve
C. Optic nerve
D. Ophthalmic nerve

42 Further assessment of this patient may also reveal:

A. Otorrhea
B. Meningism
C. Facial paresis
D. Hemianopia

43 A patient with a basal skull fracture will benefit from nursing care that:

A. Instructs the patient to blow his nose gently
B. Prevents Valsalva's maneuver
C. Fosters coughing and deep breathing
D. Implements careful insertion of a nasogastric (NG) tube

44 The presence of "raccoon's eyes" indicates:

A. Meningitis
B. Intracerebral bleed
C. Epidural hematoma
D. Anterior fossa fracture

45 A 23-year-old man who had been working out with weights at a health spa is brought to the ED because he does not feel well. While in the ED, he complains of a sudden, explosive headache. The nurse suspects:

A. Subarachnoid hemorrhage
B. Epidural hematoma
C. Basal skull fracture
D. Brain stem contusion

46 A man sustains a hemisection of the spinal cord caused by a stab wound to the right side of the back. He experiences loss of movement on the right side and loss of pain and temperature sensations on the left. This syndrome is called:

A. Brown-Séquard syndrome
B. Anterior cord syndrome
C. Partial cord syndrome
D. Central cord syndrome

SITUATION

A man who was brought to the ED by Emergency Medical Service (EMS) after a motor vehicle accident is suspected of having a spinal cord injury.

Questions 47 to 54 refer to the above situation.

47 Spine X-rays confirm a lesion at the C5 to C6 level. The nurse anticipates that the patient has:

A. Quadriplegia with intact triceps and biceps and intercostal breathing
B. Quadriplegia with gross arm movements and diaphragmatic breathing
C. Paraplegia with diaphragmatic breathing
D. Diaphragmatic and intercostal breathing with loss of intrinsic hand muscle power

48 While in the ED, the patient develops spinal shock. This condition is defined as a state of:

A. Spastic paralysis caused by a lesion of the upper motor neuron
B. Inhibition of the parasympathetic outflow
C. Sudden initiation of the facilitatory influences from higher brain centers
D. Transient reflex depression below the level of the lesion

49 Nursing assessment of the patient in spinal shock reveals all of the following findings *except*:

A. Urinary incontinence
B. Bradycardia
C. Poikilothermy
D. Hypotension

50 Optimum respiratory functioning is of major concern in the patient with spinal cord injury. Which would *not* influence the development of hypoventilation?

A. Injury below C4 results in diaphragmatic breathing and a decrease in tidal volume
B. Cervical lesions at C4 result in decreased vital capacity with incomplete loss of innervation to the diaphragm
C. Paralysis of abdominal and intercostal muscles leads to ineffective cough and retention of secretions
D. Abdominal distention from gastric dilation may restrict diaphragmatic excursion

51 During the assessment of motor function, the functioning of the patient's spinothalamic tract is determined by:

A. Applying a tuning fork to a bony prominence and asking the patient to identify the vibration
B. Asking the patient to close both eyes and touch the nose with a finger
C. Asking the patient to identify areas stimulated by pinprick
D. Testing the patient's position sense

52 Which assessment finding would indicate deterioration of this patient's respiratory status?

A. pH, 7.28; PCO_2, 36 mm Hg; HCO_3^-, 18 mEq; PO_2, 86 mm Hg
B. Inspiratory force of −20 cm
C. Measured tidal volume of 500 ml
D. Bronchial breath sounds over lung lobes

53 The phrenic nerve innervates the diaphragm at what level?

A. C2 to C3
B. C3 to C4
C. T1 to T3
D. T3 to T4

54 In the patient who has a spinal cord injury, early hypoventilation is best manifested by:

A. Poor respiratory exchange
B. The development of cyanosis
C. Shortness of breath while talking
D. ABG values

55 A patient is admitted to the ED with possible spinal cord injury between T4 and T12. Which clinical finding is *not* likely to be present?

A. Bladder and bowel incontinence
B. Paraplegia of the legs
C. Complete loss of motor power in the legs
D. Anesthesia below the truncal dermatome level, corresponding with the site of cord damage

56 If a cervical spinal cord injury is suspected, which is the best way to open the patient's airway?

A. Tilt the head forward, supporting the neck
B. Use a modified jaw-thrust maneuver
C. Logroll the patient on his side and pull down the chin
D. Perform a tracheotomy

57 Loss of motor function in the right arm and leg may indicate a lesion in the:

A. Pyramidal tract of the left hemisphere
B. Spinocerebellar tract
C. Motor nerve fibers in the anterior horn of the spinal cord
D. Spinal cord at C7

58 The most reliable technique for testing the motor strength of a patient's upper extremity is to:

A. Observe the patient for spontaneous movement
B. Test the patient's muscle reflexes
C. Ask the patient to squeeze your hands
D. Ask the patient to close his eyes and raise his arms straight in front of him

59 A patient admitted to the ED with an injury to the left cerebral hemisphere may exhibit:

A. Left hemiparesis
B. Left homonymous hemianopia
C. Deviation of the eyes to the left
D. Left hemiplegia

60 Pinpoint pupils are usually indicative of a lesion in the:

A. Pons
B. Optic nerve
C. Medulla
D. Midbrain

61 The unconscious patient with pinpoint pupils is most likely to exhibit which type of breathing pattern?

A. Apneustic breathing
B. Biot's respirations
C. Ataxic breathing
D. Cheyne-Stokes respirations

62 Which is the best means by which to assess a patient for meningeal irritation?

A. Flex the leg at the hip and knee, then straighten the knee and watch for pain and resistance
B. Stroke the lateral aspect of the sole of the foot and watch for dorsiflexion of the great toe
C. Check temperature; a reading above 102° F. (38.9° C.) indicates meningeal irritation
D. Check for papilledema

63 Which assessment finding is *not* associated with meningeal irritation?

A. Babinski's sign
B. Brudzinski's sign
C. Kernig's sign
D. Nuchal rigidity

64 Which nursing action is *not* implemented for a patient who has just been diagnosed as having viral meningitis?

A. Institute seizure precautions
B. Institute isolation precautions
C. Monitor temperature frequently
D. Control increased ICP

65 A common manifestation seen in patients with bacterial meningococcal meningitis is:

A. Petechiae
B. Hypothermia
C. Nystagmus
D. Hypertensive crisis

Answer Sheet

	A	B	C	D		A	B	C	D		A	B	C	D
1	○	○	○	○	31	○	○	○	○	61	○	○	○	○
2	○	○	○	○	32	○	○	○	○	62	○	○	○	○
3	○	○	○	○	33	○	○	○	○	63	○	○	○	○
4	○	○	○	○	34	○	○	○	○	64	○	○	○	○
5	○	○	○	○	35	○	○	○	○	65	○	○	○	○
6	○	○	○	○	36	○	○	○	○					
7	○	○	○	○	37	○	○	○	○					
8	○	○	○	○	38	○	○	○	○					
9	○	○	○	○	39	○	○	○	○					
10	○	○	○	○	40	○	○	○	○					
11	○	○	○	○	41	○	○	○	○					
12	○	○	○	○	42	○	○	○	○					
13	○	○	○	○	43	○	○	○	○					
14	○	○	○	○	44	○	○	○	○					
15	○	○	○	○	45	○	○	○	○					
16	○	○	○	○	46	○	○	○	○					
17	○	○	○	○	47	○	○	○	○					
18	○	○	○	○	48	○	○	○	○					
19	○	○	○	○	49	○	○	○	○					
20	○	○	○	○	50	○	○	○	○					
21	○	○	○	○	51	○	○	○	○					
22	○	○	○	○	52	○	○	○	○					
23	○	○	○	○	53	○	○	○	○					
24	○	○	○	○	54	○	○	○	○					
25	○	○	○	○	55	○	○	○	○					
26	○	○	○	○	56	○	○	○	○					
27	○	○	○	○	57	○	○	○	○					
28	○	○	○	○	58	○	○	○	○					
29	○	○	○	○	59	○	○	○	○					
30	○	○	○	○	60	○	○	○	○					

Answer Sheet

	A	B	C	D		A	B	C	D		A	B	C	D
1	○	○	○	○	**31**	○	○	○	○	**61**	○	○	○	○
2	○	○	○	○	**32**	○	○	○	○	**62**	○	○	○	○
3	○	○	○	○	**33**	○	○	○	○	**63**	○	○	○	○
4	○	○	○	○	**34**	○	○	○	○	**64**	○	○	○	○
5	○	○	○	○	**35**	○	○	○	○	**65**	○	○	○	○
6	○	○	○	○	**36**	○	○	○	○					
7	○	○	○	○	**37**	○	○	○	○					
8	○	○	○	○	**38**	○	○	○	○					
9	○	○	○	○	**39**	○	○	○	○					
10	○	○	○	○	**40**	○	○	○	○					
11	○	○	○	○	**41**	○	○	○	○					
12	○	○	○	○	**42**	○	○	○	○					
13	○	○	○	○	**43**	○	○	○	○					
14	○	○	○	○	**44**	○	○	○	○					
15	○	○	○	○	**45**	○	○	○	○					
16	○	○	○	○	**46**	○	○	○	○					
17	○	○	○	○	**47**	○	○	○	○					
18	○	○	○	○	**48**	○	○	○	○					
19	○	○	○	○	**49**	○	○	○	○					
20	○	○	○	○	**50**	○	○	○	○					
21	○	○	○	○	**51**	○	○	○	○					
22	○	○	○	○	**52**	○	○	○	○					
23	○	○	○	○	**53**	○	○	○	○					
24	○	○	○	○	**54**	○	○	○	○					
25	○	○	○	○	**55**	○	○	○	○					
26	○	○	○	○	**56**	○	○	○	○					
27	○	○	○	○	**57**	○	○	○	○					
28	○	○	○	○	**58**	○	○	○	○					
29	○	○	○	○	**59**	○	○	○	○					
30	○	○	○	○	**60**	○	○	○	○					

1 Correct answer—**A**

The abnormal excessive firing of brain cells causes the clinical signs and symptoms of a seizure. A portion of the brain or the entire brain can be involved. The metabolism of the involved cells is greatly increased during seizure activity. The abnormal firing of the neurons can terminate as abruptly as it begins.

2 Correct answer—**C**

Maintenance of a patent airway is the foremost nursing goal. Placing the patient in a side-lying position with the head in alignment with the body helps to prevent aspiration. An airway should be placed in the patient's mouth before a tonic phase begins. To prevent injury, objects should never be forced into the mouth during a seizure. The primary responsibility of the nurse is to stay with the patient. Summon assistance if further equipment is needed. An I.V. line may then need to be established to administer anticonvulsants. When the patient is stabilized, a complete history may then be obtained from the family.

3 Correct answer—**B**

Discontinuation of anticonvulsant therapy may be considered as a precipitating factor for seizure activity, because patients may forget to take their medication or may not understand that the medication works because medication levels are maintained in their bloodstream. Other precipitating factors include craniocerebral trauma; infections, particularly of the central nervous system (CNS); cerebral tumors; or metabolic disorders of the brain.

4 Correct answer—**A**

The patient should be placed on a cardiac monitor and carefully observed. Therapeutic blood levels of 10 to 20 mg of phenytoin can be quickly achieved by I.V. administration; however, rapid administration depresses the myocardium and can cause cardiac arrest. Obtaining a level before administration (the patient was taking this medication at home) provides the physician with a baseline level and prevents possible toxicity. Nystagmus with lateral gaze is the first sign of toxicity. Ataxia, slurred speech, diplopia, lethargy, and disturbances of coordination may result from acute overdose. I.V. phenytoin must be administered slowly at a rate no faster than 50 mg/minute in a saline solution. If given in a dextrose solution, the drug will precipitate into crystals.

5 Correct answer—**C**

Phenytoin is a myocardial depressant. Third-degree heart block and cardiac arrest produce life-threatening dysrhythmias that are most likely to occur if excessive or rapid doses of phenytoin are administered.

6 Correct answer—**B**

Phenytoin must be taken as ordered even if there is no seizure activity. The drug is effective only when therapeutic blood levels are maintained. The patient should know the signs and symptoms of toxicity. Because phenytoin is absorbed slowly from the gastrointestinal (GI) tract, daily doses can be adjusted to the patient's convenience, and missed doses can be made up safely. The patient should be encouraged to wear a medical-identification bracelet. Phenytoin's action can be potentiated by the concurrent use of aspirin, estrogen, disulfiram (Antabuse), chlordiazepoxide (Librium), and anticoagulants, especially dicumarol. Drugs that inhibit the action of phenytoin include alcohol, antihistamines, barbiturates, hypnotics, and sedatives.

7 Correct answer—**C**

With eclampsia, magnesium sulfate is the anticonvulsant of choice. Diazepam (Valium) and other sedatives should be used judiciously. Sodium nitroprusside or hydralazine may be used to control hypertension. Hydralazine is the drug of choice for controlling hypertension.

8 Correct answer—**B**

Signs and symptoms of eclampsia include hypertension, proteinuria, oliguria, and seizures. The symptoms usually occur during the third trimester but can occur up to 2 weeks postpartum. Eclampsia, most commonly seen in primagravida patients, is associated with diabetes, hypertension, and renal disease.

9 Correct answer—**B**

The drug of choice to manage status epilepticus is diazepam, because it is a rapid-acting anticonvulsant with less tendency to produce hypotension. Phenytoin and phenobarbital are indicated to prevent further seizures. Lorazepam is used for anxiety.

10 Correct answer—**B**

After seizure activity is controlled, the secondary management is to find the underlying cause of the seizure. If no one provides the ED team with this information, dextrose 50%, naloxone, and thiamine should be administered. Dextrose will reverse possible hypoglycemia, naloxone will reverse potential drug intoxication, and thiamine is administered to patients who are alcoholics and who have potential vitamin deficiency. All these conditions can result in seizure activity.

11 Correct answer—**C**

Phenytoin is the drug used for seizures resulting from head trauma because a therapeutic blood level is rapidly established. Phenytoin works by stabilizing the seizure threshold, thereby reducing seizure activity. Diazepam and phenobarbital should be avoided in the patient with head trauma because they cause sedation and will inhibit an accurate assessment of level of consciousness. Dexamethasone is used to decrease cerebral edema, and its action will be decreased by the concurrent use of phenytoin.

12 Correct answer—**C**

Jacksonian seizures are characterized by tonic-clonic movement limited to one side of the body. Grand mal seizures produce tonic-clonic movement of the entire body and loss of consciousness, followed by a postictal state of drowsiness. Petit mal seizures produce transient loss of consciousness with no postictal state. Psychomotor seizures are more common in children and are characterized by bizarre behavior with no loss of consciousness and by postictal drowsiness and amnesia about the seizure episode.

13 Correct answer—**A**

A person with jacksonian seizures develops paralysis of the affected side postictally. This transient paralysis is referred to as Todd's paralysis. Unconsciousness and incontinence are associated with grand mal seizures.

14 Correct answer—**B**

Ipsilateral pupil dilation is the earliest sign of uncal herniation. An expanding lesion of the lateral middle fossa, most often the temporal lobe, causes shifting of the inner basal temporal lobe. This area contains the uncus, which is forced through the tentorium as pressure builds. The third cranial nerve and the posterior cerebral artery on the same side of the expanding temporal lobe lesion are frequently caught between the uncus and the tentorium. Ataxic or irregular respirations are seen in the later stages of herniation. The absence of a doll's eye reflex indicates brain stem dysfunction and is a late sign of herniation. Impaired motor function is a frequent sign in various neurologic and neuromuscular diseases, such as CVA, multiple sclerosis, and myasthenia gravis.

15 Correct answer—**D**

The specific classic signs and symptoms of increased ICP involving the brain stem include widening pulse pressure, rising systolic blood pressure, and bradycardia. These three signs and symptoms, known as Cushing's response, are a compensatory mechanism for maintaining blood pressure and cerebral blood flow in the presence of rising ICP.

Vital signs such as blood pressure and pulse rate are controlled in the vital centers of the brain stem. Hypertension stimulates the baroreceptors in the carotid and aortic bodies, stimulating the vagus nerve and producing bradycardia.

16 Correct answer—**C**

Epidural hematomas occur between the skull and the dura mater. Subdural hematomas occur between the dura mater and arachnoid layer. Signs and symptoms develop more rapidly in epidural bleeding than in subdural bleeding because epidural bleeding is usually associated with arterial bleeding while subdural bleeding results from venous bleeding. Approximately 85% of patients in whom epidural hematomas develop have sustained a skull fracture, with the most common site being the temporal bone. The middle meningeal artery is located under the temporal bone and is usually the affected artery.

17 Correct answer—**B**

Hypoxemia, hypercapnia, and acidosis are potent vasodilating factors in the body's attempt to increase oxygen supply to the brain. Cerebral vasodilation causes an increase in blood volume in the brain and a subsequent increase in ICP.

18 Correct answer—**C**

Increasing plasma osmolality, which induces diffusion of water from CSF back into the plasma and extravascular space, will decrease ICP. Mannitol induces diuresis by raising the osmotic pressure of the glomerular filtrate and increasing the rate of electrolyte excretion. However, neither of these actions decreases ICP. Shifting intracellular fluid to the interstitial space will increase edema.

19 Correct answer—**D**

Valsalva's maneuver, an exertion against a closed epiglottis, which increases intrathoracic pressure, impedes venous return from the brain and increases ICP. Isometric muscle contractions, contractions that do not lengthen the muscle, cause a rise in systemic blood pressure, thus elevating ICP. Coughing and sneezing elevate intraabdominal and intrathoracic pressures. An increase in these pressures is transmitted to the spinal and intracranial subarachnoid spaces and through the veins that communicate with the dural venous sinuses and intracranial subarachnoid space. The venous return from the cranial vault is impeded, resulting in an increase in ICP. Positions that obstruct venous return from the brain include extreme flexion of the hips, Trendelenburg's position, and angulation of the neck.

20 Correct answer—**A**

Epidural monitoring, intraventricular catheters, and subarachnoid screw are the three ways to measure ICP. Although a lumbar puncture is a means of measuring ICP, it can be contraindicated in the presence of an expanding cerebral mass. A lumbar puncture will give accurate pressure readings only if CSF is flowing freely within the subarachnoid space. An expanding lesion, as well as adhesions and constrictions, will alter the flow of CSF and result in an inaccurate pressure reading. Also, with increased ICP, lumbar puncture may cause brain stem herniation by reducing spinal pressure.

21 Correct answer—**C**

Once the patient's vital signs are stabilized, cervical spine and skull X-rays must be evaluated to rule out spinal injuries and skull fractures before further diagnostic procedures or treatments, such as a CT scan (to pinpoint the area of damage), are begun.

22 Correct answer—**B**

Epidural hematomas are frequently associated with temporal fractures. The development of the hematoma causes a contralateral pineal shift. These findings, along with an ipsilateral fixed pupil and a deteriorating level of consciousness, are indicative of epidural hematomas.

23 Correct answer—**D**

Treatment of an epidural hematoma is by surgical evacuation of the hematoma and ligation of the damaged vessel. Early diagnosis and immediate surgical treatment are directly related to a good prognosis.

24 Correct answer—**B**

Although all these measures are important, maintaining oxygen supply to the brain is the primary objective in caring for a patient with a traumatic head injury. Hypoxia and carbon dioxide retention cause cerebral vasodilation and increase ICP.

25 Correct answer—**A**

All of these interventions decrease ICP. However, elevating the head of the bed 30 degrees, which allows for venous drainage by gravity, is the only nursing intervention. The other interventions require a physician's order.

26 Correct answer—**D**

A change in the patient's level of consciousness is the first sign the nurse will notice if ICP increases. It results from decreased blood supply to the cortex. Changed vital signs and temperature are late indicators, because the brain stem is not compressed until late stages of increased ICP.

27 Correct answer—**D**

Bleeding from the nose and ears is indicative of a cerebral contusion, not a concussion. A cerebral concussion is a shock to the brain's soft tissues, and a contusion involves bruising and laceration of brain tissue.

28 Correct answer—**D**

All symptoms of a concussion should subside within 24 to 48 hours. Any problems lasting longer than that time indicate a more serious injury and require reevaluation by a physician.

29 Correct answer—**D**

The sixth cranial nerve, the abducens, controls inward deviation of the eyes. The gag reflex is controlled by the ninth and tenth cranial nerves, the glossopharyngeal and vagus nerves, respectively. The third cranial nerve, the oculomotor nerve, controls pupillary constriction and dilation. Nystagmus is caused by an interruption of cerebellar function.

30 Correct answer—**B**

An X-ray of the cervical spine with a view of C7 is vitally important to determine if there is a compression injury to the spinal cord and the level at which it has occurred. The patient should not be moved to obtain the X-rays; a cross-table lateral view should be obtained.

31 Correct answer—**D**

The Glasgow Coma Scale is a standard means for assessing the patient's level of consciousness and for evaluating eye opening, verbal response, and motor response. The numeric value obtained allows the nurse to quickly observe a deterioration in the patient's neurologic status.

32 Correct answer—**A**

The RAS is responsible for maintaining consciousness by coordinating sensory input and responding, in proportion, to incoming stimuli. The hypothalamus is responsible for temperature regulation, behavior, autonomic responses, and control of the pituitary gland. The spinothalamic tract is responsible for transmitting pain and temperature to the brain. The extrapyramidal tracts regulate and control voluntary motor activity.

33 Correct answer—**B**

The Glasgow Coma Scale assigns a numeric value (from 1 to 5) to the patient's ability to open the eyes, respond verbally, and show motor response to different kinds of stimuli. Five is the best score in each area for a possible total of 15.

34 Correct answer—**B**

The brain stem and cerebrum have been damaged if decerebrate posturing is evidenced. Both control motor function. The cerebellum coordinates muscle tone with movement and maintains equilibrium. The hypothalamus does not regulate motor function.

35 Correct answer—**D**

Normally, ICP is less than 10 mm Hg. An ICP of 15 mm Hg or more is considered abnormal. Conditions responsible for an increased ICP include those that increase brain volume, such as hematomas, tumors, and cerebral edema; those that increase blood volume, such as hypercapnia; and those that increase CSF fluid, such as hydrocephalus. Head trauma, CVAs, and intracranial hemorrhage are neurologic emergencies whose underlying event is increasing ICP.

36 Correct answer—**A**

The nurse begins by providing auditory stimuli, and the patient's level of consciousness is evaluated by observing the response. When any kind of stimulation is provided, it is best to start with the minimal amount necessary to evoke a response. Speaking to the patient is the most common method of applying auditory stimuli. The response to auditory stimuli is evaluated in all patients.

37 Correct answer—**A**

The level of consciousness is the most important factor in the neurologic assessment of the patient. It is the earliest and most sensitive of indicators, providing valid information about changes in neurologic status. An alteration in consciousness is the hallmark of cerebral injury.

38 Correct answer—**A**

Alterations in the characteristics of the respiratory pattern relate to the level of brain dysfunction. Central neurogenic hyperventilation (CNH) is the respiratory pattern seen in those patients with lesions at the lower midbrain level. CNH is characterized by rapid, regular respirations with an increase in depth of respiration. The rate will exceed 24 breaths/minute. Apneustic breathing is a pattern of prolonged inspiration, with a 2- to 3-second pause at the end of inspiration. This breathing pattern occurs with lesions at the pons level. Cluster breathing, irregular breathing with periods of apnea at irregular intervals, is associated with medullary damage. Hypoventilation occurs in a patient with metabolic or drug-induced coma, respiratory depression, and increased ICP.

39 Correct answer—**C**

An epidural hematoma is caused by arterial bleeding; a subdural hematoma results from venous bleeding. A subarachnoid hemorrhage is caused by a ruptured cerebral aneurysm, which is a weakening of a vessel wall.

40 Correct answer—**B**

Bleeding with resultant ecchymosis over the mastoid bone is referred to as Battle's sign and is commonly seen in basal skull fractures involving the middle fossa. However, this finding may not be seen in the ED as it takes 24 hours to develop. A basal skull fracture may involve the anterior, middle, or posterior fossae at the base of the skull.

41 Correct answer—**B**

Basal skull fractures may also result in cranial nerve injuries. Injury to the first cranial, or olfactory, nerve is common, causing loss of the sense of smell (anosmia). Other cranial nerve injuries include those to the facial nerve (seventh), causing ipsilateral facial paralysis, and the acoustic nerve (eighth), leading to disturbances in hearing or equilibrium.

42 Correct answer—**A**

Further assessment of the patient with a basal skull fracture may reveal otorrhea or rhinorrhea of CSF. Otorrhea occurs if the dura mater is torn and the tympanic membrane is ruptured, and CSF rhinorrhea results if the tympanic membrane is intact. Drainage samples from either site will test positive for glucose.

43 Correct answer—**B**

The patient with a basal skull fracture benefits from nursing care that averts further tearing of the dura by preventing transient increases in ICP; therefore, the patient must be instructed to avoid coughing and performing Valsalva's maneuver. Also, instruct the patient not to blow the nose but to allow the fluid to drain freely. If rhinorrhea is significant, then a small loose dressing may be applied. Nothing should be put into the nose or ears, including suction catheters or NG tubes.

44 Correct answer—**D**

"Raccoon's eyes" indicate a basal skull fracture involving the anterior fossa. Bilateral ecchymoses develop from bleeding into the sinuses. Anterior fossa fractures may also result in CSF rhinorrhea if the dura mater is torn.

45 Correct answer—**A**

The patient is most likely experiencing a subarachnoid hemorrhage caused by an arteriovenous malformation and brought on by strenuous activity. Epidural hematoma, basal skull fracture, and brain stem contusion are brought on by traumatic injuries.

46 Correct answer—**A**

In Brown-Séquard syndrome, the damage is located on one side of the spinal cord. As a result, complete motor paralysis occurs on the same side (ipsilateral motor loss), with nearly complete loss of pain and temperature sensations on the opposite side below the level of the lesion (contralateral loss of pain and temperature sensations). In anterior cord syndrome, the damage is mainly concentrated in the anterior aspect of the cord. The mechanism of injury may be a forward dislocation or compression injury. Complete motor paralysis usually occurs below the level of the lesion with complete loss of pain and temperature sensations. In central cord syndrome, the mechanism of injury is usually hyperextension of the cervical spine with compression, resulting in greater motor loss of upper extremities than of lower ones. No spinal cord damage is known as partial cord syndrome.

47 Correct answer—**B**

A lesion at C5 to C6 would result in paralysis of intercostal respiration; diaphragmatic respiration continues without abdominal muscle action as the diaphragm is innervated by C2, C3, and C4. Complete loss of motor power occurs in the trunk and legs (quadriplegia), along with bladder and bowel retention.

48 Correct answer—**D**

Spinal shock is a state of transient reflex depression below the level of the lesion. The pathophysiologic process of spinal shock is incompletely understood, but the shock is the result, in part, of sudden withdrawal of facilitatory influences from higher centers. A loss of sympathetic outflow occurs if the lesion is higher than T5. Flaccidity from a lesion of the upper motor neuron results during the shock, with spasticity returning after the shock subsides.

49 Correct answer—**A**

Urinary retention, rather than incontinence, is seen in spinal shock because of bladder atony. Spinal shock may result in life-threatening symptoms, such as hypotension and bradycardia from sympathetic blockade. Poikilothermy results from the interruption of sympathetic pathways to the temperature-regulating centers in the hypothalamus.

50 Correct answer—**B**

Injury below C4 results in diaphragmatic breathing, decreased tidal volume, and a decreased vital capacity that may lead to hypoventilation. Paralysis of abdominal and intercostal muscles is present, which leads to an ineffective cough and retention of bronchial secretions. Gastric dilation and ileus lead to abdominal distention, which may restrict diaphragmatic excursions.

51 Correct answer—**C**

To assess spinothalamic tract function, the nurse should ask the patient to close both eyes and then identify areas stimulated by pinprick. The lateral spinothalamic tract conveys pain and temperature sensation, whereas the anterior spinothalamic tract conveys light touch, pressure, pain, and temperature sensation. Identifying vibrations and position assesses proprioreceptive sensation. Point-to-point testing assesses coordination.

52 Correct answer—**D**

Bronchial breath sounds over the patient's lung lobes indicate the development of pneumonia, which is most likely caused by immobility, an ineffective cough, and a decreased vital capacity. The ABG test results indicate metabolic acidosis. An inspiratory force of −20 cm and a tidal volume of 500 ml are normal values.

53 Correct answer—**B**

The phrenic nerve innervates the diaphragm at the C3 to C4 level. Respiratory paralysis is seen with complete lesions at C2 or above, caused by the loss of innervation to the diaphragm and the intercostal and abdominal muscles. A lesion at C3 or C4 will cause a weak diaphragm with absent intercostal muscle power. Diaphragmatic breathing is seen with lesions below C4.

54 Correct answer—**D**

In spinal cord injury, early hypoventilation is manifested by ABG values. Poor values indicate inadequate oxygenation and ventilation. The development of cyanosis, a late sign of hypoventilation, may not be an accurate indicator because anemic patients may never develop cyanosis. Cyanosis is also difficult to assess in the black population.

55 Correct answer—**A**

A spinal cord injury between T4 and T12 results in paraplegia involving the lower part of the body. The patient can perform all activities of daily living, achieve mobility with a wheelchair, and transfer easily. The T11 to L2 level is a particularly important area of the cord; sympathetic motor fibers exiting the spinal cord at this level innervate the trigone muscle of the bladder. Thus, injury at this level produces loss of voluntary bowel and bladder control, resulting in retention.

56 Correct answer—**B**

If a cervical spinal cord injury is suspected, the patient's airway should be opened by a modified jaw-thrust maneuver. This is the safest approach to opening the airway of a patient who has a suspected neck injury. This is accomplished by grasping one of the angles of the patient's lower jaw in each hand and lifting both hands, thus displacing the mandible forward. If the lips close, the lower lip can be retracted with the thumb. The head of the bed should not be tilted as paralysis may ensue. Pulling down the chin alone will not open the airway. A tracheotomy is not yet indicated.

57 Correct answer—**A**

Loss of motor function in the right arm and leg may indicate a lesion in the pyramidal tract of the left hemisphere. The lateral corticospinal (pyramidal) tract is the most important upper motor neuron tract. Damage to this area results in contralateral motor loss. Middle cerebral artery syndrome is by far the most common of all cerebral occlusions. If the main stem of the middle cerebral artery is occluded, a massive infarction of most of the hemisphere results.

58 Correct answer—**D**

The most reliable technique for testing upper extremity motor strength is for the nurse to ask the patient to close his eyes and raise his arms straight in front of him, palms up. The nurse should watch how well this position is maintained. By asking the patient to squeeze her hands, the nurse can assess equality of strength in hand grasps, but this is less accurate than that of arm extension. Observing for spontaneous movement does not assess strength. Testing reflexes assesses the intactness of the reflex arcs.

59 Correct answer—**C**

A patient admitted with an injury to the left cerebral hemisphere would exhibit contralateral findings, such as right hemiparesis and hemiplegia, and right homonymous hemianopia (loss of vision in the right half of both visual fields). In a left cerebral injury with right visual loss, the eyes deviate to the left to permit better visualization.

60 Correct answer—**A**

Pinpoint pupils are usually indicative of a lesion in the pons. Small, bilateral, nonreactive pupils may result from the loss of sympathetic innervation. Parasympathetic innervation remains, causing pupillary constriction. A lesion in the midbrain may result in midposition, nonreactive pupils. Bilateral fixed and dilated pupils are seen in severe cerebral anoxia.

61 Correct answer—**A**

Apneustic breathing and pinpoint pupils occur in the patient with an injury, or lesion, of the pons. In apneustic breathing, there is a prolonged inspiration with a pause at the end of the inspiratory and expiratory cycle.

62 Correct answer—**A**

Signs of meningeal irritation include Kernig's and Brudzinski's signs. Kernig's sign is elicited by flexing the upper leg at the hip to a 90-degree angle and then attempting to extend the knee. With meningitis, pain and spasm of the hamstrings occur when an attempt is made to extend the knee. Brudzinski's sign is positive when both legs flex at the hips and knees in response to passive flexion of the neck and head onto the chest. A stiff neck (nuchal rigidity) and photophobia are other symptoms of meningeal irritation.

63 Correct answer—**A**

The assessment finding of a Babinski's sign is not associated with meningeal irritation. Babinski's sign indicates pyramidal tract damage, an alteration in the motor tracts of the brain.

64 Correct answer—**B**

Isolation of the patient with viral meningitis is unnecessary. Correct nursing interventions include frequent monitoring of the temperature, because fever increases ICP, and maintaining the patient on seizure precautions, because seizure activity is common in patients with CNS infection. A major responsibility in caring for a patient with viral meningitis is the monitoring and managing of increased ICP.

65 Correct answer—**A**

A common manifestation seen in patients with bacterial meningococcal meningitis is petechiae. Petechiae, rash, purpuric lesions, or ecchymoses develop in 50% of patients. Patients with bacterial meningitis also have symptoms of fever, headache, lethargy, confusion, irritability, and stiff neck.

Selected References

Alspach J.G., and Williams, S. *Core Curriculum for Critical Care Nursing,* 3rd ed. Philadelphia: W.B. Saunders Co., 1985.

Bourg, P., et al. *Standardized Nursing Care Plans for the Emergency Department.* St. Louis: C.V. Mosby Co., 1986.

Cerullo, L.J., and Quigley, M.R. "Management of Cervical Spine Injury," *Journal of Emergency Nursing* 11:182-187, July/August 1985.

Fowler, S., et al. "Nursing Grand Rounds—Small Hopes: Care of the Patient with Head Trauma," *Nursing86* 16:52-55, May 1986.

Hickey, J. *The Clinical Practice of Neurological and Neurosurgical Nursing.* Philadelphia: J.B. Lippincott Co., 1986.

Holloway, N.M. *Emergency Department Nurses Association Core Curriculum.* Philadelphia: W.B. Saunders Co., 1985.

Manifold, S.L. "Craniocerebral Trauma: A Review of Primary and Secondary Injury and Therapeutic Modalities," *Focus on Critical Care* 13:22-35, April 1986.

Pallett, P., and O'Brien, M. *Testbook of Neurological Nursing.* Boston: Little, Brown & Co., 1985.

Richmond, T.S. "A Critical Care Challenge: The Patient with a Cervical Spinal Cord Injury," *Focus on Critical Care* 12:23-33, April 1985.

Rudy, E. *Advanced Neurological and Neurosurgical Nursing.* St. Louis: C.V. Mosby Co., 1984.

Rutkowski, B.L.C. *Neurological and Neurosurgical Nursing,* 8th ed. St. Louis: C.V. Mosby Co., 1982.

Sheehy, S.B. "Trauma Patient Guidelines," *Journal of Emergency Nursing* 11:209-210, July/August 1985.

Sheehy, S.B., and Barber, J.M. *Emergency Nursing: Principles and Practice,* 2nd ed. St. Louis: C.V. Mosby Co., 1985.

Chapter 6

Metabolic/Endocrine Emergencies Questions and Answers

You must begin with Question 1 of this chapter and progress in sequence. **Do not skip around.** Subsequent answers build on previous ones.

Patrice Case, RN, MA
Laura Gasparis, RN, MA, CCRN, CEN
Joanne Noone, RN, MSN, CCRN, CEN
Debra Toth, RN, BSN, MA Candidate

SITUATION

A 22-year-old man is unconscious when brought to the emergency department (ED). He is breathing rapidly and deeply. Although his skin is warm and dry, his pulse is 130 beats/minute and weak, and his blood pressure (BP) is 92/60 mm Hg. Blood for arterial blood gas (ABG) studies and electrolyte studies is sent to the laboratory.

Questions 1 to 15 refer to the above situation.

1 Which medications are most appropriate at this time?

A. Dextrose 50% and naloxone (Narcan)
B. Regular insulin and sodium bicarbonate
C. NPH insulin and potassium
D. Activated charcoal and naloxone

2 The ABG studies reveal pH, 7.03; PO_2, 98 mm Hg; PCO_2, 28 mm Hg; HCO_3^-, 12 mEq/liter. The SMA-6 reveals sodium level, 140 mEq/liter; potassium level, 5 mEq/liter; chloride level, 104 mEq/liter; CO_2 level, 18 mEq/liter; blood urea nitrogen (BUN), 40 mg/dl; and glucose level, 592 mg/dl. According to the patient's parents, he has a 10-year history of Type I diabetes mellitus. A diagnosis of diabetic ketoacidosis (DKA) is made. Which therapy should now be administered?

A. Dextrose 50% and naloxone
B. Regular insulin and sodium bicarbonate
C. NPH insulin and potassium
D. Activated charcoal and naloxone

3 The most appropriate I.V. fluid to infuse is:

A. 0.45% saline solution
B. 0.9% saline (normal saline) solution
C. Dextrose 5% in 0.45% saline (D_5½NS) solution
D. Dextrose 5% in normal saline (D_5NS) solution

4 The initial preferred method of insulin administration at this time is:

A. I.V. boluses of regular insulin 10 to 20 units/hour
B. I.V. bolus of 20 units regular insulin followed by a continuous drip of 4 to 8 units/hour
C. 10 units of regular insulin I.V. and 20 units of NPH insulin subcutaneously (S.C.)
D. 10 units of regular insulin I.V. and 10 units of regular insulin S.C.

5 A common, serious complication for which this patient should be monitored is:

A. Respiratory acidosis
B. Metabolic alkalosis
C. Hyperkalemia
D. Shock from dehydration

6 Three hours after admission, the patient's serum glucose level is 425 mg/dl, his pH is 7.32, his BP is 150/80 mm Hg, and his pulse is 120 beats/minute. The most appropriate fluid therapy now is:

A. 0.45% saline solution
B. Normal saline solution
C. D_5½NS solution
D. D_5NS solution

7 This patient is at risk for which complication?

A. Shock
B. Oliguria
C. Hypercalcemia
D. Hypokalemia

8 Six hours after admission, the patient's serum glucose level is 279 mg/dl. The most appropriate fluid therapy now is:

A. 0.45% saline solution
B. Normal saline solution
C. D_5½NS solution
D. Lactated Ringer's solution

9 A complication of treatment for DKA is:

A. Hyperglycemic hyperosmolar nonketotic (HHNK) coma
B. Acute renal failure
C. Cerebral edema
D. Respiratory acidosis

10 In children, signs and symptoms of DKA may mimic:

A. Hypoglycemia
B. Appendicitis
C. Sickle-cell crisis
D. Upper respiratory tract infection

11 Which EKG abnormality may be seen initially in a patient with DKA?

A. Sinus bradycardia
B. Presence of a U wave
C. ST-segment depression
D. Tall T wave

12 Which electrolyte abnormality may develop in a patient with DKA?

A. Hypomagnesemia
B. Hypophosphatemia
C. Hyperchloremia
D. Hypercalcemia

13 Which patient with insulin-dependent diabetes mellitus is most at risk for DKA?

A. The child with otitis media
B. The child who participates in a gym class
C. The child who requires insulin twice a day
D. The child who self-administers insulin

14 In a patient who has DKA and who is in the ED, which is the most effective method of determining response to insulin therapy?

A. Laboratory studies of serum glucose levels
B. Laboratory studies of serum ketone levels
C. Bedside urine glucose measurements
D. Bedside capillary glucose measurements with a glucometer

15 Which diabetic patient is most at risk for hypovolemic shock from DKA?

A. Child
B. Adolescent
C. The elderly
D. Cardiac patient

16 Precipitating factors in the development of DKA include:

A. Omission or resistance to insulin in a patient with diabetes mellitus
B. Surgery or trauma in a patient with diabetes mellitus
C. Pancreatitis
D. All of the above

17 The typical clinical presentation of the patient with DKA includes all of the following *except*:

A. Acetone breath, slow respirations
B. Altered level of consciousness, Kussmaul's respirations
C. Polyuria, signs of dehydration
D. Tachycardia, possible hypotension

18 Which initial diagnostic studies are *not* reflective of DKA?

A. Decreased PCO_2, pH, and HCO_3^-
B. Elevated serum potassium level, decreased bicarbonate level
C. Elevated urine specific gravity, elevated BUN levels
D. Decreased serum potassium level, decreased hematocrit value

19 A patient with DKA shows signs of severe intracellular dehydration. His BP is 150/80 mm Hg, sitting; and his pulse is 90 beats/minute. Which I.V. solution should be infused?

A. 0.45% saline solution
B. Normal saline solution
C. D_5NS solution
D. D_5½NS solution

20 Which is *not* appropriate for the patient with DKA?

A. Continuous administration of NPH insulin, 4 to 8 units/hour
B. Rapid administration of fluids, initially 1,000 ml/hour
C. Infusion of D_5½NS solution when serum glucose level falls to 250 mg/dl
D. Infusion of potassium, as ketosis decreases and insulin therapy is begun

21 The most obvious sign or symptom of DKA is:

A. Elevated serum potassium level
B. Elevated blood pH
C. Air hunger
D. Polyuria

SITUATION

A 68-year-old woman is brought to the ED by her son. He states that his mother has been acting funny, experiencing weakness, excessive thirst (polydipsia), and excessive urination (polyuria) for the past few days. Initial laboratory studies reveal serum glucose level of 2,000 mg/dl; no ketones are detected in the urine. A diagnosis of HHNK coma is made.

Questions 22 to 24 refer to the above situation.

22 The change in the level of consciousness of a patient with HHNK is the result of:

A. Serum osmolarity of 380 mOsm/liter
B. BUN level of 50 mg/dl
C. Serum sodium level of 125 mEq/liter
D. Nonketotic state

23 Which nursing action is *not* a priority during the initial management of this patient?

A. Administering insulin
B. Administering hypotonic saline solution
C. Monitoring of rectal temperature, notifying physician if temperature rises above 101° F. (38.3° C.)
D. Assessing neurologic status

24 The management of HHNK differs from that of DKA because the patient with HHNK requires:

A. Hypertonic fluid replacement; less insulin and potassium than for patients with DKA
B. Hypotonic fluid replacement; less insulin and potassium than for patients with DKA
C. Hypotonic fluid replacement; no insulin or potassium
D. Isotonic replacement fluid; more insulin and potassium than for patients with DKA

SITUATION

A comatose 47-year-old man is brought to the ED. The family reports that he had become confused over the last 72 hours. He had a seizure in the car on the way to the hospital. Upon arrival, the patient is minimally responsive. His respiratory rate is 32 breaths/minute; pulse, 110 beats/minute; BP, 120/90 mm Hg. Immediate laboratory work reveals an abnormal sodium level of 117 mEq/liter. The patient's chest X-ray reveals a mass in the right midlung field.

Questions 25 to 32 refer to the above situation.

25 The underlying factor responsible for this patient's change in mental status is related to:

A. Cancer of the lung with cerebral metastasis
B. Syndrome of inappropriate antidiuretic hormone (SIADH) secretion
C. Seizure activity from meningitis
D. Possible subarachnoid hemorrhage

26 Treatment of this patient is likely to include all of the following *except*:

A. Administration of furosemide (Lasix)
B. Administration of 200 to 300 ml 3% hypertonic saline solution
C. Fluid restriction
D. Administration of demeclocycline (Ledermycin) 300 mg P.O.

27 Which patient is *not* at risk for SIADH?

A. A 20-year-old patient who is transferred from a skilled nursing facility where he received prolonged positive-pressure ventilation
B. A 36-year-old patient receiving phenytoin
C. A 64-year-old patient with chronic obstructive pulmonary disease (COPD) complicated by pneumonia
D. A 70-year-old patient with carcinoma of the lung

28 An increase in antidiuretic hormone (ADH) secretion may be the result of:

A. Chlorpropamide therapy
B. Head trauma
C. Viral respiratory infection
D. All of the above

29 Which of the following laboratory findings is seen in a patient with SIADH?

A. Serum sodium level of 120 mEq/liter
B. Serum potassium level of 6 mEq/liter
C. Serum osmolarity of 350 mOsm/liter
D. Urine specific gravity of 1.003

30 Which complication occurs in the patient with SIADH?

A. Tetany
B. Seizures
C. Hypotension
D. All of the above

31 Resistance to vasopressin tannate therapy may be caused by:

A. Administration of vasopressin with calcium channel blockers
B. Mixing vasopressin with normal saline solution
C. Inadequate warming or agitation of the medication vial
D. Failure to keep medication refrigerated

32 Vasopressin therapy must be used cautiously in patients who have:

A. Liver dysfunction
B. Brain tumor
C. Angina pectoris
D. Undergone kidney transplant

SITUATION

A 16-year-old teenager is brought to the ED by his parents for symptoms of polydipsia and polyuria. His medical history was noncontributory. Immediate laboratory studies indicate a serum sodium concentration of 160 mEq/liter. The urine osmolarity is 250 mOsm/liter. A diagnosis of diabetes insipidus is made.

Questions 33 to 36 refer to the above situation.

33 Laboratory findings in a patient with diabetes insipidus are likely to show:

A. Decreased serum sodium level
B. Decreased serum osmolarity
C. Increased urine osmolarity
D. Urine specific gravity of 1.001

34 In which of the following patients is diabetes insipidus most likely to develop?

A. An elderly patient receiving thiazides and clofibrate (Atromid-S)
B. A young woman with severe pneumonia
C. A middle-aged man receiving vasopressin therapy for esophageal varices
D. A young man with a skull fracture caused by head trauma

35 Which finding is seen in diabetes insipidus?

A. Serum osmolarity level of 250 mOsm/liter
B. Serum sodium level of 165 mEq/liter
C. Urinary output of less than 600 ml in 24 hours
D. Urine specific gravity of 1.025

36 A major complication of diabetes insipidus is:

A. Hypovolemic shock
B. Seizures
C. Congestive heart failure
D. Cardiac dysrhythmias from hypokalemia

SITUATION

A 25-year-old man is brought to the ED complaining of blurred vision, headache, slurred speech, and weakness. He appears confused and somewhat lethargic. He just played an early-morning game of tennis. Immediate laboratory studies indicate a serum glucose level of 34 mg/dl.

Questions 37 and 38 refer to the above situation.

37 Emergency management of a comatose patient with hypoglycemia includes:

A. Measurement of fasting blood sugar levels and administration of sweetened orange juice via nasogastric tube
B. Measurement of fasting blood sugar levels and administration of 50 ml dextrose 50% in water I.V.
C. Administration of 50 ml of dextrose 50% I.V. push followed by glucagon injection
D. Infusion of 1 liter dextrose 10% in water followed by measurement of blood glucose levels

38 The symptoms of hypoglycemia are the result of:

A. Neuroglycopenia
B. Glycopenia
C. Decreased liver glycogenolysis
D. Decreased response of the sympathetic nervous system

SITUATION

A 66-year-old woman is brought from home to the ED by paramedics. Her BP is 104/58 mm Hg; pulse, 44 beats/minute; respiratory rate, 14 breaths/minute; and temperature, 92.4° F. (33.5° C.). No medical history is available, except for the patient's statement of not feeling "well" for the past month. Physical examination reveals a lethargic, thin woman with dry skin and periorbital and facial edema. Bilateral pulmonary congestion is noted. EKG monitoring shows sinus bradycardia. The diagnosis of impending myxedema coma is made.

Questions 39 to 43 refer to the above situation.

39 Which of the following statements is true regarding myxedema coma?

A. It is extremely advanced hypothyroidism
B. It does not occur in all patients with hypothyroidism
C. All patients who have myxedema coma are in a hypothyroid state
D. All of the above

40 This patient is likely to have which electrolyte imbalance?

A. Hyponatremia
B. Hypernatremia
C. Hypokalemia
D. Hyperkalemia

41 The patient remains hypothermic (temperature 95° F. [35° C.]). Appropriate nursing intervention includes:

A. Application of a hypothermia blanket
B. Rewarming with blankets
C. Administration of glycerin suppository every 4 hours as needed
D. All of the above

42 The treatment of myxedema coma usually does *not* include:

A. Fluid restriction
B. Thyroid hormone replacement
C. Electrolyte replacement
D. Diuretics

43 Arterial blood gas measurements are pH, 7.28; PO_2, 50 mm Hg; PCO_2, 64 mm Hg; and HCO_3^-, 20 mEq/liter. Appropriate intervention includes which therapy?

A. Administer dextrose 5% in lactated Ringer's solution I.V. at 150 ml/hour
B. Administer 35% oxygen by Venturi mask
C. Measure serum electrolyte levels immediately
D. Prepare for endotracheal intubation

SITUATION

An obese patient is transferred to the ED after ambulatory surgery. He has fever; pallor; rapid, weak pulse; signs of dehydration; headache; confusion; and restlessness. BP is 90/50 mm Hg. He has an 8-year history of Addison's disease. His laboratory data reveal a serum postassium level of 6.5 mEq/liter; white blood cell count (WBC), 15,000/mm³; serum glucose level, 55 mg/dl; and serum sodium level, 124 mEq/liter. The diagnosis of adrenal crisis is made.

Questions 44 to 50 refer to the above situation.

44 The most likely reason for the development of adrenal crisis is:

A. Obesity
B. Decreased exercise
C. Increased appetite
D. Fasting status before surgery

45 Which is the most life-threatening aspect of adrenal crisis?

A. Hypokalemia
B. Hypoglycemia
C. Vascular collapse
D. Hypernatremia

46 Which diagnostic test is the best indicator of this patient's condition?

A. Plasma carcinoembryonic antigen (CEA) level
B. 24-hour urine 17-hydroxycorticosteroid level
C. Plasma cortisol level
D. Adrenocorticotropic hormone (ACTH) infusion test

47 Which of the following is the most appropriate fluid replacement for this patient?

A. Dextrose 5% in lactated Ringer's solution at 100 ml/hour
B. D_5NS solution, 1 liter in 2 hours
C. D_5W at 200 ml/hour
D. 0.45% saline solution, 1 liter in 6 hours

48 Which medication should be ordered immediately?

A. Sodium levothyroxine (Synthroid) 0.1 mg
B. Dexamethasone (Decadron) 200 mg
C. Hydrocortisone (Cortef) 200 mg
D. Fludrocortisone (Florinef) 0.1 mg

49 Hyperkalemia can cause which of the following EKG changes?

A. T-wave depression with prolonged QT interval
B. Peaked T waves, wide QRS complexes, prolonged PR interval
C. Q-wave inversion, shortened PR interval
D. Bradycardia, bundle branch block

50 The clinical signs and symptoms of acute adrenal crisis are caused by:

A. Decreased aldosterone and cortisol
B. Decreased ADH and cortisol
C. Increased ADH and cortisol
D. Increased aldosterone and cortisol

SITUATION

A 55-year-old woman is admitted to the ED with a temperature of 105° F. (40.5° C.); BP, 180/110 mm Hg; pulse, 120 beats/minute; respirations, 36 breaths/minute. She shows signs of dehydration and complains of muscle weakness and bone pain for the past week. She has a history of Graves' disease; the diagnosis of thyroid crisis is made.

Questions 51 to 55 refer to the above situation.

51 This patient should be monitored for:

A. Hypocalcemia and hypoglycemia
B. Hyponatremia and hyperglycemia
C. Hypernatremia and hypokalemia
D. Metabolic alkalosis

52 Which of the following drugs may be used in treating this patient who is found to be iodine sensitive?

A. ACTH
B. Sodium levothyroxine
C. Lithium (Lithobid)
D. Phenytoin (Dilantin)

53 Which nursing measure is *not* appropriate in controlling pyrexia?

A. Administration of aspirin
B. Administration of muscle relaxants to control shivering
C. Application of ice packs to axilla and groin
D. Use of hypothermia blanket with rectal probe

54 Which of the following is *not* useful in determining thyroid function?

A. Serum protein-bound iodine (PBI)
B. Radioactive iodine (RAI) uptake
C. Thyroid-stimulating hormone (TSH)
D. Urine 17-ketosteroids

55 The patient begins to complain of bone pain and thirst; she displays a decreased level of consciousness, and the muscles are hypotonic. Which condition do these signs and symptoms suggest?

A. Dehydration
B. Hypokalemia
C. Hyponatremia
D. Hypercalcemia

SITUATION

After fainting, a 65-year-old woman is brought to the ED by ambulance. Physical examination reveals central-type obesity with a fatty buffalo hump in the neck; hirsutism; thin, fragile extremities with areas of ecchymosis; hypertension; and mild congestive heart failure. She has had extreme weakness and fatigue in the past month and altered sleep patterns.

Questions 56 to 60 refer to the above situation.

56 This patient's signs and symptoms are characteristic of:

A. Conn's syndrome
B. Cushing's syndrome
C. Diabetes insipidus
D. Myxedema coma

57 Which statement is true regarding the pathophysiologic process of this patient's condition?

A. It is caused by removal of the pituitary gland
B. It is a disorder of the posterior lobe of the pituitary gland that is caused by a deficiency of vasopressin
C. The clinical presentation reflects excessive adrenocortical activity
D. The clinical presentation reflects deficient adrenocortical activity

58 This patient should be monitored for:

A. Hyperglycemia
B. Hypokalemia
C. Hypernatremia
D. All of the above

59 The patient's condition produces anti-inflammatory effects. Which nursing diagnosis would reflect this assessment?

A. Self-care deficit related to weakness
B. Susceptibility to injury and infection related to altered metabolism
C. Altered body image related to physical appearance
D. Sleep pattern disturbance related to anxiety

60 What would a patient with increased levels of mineralocorticoids and glucocorticoids exhibit?

A. Increased heart rate with atrial premature complexes (APCs)
B. Decreased serum osmolarity
C. Elevated calcitonin level
D. Chvostek's sign

Answer Sheet

	A	B	C	D		A	B	C	D
1	○	○	○	○	**31**	○	○	○	○
2	○	○	○	○	**32**	○	○	○	○
3	○	○	○	○	**33**	○	○	○	○
4	○	○	○	○	**34**	○	○	○	○
5	○	○	○	○	**35**	○	○	○	○
6	○	○	○	○	**36**	○	○	○	○
7	○	○	○	○	**37**	○	○	○	○
8	○	○	○	○	**38**	○	○	○	○
9	○	○	○	○	**39**	○	○	○	○
10	○	○	○	○	**40**	○	○	○	○
11	○	○	○	○	**41**	○	○	○	○
12	○	○	○	○	**42**	○	○	○	○
13	○	○	○	○	**43**	○	○	○	○
14	○	○	○	○	**44**	○	○	○	○
15	○	○	○	○	**45**	○	○	○	○
16	○	○	○	○	**46**	○	○	○	○
17	○	○	○	○	**47**	○	○	○	○
18	○	○	○	○	**48**	○	○	○	○
19	○	○	○	○	**49**	○	○	○	○
20	○	○	○	○	**50**	○	○	○	○
21	○	○	○	○	**51**	○	○	○	○
22	○	○	○	○	**52**	○	○	○	○
23	○	○	○	○	**53**	○	○	○	○
24	○	○	○	○	**54**	○	○	○	○
25	○	○	○	○	**55**	○	○	○	○
26	○	○	○	○	**56**	○	○	○	○
27	○	○	○	○	**57**	○	○	○	○
28	○	○	○	○	**58**	○	○	○	○
29	○	○	○	○	**59**	○	○	○	○
30	○	○	○	○	**60**	○	○	○	○

Answer Sheet

	A	B	C	D		A	B	C	D
1	○	○	○	○	31	○	○	○	○
2	○	○	○	○	32	○	○	○	○
3	○	○	○	○	33	○	○	○	○
4	○	○	○	○	34	○	○	○	○
5	○	○	○	○	35	○	○	○	○
6	○	○	○	○	36	○	○	○	○
7	○	○	○	○	37	○	○	○	○
8	○	○	○	○	38	○	○	○	○
9	○	○	○	○	39	○	○	○	○
10	○	○	○	○	40	○	○	○	○
11	○	○	○	○	41	○	○	○	○
12	○	○	○	○	42	○	○	○	○
13	○	○	○	○	43	○	○	○	○
14	○	○	○	○	44	○	○	○	○
15	○	○	○	○	45	○	○	○	○
16	○	○	○	○	46	○	○	○	○
17	○	○	○	○	47	○	○	○	○
18	○	○	○	○	48	○	○	○	○
19	○	○	○	○	49	○	○	○	○
20	○	○	○	○	50	○	○	○	○
21	○	○	○	○	51	○	○	○	○
22	○	○	○	○	52	○	○	○	○
23	○	○	○	○	53	○	○	○	○
24	○	○	○	○	54	○	○	○	○
25	○	○	○	○	55	○	○	○	○
26	○	○	○	○	56	○	○	○	○
27	○	○	○	○	57	○	○	○	○
28	○	○	○	○	58	○	○	○	○
29	○	○	○	○	59	○	○	○	○
30	○	○	○	○	60	○	○	○	○

1 Correct answer—**A**

When an ED patient is unconscious and the cause is unknown, it is appropriate to administer one ampule of dextrose 50% and 0.8 mg naloxone. Dextrose is administered in case the patient is in insulin shock, a condition more dangerous than DKA. Naloxone is administered to reverse respiratory depression, in case an overdose of narcotics caused the unconscious state. Administering insulin to an unconscious patient before establishing the cause of unconsciousness could be harmful because it may result in furthering hypoglycemia.

2 Correct answer—**B**

Regular insulin and sodium bicarbonate should be administered to a patient whose serum glucose level is 592 mg/dl and pH is 7.03. Regular insulin is preferable to NPH insulin because of its rapid onset of action; sodium bicarbonate should be administered to a DKA patient if the pH falls below 7.10. A patient with DKA usually has a normal or slightly elevated serum potassium level; therefore, potassium is not indicated. Naloxone, dextrose, and activated charcoal are not indicated in the treatment of DKA.

3 Correct answer—**B**

Tachycardia and hypotension indicate intravascular volume depletion. The most appropriate therapy at present is saline. Usually, 1 liter of normal saline solution is infused every hour for 2 to 3 hours, until BP returns to normal or urine output improves. Hypertonic solutions such as D_5½NS and D_5NS, and a hypotonic solution such as 0.45% saline are inappropriate. Hypertonic solutions would cause further cellular depletion, and a hypotonic solution would cause further intravascular volume loss as fluid shifts into the cell.

4 Correct answer—**B**

The initial preferred method of insulin administration at this time is an I.V. bolus of regular insulin, 20 units, followed by a continuous infusion of 4 to 8 units/hour. The insulin should be diluted in a glass bottle, because it will bind to plastic containers. The S.C. route should be avoided in hypotensive patients because absorption is variable. Continuous infusion maintains a steady blood insulin level.

5 Correct answer—**D**

A common serious complication of DKA is shock from dehydration. An elevated serum glucose level results in intracellular dehydration and intravascular depletion. Hyperglycemia increases the serum osmolarity, thereby causing a shift of intracellular water into the intravascular space, producing intracellular dehydration. An increased serum osmolarity produces an osmotic diuresis and polyuria (excessive urination).

6 Correct answer—**A**

A BP of 150/80 mm Hg indicates a reversal of intravascular fluid depletion. Administration of a hypotonic solution, such as 0.45% saline solution, will promote intracellular hydration. Usually, 1 liter of 0.45% saline solution is given over 4 to 6 hours, until oral intake is reestablished and the patient appears clinically well hydrated.

7 Correct answer—**D**

After initiation of therapy, hypokalemia usually results from correction of acidosis or from insulin therapy. Once intravascular fluid depletion has been reversed, 20 to 40 mEq of potassium should be added to each liter of I.V. fluid.

8 Correct answer—**C**

Once the serum glucose level falls to between 250 and 300 mg/dl, D_5½NS should be administered as the I.V. solution to prevent hypoglycemia, hypokalemia, and cerebral edema.

9 Correct answer—**C**

Cerebral edema can result from overzealous fluid replacement and administration of sodium bicarbonate. Although a rare complication, it is most commonly seen in children and adolescents during the first day of treatment. Mannitol, an osmotic diuretic, is the treatment of choice.

10 Correct answer—**B**

Children with DKA may erroneously be thought to have appendicitis or urinary tract infection. The abdominal pain associated with DKA is so severe that it mimics an acute surgical abdomen. The symptom of polyuria may cause DKA to be mistaken for a urinary tract infection.

11 Correct answer—**D**

A T wave will be seen. Hyperkalemia may initially be present in the patient with DKA. Metabolic acidosis causes potassium to shift out of the cell, thereby increasing serum levels. Hyperkalemia is reflected on the EKG by tall T waves, the absence of a P wave, and a wide QRS complex. As the acidosis is reversed, potassium returns to the cell and a hypokalemic state may result from osmotic diuresis. ST-segment depression and a U wave indicate hypokalemia. The patient with DKA is in sinus tachycardia because of hypovolemia.

12 Correct answer—**B**

Hypophosphatemia, manifested by muscle weakness, may occur in DKA as a result of total body phosphate depletion because of diuresis and acidosis. Initial phosphate measurements may be normal or high, as seen with potassium measurements, but may drop after therapy. Both phosphate and potassium may be replaced by administration of I.V. potassium phosphate.

13 Correct answer—**A**

Children at risk for DKA are those who have infections, are under emotional stress, or are noncompliant with therapy. Young children most commonly develop infections, while adolescents tend to suffer more from emotional stress and are noncompliant with therapy. An increase in activity may precipitate hypoglycemia by lowering insulin requirements.

14 Correct answer—**D**

In the patient with DKA who is in the ED, the most effective method of determining the response to insulin therapy is bedside capillary measurements using a glucometer. This provides instantaneous results; sending serum to the laboratory will provide values in 1 or 2 hours. Urine measurements are inconsistent because urine glucose thresholds are variable, and glycosuria is usually present when the serum glucose level is above 180 mg/dl.

15 Correct answer—**A**

Children with DKA are more at risk for hypovolemic shock because, compared with adults, relatively less fluid loss can result in dehydration. Children with DKA can lose up to 10% of their body weight. Children and adolescents have a higher risk of developing cerebral edema during fluid resuscitation. The elderly and cardiac patients are at an increased risk of developing pulmonary edema.

16 Correct answer—**D**

Precipitating factors in the development of DKA include omission or resistance to insulin in the diabetic patient, surgery or trauma in the diabetic patient, and pancreatitis, which interferes with insulin production and release. These conditions produce stress, thereby increasing glucocorticoid release, which results in elevated blood glucose levels.

17 Correct answer—**A**

The clinical presentation of the patient with DKA includes altered level of consciousness, poor skin turgor, hypotension, and tachycardia, which are the result of dehydration. Hyperglycemia promotes an osmotic diuresis, producing polyuria, polydipsia, and cellular and intravascular fluid depletion. The breakdown of body fats releases excessive ketones, producing metabolic acidosis. An acetone breath odor is present. An increase in the rate and depth of respirations compensates for the acidosis by blowing off carbon dioxide; this is known as Kussmaul's respirations.

18 Correct answer—**D**

Initial diagnostic studies of the patient with DKA reveal decreased arterial pH, HCO_3^-, and CO_2 levels because of the metabolic acidosis with respiratory compensation. The BUN and hematocrit levels and the urine specific gravity increase as a result of dehydration. Potassium shifts from the cells into the intravascular fluid, with a corresponding hydrogen shift into cells. This compensatory mechanism is an attempt to buffer the acidosis, which produces an elevated potassium level.

19 Correct answer—**A**

Administration of a hypotonic solution, such as 0.45% saline solution, will promote intracellular hydration. An isotonic solution, such as normal saline solution, would promote intravascular hydration, which is not required by the patient at this time. Hypertonic solutions such as D_5½NS or D_5NS would shift fluid from the intracellular compartment into the intravascular compartment, thus promoting further intracellular dehydration.

20 Correct answer—**A**

Specific care for the patient with DKA strives to restore fluid balance; to restore normal carbohydrate, fat, and protein metabolism; and to maintain electrolyte balance and function of related systems. During restoration of fluid balance, rapid administration may be ordered, up to 1,000 ml/hour initially. When the patient's serum glucose level falls to 250 mg/dl, the initial infusions of 0.45% saline or normal saline solution should be changed to D_5½NS to prevent hypoglycemia, hypokalemia, and cerebral edema. To restore normal carbohydrate, fat, and protein metabolism, rapid-acting insulin (regular) is administered. Continuous I.V. infusion, 4 to 8 units/hour, is the preferred method; alternatives include loading doses, I.M., or I.V.; or I.V. bolus, 10 to 25 units/hour. During treatment, electrolyte levels, especially potassium, should be monitored.

21 Correct answer—**D**

Polyuria is the most obvious symptom observed in the patient with DKA. It initially results from the osmotic diuretic effect of hyperglycemia. Although the ketone-induced metabolic acidosis causes a shift of potassium into the serum, the resulting elevated serum potassium level is not so obvious. Metabolic acidosis decreases blood pH; Kussmaul's respirations compensate for this.

22 Correct answer—**A**

Hyperglycemia results in an elevated plasma osmolarity. This hyperosmolar state causes the brain cells to become dehydrated, thereby producing a change in the level of consciousness. A BUN level of 50 mg/dl would not alter the patient's level of consciousness. A serum sodium level of 125 mEq/liters could cause a change in mental status, but the severe state of dehydration from the osmotic diuresis also results in hypernatremia.

23 Correct answer—**C**

HHNK frequently is precipitated by a situation such as prolonged administration of total parenteral nutrition, pneumonia, burns, cerebrovascular accident, or recent surgery. Although temperature assessment is an important component of these states, it is not appropriate in initial management. Initially, the patient should be rehydrated with a hypotonic solution, such as 0.45% saline solution if BP is stable, or normal saline solution if intravascular depletion is present. Frequent neurologic assessments are necessary, because cerebral intracellular dehydration results in mental status changes. The serum glucose level should be normalized by insulin administration.

24 Correct answer—**B**

Hypotonic, 0.45% saline, fluid replacement is preferable to isotonic, 0.9% saline, because patients with HHNK have marked hyperosmolarity. Because of this severely dehydrated state, as much as 4 to 6 liters may be required in the first 10 hours. In the absence of acidosis, potassium loss in the urine is greatly decreased during the initial stages of glycosuria. Less insulin is generally required to reduce the hyperglycemia in patients with HHNK as compared with those with DKA.

25 Correct answer—**B**

Hyponatremia and altered mental status are symptoms of SIADH. Subarachnoid hemorrhage is characterized by an acute onset of headache and change in mental status. It may be associated with hyponatremia and may cause SIADH. The chest X-ray abnormalities of a mass in the right lung field have most likely resulted in SIADH; many oat-cell carcinomas of the lung produce ADH. Cerebral metastasis usually produces neurologic dysfunction of one area or one side of the body. Acute purulent meningitis could cause an altered mental status without such dysfunction, but the lack of fever or elevated white blood cell (WBC) count makes meningitis a less likely diagnosis.

26 Correct answer—**D**

The hyponatremia and resultant decreased osmolarity are responsible for patient seizures. The goal is to raise the serum sodium level to at least 125 mEq/liter to avoid neurologic symptoms. At this level, the patient's mental status should improve. Administration of furosemide will produce diuresis; hypertonic saline solution also is administered and fluids are restricted. The use of demeclocycline and other drugs that block the effect of antidiuretic hormone (ADH) on the renal tubules are not appropriate for the acute treatment of SIADH but may be appropriate for long-term therapy.

27 Correct answer—**B**

Carcinoma of the lung is the most common cause of SIADH; oat-cell carcinoma accounts for 80% of all cases of SIADH. Vasopressin is synthesized, stored, and released from the tumor tissue. Positive-pressure ventilation has been associated with SIADH, probably by causing a reduction in left atrial filling, which stimulates central ADH release. Pneumonia, tuberculosis, lung abscesses, and empyema also have been associated. The probable mechanism is the release of ADH from the inflamed pulmonary tissue. Phenytoin (Dilantin) has not been associated with SIADH; however, many other drugs have been, including chlorpropamide, vincristine, vinblastine, cyclophosphamide, and tricyclic antidepressants.

28 Correct answer—**D**

SIADH is caused by increased secretion of ADH by the posterior pituitary gland. Precipitating factors include tuberculous meningitis; extracranial malignant tumors, especially bronchogenic and pancreatic tumors; skull fractures; medications, such as chlorpropamide, clofibrate, and thiazides; and viral respiratory infections.

29 Correct answer—**A**

An increase in ADH secretion promotes excessive water retention by the kidneys. This lowers the serum sodium level and produces a marked decrease in serum osmolarity. The normal range for serum osmolarity is between 275 and 295 mOsm/liter. Dilutional hypokalemia also results. Urine output decreases as a result of increased reabsorption of water. The concentrated urine that is produced has high specific gravity and osmolarity.

30 Correct answer—**B**

Seizures may occur in the patient with SIADH. The clinical manifestations of SIADH are from excessive water retention, which leads to overhydration and water intoxication. Water intoxication dilutes serum sodium levels, producing hyponatremia, which results in neurologic changes. The manifestations of hyponatremia and water intoxication vary from a mild headache to seizures, coma, and death.

31 Correct answer—**C**

The mainstay of management in diabetes insipidus is the administration of vasopressin (Pitressin), because the patient with diabetes insipidus is deficient in ADH, or vasopressin. If Pitressin Tannate is prescribed, the vial must be warmed under hot water for several minutes and vigorously shaken. Other forms of ADH therapy include aqueous pitressin, a shorter-acting preparation that lasts approximately 4 hours, and lysine vasopressin, a nasal spray.

32 Correct answer—**C**

Vasopressin therapy must be used cautiously in patients with heart disease because its vasoconstrictive properties may precipitate myocardial ischemia. Vasopressin increases water reabsorption by the renal tubules and constriction of the smooth muscle of the arterioles.

33 Correct answer—**D**

Laboratory findings will show a urine specific gravity between 1.001 and 1.005. Diabetes insipidus results from a defect in the release or synthesis of ADH within the pituitary or a defect in renal tubular response to ADH. In diabetes insipidus, there is an impaired renal conservation of water; therefore, little water reabsorption occurs. As water is lost from the body, the serum sodium level rises, resulting in an increased serum osmolarity. As the kidneys fail to conserve water, the urine remains very dilute, resulting in a decreased urine osmolarity and a specific gravity between 1.001 and 1.005.

34 Correct answer—**D**

Diabetes insipidus develops from many causes. It is seen most commonly in neurosurgical patients. The second major cause is head trauma, especially basal skull fractures. Other precipitating factors include inflammatory or degenerative conditions, such as tubercular meningitis, syphilis, sarcoidosis, Hodgkin's disease, and tumors. Severe pneumonia and therapy with thiazides and vasopressin predispose the patient to SIADH.

35 Correct answer—**B**

Diabetes insipidus is a clinical syndrome characterized by an excessive urine output. Without ADH, the renal tubules are unable to reabsorb water, thereby producing polyuria (6 to 24 liters/day). The urine remains very dilute, with a specific gravity below 1.005. As water is lost from the body, the serum sodium level increases and results in an increased serum osmolarity (normal range is 275 to 295 mOsm/liter).

36 Correct answer—**A**

Diabetes insipidus can be complicated by severe volume depletion and dehydration, resulting in hypovolemic shock. The appropriate nursing intervention is assessment for rapidly developing hypovolemia. Meticulous recording of fluid intake and output, monitoring of vital signs, and daily weighing of the patient are mandatory.

37 Correct answer—**C**

Emergency management for hypoglycemic coma includes the administration of 50 ml of a dextrose 50% I.V. push followed by glucagon injection. If there is doubt as to whether hypoglycemia or hyperglycemia exists in a comatose patient, a serum glucose level should be obtained by finger stick. A fasting blood sugar level measurement is not feasible because one does not know whether or not the patient is fasting.

38 Correct answer—**A**

The symptoms of hypoglycemia are the result of neurologic responses. During hypoglycemia, insulin-antagonist hormones such as epinephrine are released, causing tachycardia, diaphoresis, tremors, and nervousness, also referred to as neuroglycopenia.

39 Correct answer—**D**

Myxedema occurs in patients with moderate to severe hypothyroidism. If the hypothyroidism is allowed to progress, the patient's condition will deteriorate and coma will eventually ensue. Myxedema coma is extremely advanced hypothyroidism; all persons who develop myxedema coma are in a hypothyroid state, but not all patients with hypothyroidism have myxedema.

40 Correct answer—**A**

Hyponatremia is caused by impairment of water excretion, which is dilutional in nature. The potassium level of patients with myxedema is usually normal, unless there is some other underlying pathologic process.

41 Correct answer—**B**

Rewarming should take place gradually, using only blankets or sheets. The use of a hypothermia blanket is strongly contraindicated because rapid rewarming can precipitate vasodilation, which can cause cardiac dysrhythmias, circulatory collapse, or death. Once thyroid replacement has begun, the body will begin to compensate and slowly return to a normal temperature. No benefit occurs from glycerin suppositories in this condition.

42 Correct answer—**D**

Fluid restriction may be indicated in myxedema coma to correct hyponatremia. If the hyponatremia is severe (less than 115 mEq/liter), normal saline solution may be necessary to elevate the serum sodium level. Thyroid hormone replacement is essential to correct the decreased secretion of thyroid hormone. Diuretic therapy may cause sodium loss, thus lowering levels further.

43 Correct answer—**D**

In this case, the patient's CO_2 value is 64 mm Hg, indicating acute respiratory acidosis; thus, the appropriate nursing intervention at this time would be to set up for endotracheal intubation. The initial assessment noted bilateral pulmonary congestion. Myxedema coma causes changes in the thoracic ventilatory capacity and respiratory center. Pleural effusion and ascites may be present. The ED nurse must carefully assess the respiratory system to monitor the need for ventilatory assistance. ABG study results usually demonstrate respiratory acidosis with CO_2 narcosis.

44 Correct answer—**D**

The patient has a history of Addison's disease, which can be controlled by corticosteroids. However, because he had been fasting and did not take his medication, the blood level of corticosteroids decreased. Abrupt discontinuation of steroid therapy precipated the adrenal crisis.

45 Correct answer—**C**

The most serious threat in adrenal crisis is peripheral vascular collapse. A patient may lose as much as 20% of extracellular fluid volume. Therefore, the first goal of emergency treatment is fluid replacement.

46 Correct answer—**C**

The most definitive diagnostic test for adrenal crisis is measurement of plasma cortisol levels. Abnormally low levels indicate adrenocortical insufficiency. ACTH and 24-hour urine 17-hydroxycorticosteroid level measurements are used in the diagnosis of adrenal disorders. However, they are contraindicated for a patient with adrenal crisis because of the potentially life-threatening delay associated with the tests. CEA levels are used in the diagnosis of cancer or abnormal cells in the body.

47 Correct answer—**B**

To combat fluid deficit, an I.V. of D_5NS should be infused. The infusion rate should be extremely rapid, usually within 1 to 2 hours, barring complications such as cardiac or renal disease. Fluid replacement will raise the blood pressure by volume expansion and will contribute needed glucose and sodium. After the first liter, the patient may require additional fluids at a rate of 1 liter every 3 to 4 hours. A 0.45% saline solution and dextrose 5% in lactated Ringer's solution are inappropriate because they do not contain enough sodium, which is needed to correct the hyponatremia seen in adrenal crisis.

48 Correct answer—**C**

Hydrocortisone, a soluble cortisol replacement, usually is used to treat adrenal crisis. This drug replaces the glucocorticoids that the patient has lost. The usual dosage is 100 to 200 mg I.V. immediately, then every 6 hours. Sodium levothyroxine is used for thyroid disease. Dexamethasone and fludrocortisone, mineralocorticoid replacements, may be used to treat adrenal crisis but are not urgently required because saline solution and hydrocortisone adequately compensate for lost mineralocorticoids.

49 Correct answer—**B**

When adrenal crisis is complicated by hyperkalemia, the EKG will show a prolonged PR interval, a wide QRS complex, and a tall, tented T wave. It may cause bradycardia but is not associated with a bundle branch block or T-wave depression.

50 Correct answer—**A**

Decreases of both cortisol and aldosterone secretion by the adrenal cortex precipate adrenal crisis, acute adrenocortisol insufficiency. ADH is secreted by the posterior pituitary and has no significance in adrenal crisis.

51 Correct answer—**B**

Excessive thyroid hormone appears to produce an increase in glycogenolysis and rapid intestinal glucose absorption. Also, the increased adrenergic activity may cause insulin resistance and impair insulin secretion, resulting in hyperglycemia. As a result of diaphoresis in patients with high fever who may consume large quantities of water without adequate salt intake, water toxicity or dilutional hyponatremia may be induced.

52 Correct answer—**C**

For patients who are iodine-sensitive, lithium is used to inhibit thyroid hormone release. Sodium levothyroxine is used for thyroid hormone replacement. ACTH is used mainly in the treatment of adrenal diseases.

53 Correct answer—**A**

Aspirin should be avoided because salicylates are thought to interfere with the binding of T_3 and T_4 to circulating thyroid-binding protein. The increase of free T_3 and T_4 may exacerbate the already existing hyperthyroidism. A nonaspirin pyretic should be used in thyroid storm. The other choices are acceptable forms of treating pyrexia.

54 Correct answer—**D**

Measurement of 24-hour urine 17-ketosteroids is used to assess adrenal function. PBI, TSH, and RAI uptake assess thyroid function.

55 Correct answer—**D**

Bone pain, muscle weakness, and hypotonic muscles are symptoms of hypercalcemia, which is caused by hypermetabolism of the bone. Hypercalcemia also causes thirst, lethargy, and drowsiness, which may progress to stupor and coma. Thirst may occur in patients with the other conditions, but they seldom present the other stated signs and symptoms.

56 Correct answer—**B**

These clinical manifestations are a classic presentation of Cushing's syndrome with associated protein catabolic, glyconeogenic, mineralocorticoid, androgenic, and behavioral effects.

57 Correct answer—**C**

Cushing's syndrome is the opposite of Addison's disease. This clinical presentation reflects excessive, rather than deficient, adrenocortical activity. The syndrome may result from excessive administration of cortisone or ACTH or from hyperplasia of the adrenal cortex.

58 Correct answer—**D**

Patients with Cushing's syndrome should be monitored for mineralocorticoid effects, including increased serum sodium levels, decreased serum potassium levels, hypertension, and edema. The increased blood glucose level is a glyconeogenic effect manifested by glucose intolerance.

59 Correct answer—**B**

The anti-inflammatory effects of excessive glucocorticoids produce increased susceptibility to infection and mask infections that do occur. Also, the continual protein catabolism results in muscle weakness. The risk of soft tissue injuries and fractures, caused by progressive osteoporosis, is increased.

60 Correct answer—**A**

In patients with Cushing's syndrome, hypokalemia produces an increased heart rate, frequently with APCs. Also, an increased serum aldosterone level results in an increased serum osmolarity and produces hypernatremia. Chvostek's sign, a facial twitch in response to tapping on the side of a patient's face, occurs with hypocalcemia.

Selected References

Adams, C. "Pulling Your Patient Through an Adrenal Crisis," *RN* 46:36-38, October 1983.

Alspach, J., and Williams, S. *Core Curriculum for Critical Care Nursing,* 3rd ed. Philadelphia: W.B. Saunders Co., 1985.

Bates, B. *A Guide to Physical Examination,* 3rd ed. Philadelphia: J.B. Lippincott Co., 1983.

Bolinger, R.E. "Hypoglycemia," *Critical Care Quarterly* 3:99, 109, September 1980.

Bondy, P.K., and Rosenburg, L.E. *Metabolic Control of Disease,* 8th ed. Philadelphia: W.B. Saunders Co., 1980.

Bruce, G. "The Somogyi Phenomenon: Insulin-Induced Posthypoglycemic Hyperglycemia, Part 1," *Heart and Lung* 7:463-466, May/June 1978.

Brunner, L., and Suddarth, D. *The Lippincott Manual of Nursing Practice,* 3rd ed. Philadelphia: J.B. Lippincott Co., 1982.

Campbell, J.W., and Frisse, M. *Manual of Medical Therapeutics,* 24th ed. Boston: Little, Brown & Co., 1983.

Cataland, S. "Hypoglycemia—A Spectrum of Problems, Part 1," *Heart & Lung* 7:455-462, May/June 1978.

Danowski, T.S. "Cushing's Syndrome," *Hospital Medicine* 21:155-157,160, April 1985.

Evangelisti, J.T., and Thorpe, C.J. "Thyroid Storm—A Nursing Crisis (Care Plan)," *Heart and Lung* 12:189-194, March 1983.

Fairchild, R.S. "Diabetes Insipidus: A Review," *Critical Care Quarterly* 3:111-118, September 1980.

Fletcher, B. *Quick Reference to Critical Care Nursing.* Philadelphia: J.B. Lippincott Co., 1982.

Greenspan, F., and Forsham, P., eds. *Basic and Clinical Endocrinology.* Los Altos, Calif.: Lange Medical Pubns., 1983.

Guthrie, D., and Guthrie, R. *Nursing Management of Diabetes,* 2nd ed. St. Louis: C.V. Mosby Co., 1982.

Guyton, A. *A Textbook of Medical Physiology,* 6th ed. Philadelphia: W.B. Saunders Co., 1981.

Hellman, R. "The Evaluation and Management of Hyperthyroid Crises," *Critical Care Quarterly* 3:77-92, September 1980.

Kinney, M. ed. *AACN's Clinical Reference for Critical Care Nursing.* New York: McGraw-Hill Book Co., 1981.

Kyner, N.L. "Diabetic Ketoacidosis," *Critical Care Quarterly* 3:65-75, 1980.

Larson, C. "The Critical Path of Adrenocortical Insufficiency," *Nursing84* 14:66-69, October 1984.

Larson, E.L., and Vasquez, M. *Critical Care Nursing.* Philadelphia: W.B. Saunders Co., 1983.

Lipman, T.H. "Assessment of the Child with Diabetic Ketoacidosis," *Dimensions of Critical Care Nursing* 6:82-93, March/April 1987.

Meek, J. "Myxedema Coma," *Critical Care Nurse* 3:67-75, May/June 1983.

Murray, P. "When Hyperglycemia Goes Critical," *RN* 46:56-60, March 1983.

Niedringhaus, L. "Acute Adrenal Crisis," *Focus on Critical Care* 10:30-36, February 1983.

Payne, N. "Emergency Care of the Patient with Myxedema Coma," *Journal of Emergency Nursing* 12:343-347, November/December 1986.

Rice, V. "Problems of Water Regulation: Diabetes Insipidus and Syndrome of Inappropriate Anti-diuretic Hormone," *Critical Care Nurse* 3:63-82, January/February 1983.

Sheehy, S.B., and Barber, J. *Emergency Nursing: Principles and Practice,* 2nd ed. St. Louis: C.V. Mosby Co., 1985.

Sommers, M. "Nonketotic Hyperosmolar Coma (Care Plan)," *Critical Care Nurse* 3:58-61, January/February 1983.

Winters, B. "Nursing Implications of Hyperosmolar Coma," *Heart and Lung* 12:439-446, July 1983.

[illegible] *Wyeth* [illegible]

[illegible] *Mag* [illegible]

[illegible] 1985.

[illegible] 1986.

[illegible]

[illegible]

[illegible]

[illegible]

Chapter 7

Renal/Genitourinary Emergencies Questions and Answers

You must begin with Question 1 of this chapter and progress in sequence. **Do not skip around.** Subsequent answers build on previous ones.

Joanne Noone, RN, MSN, CCRN, CEN
Catherine Paradiso, RN, MSN, CCRN, CEN

SITUATION

A 24-year-old man is brought to the emergency department (ED), having sustained blunt trauma to the left kidney during a boxing match. He is awake and alert. His chief complaint is flank tenderness. His urinalysis reveals microscopic hematuria. All other laboratory data are within normal limits. Vital signs are blood pressure (BP), 130/70 mm Hg; pulse, 76 beats/minute; respirations, 20 breaths/minute. He will be admitted to a medical/surgical unit when a bed is available.

Questions 1 to 5 refer to the above situation.

1 Which assessment findings indicate renal trauma?

A. Severe, colicky flank pain and diaphoresis
B. Flank tenderness and hematuria
C. Severe flank pain and urethral bleeding
D. Severe flank pain and no urine output

2 Which type of injury results from blunt renal trauma and can be resolved without surgery?

A. Contusion
B. Rupture of a major renal artery
C. Renal pedicle injuries
D. None of the above

3 Ecchymosis around the area of the patient's left flank can indicate:

A. Pulled muscles in the flank area
B. Fractured ilium bone
C. Retroperitoneal bleeding
D. All of the above

4 The physician determines that the patient has a renal contusion. Which best describes the necessary treatment?

A. Immediate surgery
B. Patient lies on affected side to apply pressure
C. Percutaneous evacuation of blood from the abdominal cavity
D. No treatment other than observation for worsening of the injury

5 If the patient has increased pain, the nurse should first:

A. Administer narcotics
B. Draw blood for electrolyte studies, blood urea nitrogen (BUN) level, and glucose level
C. Draw blood to determine a hematocrit value
D. Take the blood pressure

6 Renal trauma should be suspected if which of the following findings is present?

A. Positive Chvostek's sign
B. Oliguria
C. Hematoma in flank area
D. Dysuria

7 Trauma to the kidneys should be suspected in which of the following injuries?

A. Chest trauma
B. Fracture of pelvis
C. Deceleration injury
D. All of the above

8 Renal trauma is best diagnosed by which of the following tests?

A. X-ray of kidneys, ureters, bladder (KUB)
B. Abdominal computed tomography (CT) scan
C. Intravenous pyelogram (IVP)
D. Peritoneal tap

SITUATION

Unable to urinate for 2 days, a 62-year-old man comes to the ED. His history reveals no renal dysfunction but does indicate history of benign prostatic hypertrophy. He is slightly confused and complains of nausea, vomiting, and swollen ankles. Laboratory reports show a BUN level of 38 mg/dl and serum creatinine level of 4 mg/dl.

Questions 9 to 13 refer to the above situation.

9 This patient's signs and symptoms are characteristic of:

A. Postrenal acute renal failure (ARF)
B. Congestive heart failure
C. Glomerulonephritis
D. Chronic renal failure

10 The hallmark symptom of this problem is:

A. Edema
B. Rising BUN and creatinine levels
C. Anuria
D. Confusion

11 The test most likely to be used in initially diagnosing this patient's condition is:

A. KUB
B. Abdominal CT scan
C. IVP
D. Peritoneal tap

12 An indwelling (Foley) catheter is inserted, and 2,500 ml of urine is drained. The most important intervention at this time is:

A. Clamping the catheter
B. Fluid replacement
C. Diuretic administration
D. Emergency surgical consultation

13 An intravenous (I.V.) line is inserted. The most appropriate solution and rate of administration is:

A. Dextrose 5% in water (D_5W) at keep-vein-open rate
B. 3% saline solution at 20 ml/hour
C. Normal saline solution with potassium at 30 ml/hour
D. Dextrose 5% in 0.45% saline solution with potassium at 160 ml/hour

14 The most appropriate treatment for a zipper injury is:

A. Delicately unzip after giving local anesthesia
B. Delicately unzip using no anesthesia
C. Cut zipper around injury, allowing track to separate
D. Perform circumcision to remove injured foreskin

SITUATION

A 35-year-old woman comes to the ED complaining of nausea, vomiting, malaise, and a decrease in urine output. She recently completed a 2-week course of cephradine (Velosef) for a urinary tract infection (UTI). Urinalysis reveals a sodium level of 40 mEq/liter with a urine specific gravity of 1.010. Urine sediment includes casts, with few red blood cells (RBCs) or white blood cells (WBCs). BUN level is 40 mg/dl with a serum creatinine level of 4 mg/dl.

Questions 15 to 19 refer to the above situation.

15 This patient's clinical presentation suggests which condition?

A. Recurrence of UTI
B. Dehydration from vomiting
C. Allergic drug reaction
D. Acute tubular necrosis (ATN)

16 The most accurate indicator of the patient's renal function is the:

A. Creatinine level
B. BUN level
C. Urine sodium level
D. Urine specific gravity

17 An indirect measurement of the patient's glomerular filtration rate (GFR) is the:

A. Creatinine clearance
B. BUN level
C. Urine sodium level
D. Urine specific gravity

18 Treatment of this condition should include:

A. Antibiotic therapy with penicillins or aminoglycosides
B. Fluid restriction
C. Furosemide (Lasix) administration
D. Electrolyte replacement

19 The patient should also be monitored for:

A. Hypernatremia
B. Metabolic alkalosis
C. Hyperkalemia
D. Hypercalcemia

SITUATION

A male patient is admitted to the ED complaining of sudden onset of pain to the testicular area, especially upon elevation of the scrotum. The pain radiates to the flank area and is accompanied by nausea, vomiting, and testicular edema.

Questions 20 to 22 refer to the above situation.

20 This patient's signs and symptoms suggest which of the following conditions?

A. Testicular tumor
B. Priapism
C. Acute epididymitis
D. Testicular torsion

21 This condition is most frequently observed in which of the following age groups?

A. Childhood and adolescence
B. Young adulthood
C. Middle age
D. Old age

22 Treatment of this problem should include:

A. Antibiotic therapy
B. Ice packs and manipulation
C. Immediate orchiectomy
D. Sedation

SITUATION

A 52-year-old diabetic man has a year-old history of chronic renal failure, which is treated with continuous ambulatory peritoneal dialysis. On admission to the ED he is unconscious; his BP is 190/100 mm Hg; serum potassium level, 7.8 mEq/liter; BUN level, 200 mg/dl; and creatinine level, 10 mg/dl. Available medical records from 2 years ago indicate he was receiving NPH insulin, 28 units daily.

Questions 23 to 28 refer to the above situation.

23 End-stage renal disease (ESRD) develops when:

A. The creatinine level reaches 4 mg/dl
B. 90% of the nephrons are destroyed
C. The kidneys can no longer concentrate urine
D. The kidneys can no longer absorb sodium

24 This patient's hyperkalemia should be treated with:

A. Ion-exchange resin
B. Sodium bicarbonate
C. Calcium chloride
D. All of the above

25 When compared to 2 years ago, which statement *most* likely describes the current status of this patient's diabetes, as a result of ESRD?

A. Insulin requirements have decreased
B. Insulin requirements have increased
C. Blood glucose control is poorer
D. Symptoms of diabetic neuropathy have increased

26 The patient has pulmonary edema, and peritoneal dialysis is indicated. What percentage of glucose is appropriate in the dialysate solution?

A. 0.45%
B. 1.5%
C. 2.5%
D. 4.25%

27 As a result of using the dialysate solution indicated, the patient should be monitored for:

A. Overhydration
B. Hyperkalemia
C. Hypercalcemia
D. Hyperglycemia

28 Patients with chronic renal failure should be monitored for the development of:

A. Coagulopathies
B. Heart block
C. Hypotension
D. Metabolic alkalosis

29 Which statement is true regarding trauma to the urethra?

A. Most frequently seen in women
B. Frequently occurs in fracture of pelvis
C. Diagnosed by IVP
D. The patient should not be allowed to void

30 Which statement is true regarding the assessment or treatment of urethral trauma?

A. The patient is encouraged to void to prevent urinary retention
B. A Foley catheter is inserted as soon as possible to maintain a patent urethra
C. A suprapubic catheter may be inserted to divert urine
D. The patient is usually incontinent of urine because the sphincter is damaged

SITUATION

A 58-year-old man arrives in the ED diaphoretic and complaining of severe pain in the right side. He states, "I was walking my dog and all of a sudden I got this horrible pain." Assessment findings reveal the following: BP, 160/70 mm Hg; pulse, 124 beats/minute and regular; temperature, 98.6° F. (37° C.); and respirations, 24 breaths/minute. His abdomen, when palpated, reveals tenderness in the right flank. Urinalysis reveals elevated RBC. The patient has a history of hypertension and no known allergies. A diagnosis of renal calculi is made, and a urologic consultation is called.

Questions 31 to 37 refer to the above situation.

31 A patient with which medical history is more likely to develop renal calculi?

A. UTI
B. Hypothyroidism
C. Hyperparathyroidism
D. Chronic renal failure

32 When a patient complains of flank pain, which question will yield the most valuable information?

A. "When did the pain start?"
B. "Is the pain steady, or does it increase and decrease in severity?"
C. "What helps to relieve your pain?"
D. "Does the pain radiate anywhere?"

33 Which nursing action should be the priority for a patient with renal colic?

A. Strain urine
B. Push fluids
C. Monitor fluid intake and output
D. Relieve pain

34 Which diagnostic test is indicated in diagnosing this patient's condition?

A. IVP
B. Retrograde urogram
C. KUB
D. Abdominal ultrasound

35 If a kidney is partially obstructed by a calculus, the patient's urine output will:

A. Increase
B. Decrease
C. Remain the same
D. Stop completely

36 Which medication should be avoided if renal calculi are suspected?

A. Atropine
B. Furosemide (Lasix)
C. Antacids
D. Antibiotics

37 The patient should also be monitored for:

A. Hypocalcemia
B. Hypophosphatemia
C. Hypertension
D. Bladder injury

38 Which is considered a true urologic emergency?

A. Pyelonephritis
B. Testicular tumor
C. Phimosis
D. Acute epididymitis

39 A hard scrotal mass that cannot be transilluminated would most likely be:

A. Hydrocele
B. Spermatocele
C. Testicular tumor
D. Epididymitis

40 An IVP is contraindicated for a patient with which condition?

A. Renal trauma
B. Urethral trauma
C. Pyelonephritis
D. ARF

41 Decreased renal perfusion can be differentiated from ATN because only in the former will there be a:

A. Serum creatinine level of 4 mg/dl
B. Urine sodium level of 15 mEq/liter
C. Urine output of 350 ml/24 hours
D. Urine specific gravity of 1.010

SITUATION

A 26-year-old woman arrives in the ED complaining of dysuria, fever (101° F. [38.3° C.]), and urinary frequency. These symptoms have been present for 36 hours. Suprapubic tenderness is present, but there is no flank pain. No history of UTI or urologic instrumentation is evident. She had sexual intercourse 12 hours before the onset of symptoms. She has no significant medical history and takes no medications. Her complete blood count (CBC), serum electrolyte, BUN, and glucose levels are normal. A tentative diagnosis of UTI is made, and urine specimens for analysis and culture are sent to the laboratory.

Questions 42 to 47 refer to the above situation.

42 Which set of assessment data indicates a UTI?

A. Dysuria, fever, many bacteria in the urine, urinary frequency
B. Dysuria, low WBC count, acetone in the urine
C. Dysuria, many platelets, and glucose in the urine
D. Dysuria, and acetone and protein in the urine

43 Before the patient is discharged, what information should the nurse teach regarding a UTI?

A. A UTI is not a serious illness; therefore, there is no need to be anxious
B. The patient must be sure to take the full course of antibiotic therapy ordered
C. The patient should not have sexual relations for 6 weeks to avoid the risk of contaminating her partner
D. Now that the patient has a history of UTI, she should have a routine urinalysis every 3 months

44 If a patient has hematuria, which study is necessary?

A. The number of RBCs in the urine
B. The presence or absence of RBC casts in the urine
C. The number of leukocytes in the urine
D. A Gram stain of the urine

45 When taking the health history, about what should the nurse inquire?

A. Prior surgery or instrumentation of the genitourinary tract
B. Presence of hypoparathyroidism
C. Occurrence of venereal disease
D. Birth control methods used

46 Which organism is the most common cause of UTI?

A. *Staphylococcus saprophyticus*
B. *Klebsiella* species
C. *Proteus* species
D. *Escherichia coli*

47 Which statement is *true* regarding the treatment of UTI?

A. To prevent the spread of infection, the patient should not be catheterized to obtain a urine specimen
B. Bladder discomfort should be treated with phenazopyridine (Pyridium)
C. The patient should be encouraged to drink coffee and tea to aid in diuresis
D. If antibiotic therapy has been instituted, no sexual restrictions are necessary

48 Anuria is a symptom of:

A. Urethral injury
B. Bladder injury
C. Postrenal ARF
D. All of the above

49 Trauma to the ureters is best treated by:

A. Surgical repair
B. Insertion of a Foley catheter
C. Insertion of a suprapubic catheter
D. Bed rest and monitoring of urine output

50 Fracture of the penis is usually treated by:

A. Insertion of a suprapubic catheter
B. Surgical repair
C. Splinting
D. Casting

51 A common, nonspecific sign of genitourinary trauma is:

A. Flank pain
B. Hypotension
C. Urinary retention
D. Hematuria

52 Signs and symptoms of epididymitis may be confused with those of:

A. Testicular torsion
B. Priapism
C. UTI
D. Pyelonephritis

SITUATION

A 35-year-old man comes to the ED with severe pain in the right flank. It began 2 hours ago, spontaneously abated, and then recurred. The pain is severe, sharp, and radiates to the groin. Physical examination reveals tenderness in the right costovertebral angle. Pulse is 110 beats/minute; BP, 150/94 mm Hg; temperature, 100° F. (37.8° C.); respirations, 24 breaths/minute. Laboratory results are as follows: WBC, 10,000 mm³; hemoglobin and hematocrit levels, normal; serum electrolyte, BUN, and glucose levels are normal; and urinalysis reveals RBC count greater than 100 high-powered field. A Foley catheter is inserted, and 800 ml of urine is obtained. The patient is sent for an emergency IVP.

Questions 53 to 58 refer to the above situation.

53 The management of patients with obstructive uropathy is primarily directed towards:

A. Preventing ARF
B. Correcting acidosis
C. Decompressing the urinary tract above the level of the obstruction
D. Decompressing the urinary bladder to relieve pressure on the obstructed area

54 Which urinalysis finding is consistent with obstructive uropathy?

A. Normal urinalysis
B. Proteinuria of 3.5 grams in 24 hours
C. Acetone 2+
D. Glycosuria 2%

55 Which action is most appropriate for the nurse to take when urine has not drained from a patient's catheter for 2 hours?

A. Summon the physician because the patient probably is in ARF
B. Check the catheter for patency
C. Have the patient change position
D. Assume that the obstruction has become worse and summon the physician

56 The IVP reveals 100% obstruction of the right ureter with severe hydronephrosis in the right kidney. The physician determines the need for percutaneous nephrostomy. Which is the *most* appropriate explanation for the nurse to tell the patient?

A. The nephrostomy will cure the uropathy
B. Urine will temporarily drain through a tube in the patient's right side
C. The procedure is necessary to prevent renal failure
D. All of the above

57 The initial goal in caring for this patient is:

A. Relief of pain
B. Reduction of blood pressure
C. Prevention of cardiac dysrhythmias
D. Maintenance of normal fluid and electrolyte balance

58 Which test will provide the health care team with the most valuable diagnostic information?

A. Abdominal X-ray
B. Renal ultrasound
C. Renal arteriography
D. IVP

SITUATION

A 56-year-old man is admitted to the ED with the chief complaint of shortness of breath. He has a history of congestive heart failure, myocardial infarction, and hypertension. Assessment findings reveal the following: BP, 220/110 mm Hg; pulse, 100 beats/minute, full and bounding; respirations, 34 breaths/minute, deep, fast, and very labored. Auscultation reveals pericardial friction rub and rales in both lung bases, and the EKG reveals normal sinus rhythm with tall tented T waves. Edema is noted in hands, feet, periorbital areas, and sacrum. Jugular veins are distended. Foley catheterization yields 20 ml of dark amber urine. Arterial blood gas studies show pH, 7.25; PO_2, 60 mm Hg; PCO_2, 36 mm Hg; and HCO_3^-, 14 mEq/liter. Laboratory results reveal a BUN level of 50 mg/dl and a serum creatinine level of 5.5 mg/dl. A diagnosis of ARF is made by the physician.

Questions 59 to 62 refer to the above situation.

59 Prerenal azotemia results from all of the following *except*:

A. Fluid volume that shifts from the intravascular space to the interstitial space
B. Hemorrhage
C. Calcium oxalate calculi that become lodged in a ureter
D. Hypotension

60 When a patient with ARF exhibits a pericardial friction rub, the nurse should immediately:

A. Notify the physician because the patient will need hemodialysis
B. Assess for a pulsus paradoxus
C. Administer oxygen
D. Administer furosemide (Lasix)

61 The physician determines that hemodialysis is necessary for this patient. The nurse should explain to the patient that:

A. Because his kidneys no longer function, he is now in ARF and will need dialysis for the rest of his life
B. His kidneys do not function, but dialysis will repair them
C. When hemodialysis removes fluid and toxins that his kidneys cannot, he will be able to breathe easier
D. Hemodialysis will not remove all toxins

62 Tall tented T waves on the EKG are indicative of:

A. Hypercalcemia
B. Hypochloremia
C. Hypophosphatemia
D. Hyperkalemia

SITUATION

A 24-year-old man who was involved in a head-on automobile accident is brought to the ED. The dashboard and steering wheel were pinned against his abdomen and legs for 1 hour before rescue workers were able to release him. He is conscious and in severe abdominal and pelvic pain. His vital signs are stable: BP, 120/70 mm Hg; pulse, 86 beats/minute; respirations, 22 breaths/minute. His penis and testes are swollen and painful. Blood is oozing from his urethra. The diagnosis of pelvic fracture with genitourinary trauma is made, and a urologist is summoned.

Questions 63 to 67 refer to the above situation.

63 Rupture of the bladder is more likely to occur:

A. When the bladder is full
B. In women
C. In straddle injuries
D. In injuries to the lower chest

64 The patient with bladder rupture should also be assessed for:

A. Ruptured spleen
B. Pancreatitis
C. Rectal injury
D. Spinal cord injury

65 The patient with bladder rupture will probably exhibit which of the following signs and symptoms?

A. Pyuria, fever
B. Hematuria, fever
C. Pyuria, severe pelvic pain
D. Hematuria, pelvic discomfort, difficulty in voiding

66 Besides relief of pain, which nursing action should be included in the care plan for a patient who has sustained trauma to the testes?

A. Apply ice packs, elevate the testes
B. Apply heat packs, elevate the testes
C. Apply heat packs, leave the testes in their natural position to avoid further trauma
D. Apply ice packs, leave the testes in their natural position to avoid further trauma

67 Which symptom is present when the urethra is completely transected?

A. Hematuria
B. Emptying of bladder contents into the peritoneum
C. Urethral bleeding
D. Severe colicky pain

Answer Sheet

	A	B	C	D		A	B	C	D		A	B	C	D
1	○	○	○	○	**31**	○	○	○	○	**61**	○	○	○	○
2	○	○	○	○	**32**	○	○	○	○	**62**	○	○	○	○
3	○	○	○	○	**33**	○	○	○	○	**63**	○	○	○	○
4	○	○	○	○	**34**	○	○	○	○	**64**	○	○	○	○
5	○	○	○	○	**35**	○	○	○	○	**65**	○	○	○	○
6	○	○	○	○	**36**	○	○	○	○	**66**	○	○	○	○
7	○	○	○	○	**37**	○	○	○	○	**67**	○	○	○	○
8	○	○	○	○	**38**	○	○	○	○					
9	○	○	○	○	**39**	○	○	○	○					
10	○	○	○	○	**40**	○	○	○	○					
11	○	○	○	○	**41**	○	○	○	○					
12	○	○	○	○	**42**	○	○	○	○					
13	○	○	○	○	**43**	○	○	○	○					
14	○	○	○	○	**44**	○	○	○	○					
15	○	○	○	○	**45**	○	○	○	○					
16	○	○	○	○	**46**	○	○	○	○					
17	○	○	○	○	**47**	○	○	○	○					
18	○	○	○	○	**48**	○	○	○	○					
19	○	○	○	○	**49**	○	○	○	○					
20	○	○	○	○	**50**	○	○	○	○					
21	○	○	○	○	**51**	○	○	○	○					
22	○	○	○	○	**52**	○	○	○	○					
23	○	○	○	○	**53**	○	○	○	○					
24	○	○	○	○	**54**	○	○	○	○					
25	○	○	○	○	**55**	○	○	○	○					
26	○	○	○	○	**56**	○	○	○	○					
27	○	○	○	○	**57**	○	○	○	○					
28	○	○	○	○	**58**	○	○	○	○					
29	○	○	○	○	**59**	○	○	○	○					
30	○	○	○	○	**60**	○	○	○	○					

Answer Sheet

	A	B	C	D		A	B	C	D		A	B	C	D
1	○	○	○	○	**31**	○	○	○	○	**61**	○	○	○	○
2	○	○	○	○	**32**	○	○	○	○	**62**	○	○	○	○
3	○	○	○	○	**33**	○	○	○	○	**63**	○	○	○	○
4	○	○	○	○	**34**	○	○	○	○	**64**	○	○	○	○
5	○	○	○	○	**35**	○	○	○	○	**65**	○	○	○	○
6	○	○	○	○	**36**	○	○	○	○	**66**	○	○	○	○
7	○	○	○	○	**37**	○	○	○	○	**67**	○	○	○	○
8	○	○	○	○	**38**	○	○	○	○					
9	○	○	○	○	**39**	○	○	○	○					
10	○	○	○	○	**40**	○	○	○	○					
11	○	○	○	○	**41**	○	○	○	○					
12	○	○	○	○	**42**	○	○	○	○					
13	○	○	○	○	**43**	○	○	○	○					
14	○	○	○	○	**44**	○	○	○	○					
15	○	○	○	○	**45**	○	○	○	○					
16	○	○	○	○	**46**	○	○	○	○					
17	○	○	○	○	**47**	○	○	○	○					
18	○	○	○	○	**48**	○	○	○	○					
19	○	○	○	○	**49**	○	○	○	○					
20	○	○	○	○	**50**	○	○	○	○					
21	○	○	○	○	**51**	○	○	○	○					
22	○	○	○	○	**52**	○	○	○	○					
23	○	○	○	○	**53**	○	○	○	○					
24	○	○	○	○	**54**	○	○	○	○					
25	○	○	○	○	**55**	○	○	○	○					
26	○	○	○	○	**56**	○	○	○	○					
27	○	○	○	○	**57**	○	○	○	○					
28	○	○	○	○	**58**	○	○	○	○					
29	○	○	○	○	**59**	○	○	○	○					
30	○	○	○	○	**60**	○	○	○	○					

1 Correct answer—**B**

Hematuria and flank tenderness indicate renal trauma. Minor contusions are associated with microscopic hematuria, whereas gross blood in the urine is consistent with major renal damage. Flank tenderness may reflect hemorrhage or extravasation of urine. Colicky pain is associated with obstruction rather than trauma. Bleeding from the urethra is a manifestation of urethral trauma, and urine output will not initially change as a result of trauma.

2 Correct answer—**A**

Minor renal injuries include contusion of the kidney as well as disruption of the fornix and lacerations that do not extend beyond the renal cortex. Life-threatening renal injuries include deep cortical lacerations, renal pedicle injury, or renal pelvis injury. Disruption of a major renal artery causes massive bleeding and warrants surgical intervention.

3 Correct answer—**C**

When trauma causes rupture of the renal vasculature, bleeding into the retroperitoneal space occurs. The amount of bleeding depends on the degree of injury. This condition may be so severe that the patient succumbs to shock, resulting from hemorrhage.

4 Correct answer—**D**

Renal contusions are minor injuries and require no immediate treatment.

5 Correct answer—**D**

The nurse should first take the patient's blood pressure. A hematoma in the kidney may expand, causing an increase in pain or tenderness. Bleeding should be suspected if hypotension is present. Although it is appropriate to draw blood for a hematocrit level, the *first* action should be an assessment of vital signs. Drawing blood for serum electrolyte levels, BUN level, and glucose level will yield information of no value in this situation. Narcotics may be given for pain, but again, narcotics administration is not the primary intervention for bleeding. In some instances, narcotics will be withheld to avoid masking symptoms, such as increased pain.

6 Correct answer—**C**

Renal trauma should be suspected if a hematoma exists in the flank area. Other signs and symptoms include frank or microscopic hematuria, flank pain that increases with movement and may radiate to the groin, and abdominal rigidity. Hypotension and hypovolemic shock may result if significant blood loss occurs. Swelling or a mass in the flank area may present on palpation. Chvostek's sign, facial twitching elicited by tapping the facial nerve, indicates hypocalcemia. Oliguria is seen in acute prerenal and intrarenal failure. Dysuria, painful urination, is a sign of urinary tract infections (UTI) and renal calculi.

7 Correct answer—**D**

Trauma to the kidneys should be suspected in chest trauma, fracture of the pelvis, and deceleration injuries. Chest trauma can cause kidney injuries, especially if the lower ribs have been fractured. Deceleration injuries, such as those caused by motor vehicle accidents and contact sports, most commonly cause renal trauma. Although most kidney injuries are from blunt trauma, penetrating trauma, such as gunshot or stab wounds, may also result in renal trauma.

8 Correct answer—**B**

Renal trauma is best diagnosed by an abdominal CT scan. An IVP may be diagnostic also, because positive findings include extravasation or delayed excretion of contrast media, distortion of the renal silhouette, or no visualization of the affected kidney. Before this test, the patient should be checked for any allergy to contrast media or iodine. Hydrocortisone sodium (Solu-Cortef) and diphenhydramine (Benadryl) should be available if the allergy history is unknown. A KUB may also help determine renal injury and will demonstrate an enlarged kidney shadow on the affected side. A peritoneal tap is indicated if trauma to bowels is suspected.

9 Correct answer—**A**

The patient has signs and symptoms consistent with postrenal ARF. Postrenal ARF occurs when there is an obstruction to the flow of urine and most commonly results from renal calculi, prostatic hypertrophy, or tumors of the bladder, pelvis, or prostate gland. BUN and creatinine levels rise because metabolic waste products cannot be eliminated from the body.

10 Correct answer—**C**

The hallmark symptom of a complete obstruction causing postrenal ARF is anuria, the absence of urine output. Conversely, prerenal and intrarenal ARF are characterized by oliguria, a urine output of less than 400 ml in 24 hours. Later in the course of intrarenal ARF, polyuria develops. Other signs and symptoms of postrenal ARF are the result of hypervolemia and uremia: edema, shortness of breath, nausea, vomiting, and confusion.

11 Correct answer—**A**

KUB will most likely diagnose the patient's condition, demonstrating enlargement of the structures distended with urine from the obstruction. Ultrasonography may also be used to diagnose postrenal obstruction.

12 Correct answer—**B**

After drainage of 2,500 ml of urine, be sure to replace lost fluid. Once the obstruction is removed, diuresis of dilute urine high in electrolytes results. If fluids are not replaced, dehydration and electrolyte imbalance may occur. The Foley catheter should be clamped after 800 ml of fluid drains. Emergency surgical consultation is not indicated, because the obstruction has been temporarily relieved.

13 Correct answer—**D**

The most appropriate solution for fluid replacement is dextrose 5% in 0.45% saline solution. Sodium and potassium must be replaced as per serum results. A 0.45% saline solution is hypotonic and is used to replace total fluid volume (intravascular and intracellular). Replace two-thirds of lost urine over 24 hours, plus another 30 ml/hour for insensible water loss.

14 Correct answer—**C**

The best treatment for a zipper injury is to cut the zipper around the injury, allowing the zipper track to separate. No further tissue trauma should ensue. Another method is to delicately unzip, using petrolatum as a lubricant. Local anesthesia should be avoided because edema will result. Cutting the skin or performing a circumcision may cause extensive scarring or may damage the urethra if the congenital abnormality of epispadias (urethra located at top of glans) or hypospadias (urethra located at bottom of glans) is present.

15 Correct answer—**D**

This patient has the signs and symptoms of ATN, a form of ARF resulting from drug-induced nephrotoxicity. When intrarenal damage occurs, the kidneys can no longer reabsorb sodium and concentrate urine. The urine sodium level will be above 40 mEq/liter, and urine specific gravity will be a plasmalike 1.010. Casts, cellular debris from the damage, appear in the urine, because the renal tubules have been damaged. BUN and creatinine levels rise as metabolic wastes accumulate, producing the symptoms of nausea, vomiting, and malaise.

16 Correct answer—**A**

The serum creatinine level is the most accurate indicator of this patient's renal function. Creatinine is the end product of muscle metabolism and is produced at a constant rate. Creatinine is also excreted by the kidneys at a constant rate with no reabsorption. The normal serum creatinine level is 1 to 2 mg/dl. BUN, the end product of protein metabolism, is a less accurate indicator than serum creatinine, because BUN is excreted as well as reabsorbed; it is also not produced at a constant rate, and is elevated in high-protein diets, with blood in the gastrointestinal tract, and in dehydration. Normal BUN is 10 to 20 mg/dl. The urine sodium level provides information about the kidney's ability to reabsorb sodium. The urine specific gravity provides information on the kidney's ability to concentrate urine.

17 Correct answer—**A**

An indirect measurement of the patient's GFR is the creatinine clearance. Creatinine is produced and excreted at a constant rate. Creatinine clearance is the specific test for determining GFR and involves obtaining a 24-hour urine collection and a serum creatinine specimen. Normal GFR (and creatinine clearance) is 125 ml/minute.

18 Correct answer—**B**

The patient requires fluid restriction because of impaired kidney function, causing hypervolemia and oliguria. Penicillins and aminoglycosides are not indicated because there are no symptoms of infection. These antibiotics are nephrotoxic. Lasix administration and fluid replacement are indicated in prerenal conditions; in this situation, such therapy could compound nephrotoxicity. The patient is very likely retaining electrolytes and does not require their replacement at this time.

19 Correct answer—**C**

The patient should also be monitored for hyperkalemia because of decreased renal excretion. Hyperkalemia occurs when the serum potassium level rises above 5 mEq/liter. Tall T waves and cardiac dysrhythmias appear on electrocardiogram (EKG). Symptoms include nausea, vomiting, and weakness. Other electrolyte abnormalities seen in ATN are hyponatremia, as a result of the kidney's inability to reabsorb sodium, and hypocalcemia and hyperphosphatemia (after about a week) from decreased vitamin D utilization. Metabolic acidosis occurs because of the inability to excrete hydrogen ions.

20 Correct answer—**D**

This patient's signs and symptoms suggest testicular torsion, twisting of the spermatic cord. If untreated for more than 4 hours, testicular ischemia may result. The pain is severe and increases upon elevation of the testis. Acute epididymitis, infection of the male reproductive system, can be confused with testicular torsion; however, pain from epididymitis is relieved by elevating the scrotum. Testicular tumor may be suspected if a hard, testicular mass is palpated; pain may or may not be present. Priapism is an involuntary, painful erection.

21 Correct answer—**A**

Testicular torsion is most frequently observed in childhood and adolescence, but it is also seen in young adulthood. It is believed to be caused by a congenital abnormality of the spermatic cord.

22 Correct answer—**B**

Treatment of testicular torsion includes ice packs to reduce edema and manual manipulation to reduce the torsion. An emergency urologic consultation is indicated. Surgery may be required if manipulation by the urologist is unsuccessful.

23 Correct answer—**B**

End-stage renal disease develops when 90% of the nephrons are destroyed. Functional nephrons hypertrophy to maintain integrity of the renal system. The serum creatinine level will be approximately 10 mg/dl when ESRD occurs.

24 Correct answer—**D**

Hyperkalemia can be treated with ion-exchange resins, sodium bicarbonate, calcium chloride, and insulin and 50% dextrose. Ion-exchange resins, such as sodium polystyrene sulfonate (Kayexalate), exchange sodium for potassium ions in the intestine. Sodium bicarbonate temporarily shifts potassium back into the cells by creating alkalosis. Calcium chloride or calcium gluconate do not decrease the serum potassium level, but do protect the heart from the adverse effects of hyperkalemia and enhance contraction. Insulin and 50% dextrose also decrease the serum potassium level by temporarily shifting potassium into the cell. Potassium enters the cell along with glucose; insulin helps glucose enter the cell.

25 Correct answer—**A**

This patient's insulin requirements have most likely decreased over the past 2 years. Insulin requirements during the last year of ESRD, before dialysis, decrease by 40% to 50%. Peripheral tissues become resistant to insulin, and its half-life is increased. That usually improves after dialysis is instituted. Blood glucose control and diabetic neuropathy are unaffected by ESRD.

26 Correct answer—**D**

A 4.25% glucose dialysate solution is indicated for the treatment of pulmonary edema. In peritoneal dialysis, glucose creates a hyperosmolar condition in the peritoneal cavity, drawing fluid from the intravascular space. A 4.25% glucose dialysate has an osmolality of 486 mOsm/liter, compared with a normal serum osmolality of 285 to 295 mOsm/liter. Higher glucose concentrations draw off more fluid, whereas lower concentrations do not remove sufficient fluid to be of benefit.

27 Correct answer—**D**

The patient should be monitored for hyperglycemia while being dialyzed with a 4.25% glucose dialysate because of its high glucose concentration. That is especially warranted in diabetic patients. If too much fluid is drawn off, hypovolemia may occur. Dialysis will help to correct hyperkalemia. A slight hypocalcemia may result from peritoneal dialysis because protein and calcium are drawn off.

28 Correct answer—**A**

Patients with chronic renal failure should be monitored for the development of coagulopathies. Platelet function and the clotting mechanism are impaired by uremia. Hypocalcemia increases the fragility of capillary membranes. The patient with chronic renal failure is anemic from decreased erythropoiesis. All these problems place the patient with chronic renal failure at risk for hemorrhage. Bradycardia, hypertension, and metabolic acidosis are also present.

29 Correct answer—**D**

Do not allow the patient to void if urethral trauma is suspected. Urine may extravasate into the peritoneum, causing pain and inflammation. Urethral injuries more commonly occur in men and are associated with straddle injuries. Urethral trauma can be diagnosed by KUB or a retrograde urethrogram.

30 Correct answer—**C**

A suprapubic catheter may be inserted to divert urine in urethral trauma. Do not insert a Foley catheter. An emergency urologic consultation is required. The urologist will either insert a Foley catheter or suprapubic catheter. Before the urologist arrives, the nurse should discourage voiding, because extravasation of urine may occur. The patient usually cannot void, although he may have the desire to, because sphincter damage may have occurred.

31 Correct answer—**C**

A patient with hyperparathyroidism will have an excess of parathyroid hormone, or parathormone, in the serum. That will pull calcium from the bone into the blood as well as increase renal tubular reabsorption of calcium. Excess calcium in the urine contributes to calculus formation. Patients with bone carcinoma are also at risk for renal calculus formation, because bone lesions may release calcium into the blood.

32 Correct answer—**B**

When a patient has flank pain, it must be determined if the pain is colicky or noncolicky. Colic is associated with renal pelvis or ureter problems. Renal colic is acute and has a sudden, severe onset. The patient experiences crescendo-decrescendo variations in the pain. Acute noncolicky pain is steady; onset and severity will vary from patient to patient.

33 Correct answer—**D**

This patient's most immediate need is pain relief. Straining urine, pushing fluids, and monitoring intake and output should all be included in the plan of care.

34 Correct answer—**A**

The IVP is most helpful in identifying the location and size of the calculus. If obstruction is present, the IVP is also helpful in identifying the extent.

35 Correct answer—**C**

When a kidney is partially obstructed, urine output remains virtually the same. Because urine output and urine constituents are unchanged, the diagnosis may be delayed unless other symptoms are present.

36 Correct answer—**A**

Atropine causes urinary retention and should be avoided if renal calculi are suspected. The patient with renal calculi is most likely dehydrated from vomiting, fever, and diaphoresis. I.V. fluids are necessary for rehydration and to aid in the passage of calculi. Atropine would interfere with this process.

37 Correct answer—**B**

The patient should be monitored for hypophosphatemia. Symptoms of renal calculi include nausea, vomiting, abdominal distention, severe flank pain that may radiate, fever, tachycardia, and hypotension. The patient may also have dysuria, urethral injury, hematuria, and urinary urgency. Further monitoring would include the observation of phosphate and calcium imbalances, because these have a reciprocal relationship. This patient has hyperparathyroidism, which results in hypercalcemia and hypophosphatemia. The symptoms of both of these imbalances include malaise, muscle weakness, and lethargy.

38 Correct answer—**B**

Testicular tumor is a true urologic emergency because of the high incidence of metastasis. An immediate orchiectomy is necessary. Pyelonephritis is an infection of the kidney. Phimosis is a contraction of the foreskin, treated by circumcision. Acute epididymitis, an infection of the male reproductive system, is treated antimicrobially.

39 Correct answer—**C**

A hard scrotal mass that does not transilluminate would most likely be a testicular tumor. In transillumination, a light beam is shone through the scrotum, resulting in a red glow emanating through the skin. This glow is not present in masses resulting from blood or tissue. If the mass is filled with fluid, as in hydrocele or spermatocele, it will transilluminate. Epididymitis does not produce a mass, although the scrotum is edematous.

40 Correct answer—**D**

An IVP is contraindicated in ARF because the contrast media has an osmotic and nephrotoxic effect and can further compromise renal function. An IVP is indicated in renal trauma; it does not aid diagnosis of urethral trauma or pyelonephritis.

41 Correct answer—**B**

Decreased renal perfusion can be differentiated from ATN by a urine sodium level of 15 mEq/liter. In decreased renal perfusion, the kidneys reabsorb sodium and water in an effort to increase intravascular volume. The urine sodium level will be below 20 mEq/liter. Urine will be concentrated, resulting in a urine specific gravity above 1.010. In ATN, the damaged kidney loses its ability to reabsorb sodium, reflected by a urine sodium level of 40 mEq/liter. Because the urine is plasmalike, the urine specific gravity will be 1.010. The creatinine level will be elevated above 2 mg/dl. A low urine output is characteristic of both decreased renal perfusion and the early phase of ATN.

42 Correct answer—**A**

Dysuria, fever, many bacteria in the urine, and urinary frequency best describe the group of symptoms associated with UTI. Dysuria results from decreased bladder compliance and inflammation of the genitourinary mucosa. Normally the stretching reflex is stimulated at 350 to 400 ml, thereby producing the urge to urinate. Inflammation decreases bladder elasticity, producing pain with minimal distention. Fever is the body's normal response to infection. The urinalysis will reveal many WBCs and must be followed up by a culture and sensitivity report.

43 Correct answer—**B**

Antibiotic therapy is the only treatment for UTI. The patient must understand the significance of the treatment. She must also be taught not to stop the medication when symptoms are relieved, but to continue the full course. The danger of UTI is that, if left untreated, it can ascend to the kidneys. This is a severe complication and must be avoided. The patient should not be released from the ED without this information. Sexual relations should be avoided during the course of antibiotic therapy to avoid reinfection. Routine urinalysis is not indicated.

44 Correct answer—**B**

When hematuria is present, the existence or absence of RBC casts in the urine must be known. That will identify the source of bleeding in the urinary tract. If RBC casts are present, the source of bleeding is glomerular. If the RBCs in the urine are of normal contour, the bleeding is from the urinary tract. No RBC casts will be seen in UTI. This differentiation should be made, because the treatment plan will differ significantly.

45 Correct answer—**A**

History of surgery or instrumentation is associated with the development of UTI. A history of hypoparathyroidism, venereal disease, or type of birth control bear no significance to existing UTI.

46 Correct answer—**D**

E. coli is the most common causative agent of UTI. Found in the anal area, it is transported to the urethra and ascends the urinary tract. Whereas the other microbes may cause UTI, *E. coli* is, by far, the most common. *S. saprophyticus* is seen in increasing frequency, but its incidence has not surpassed that of *E. coli*.

47 Correct answer—**B**

Bladder discomfort in UTIs should be treated with the antispasmodic agent phenazopyridine (Pyridium). Catheterization may be necessary in a menstruating patient to obtain a true urine specimen. Coffee and tea are bladder irritants and may increase bladder discomfort, as will sexual intercourse in the female patient.

48 Correct answer—**D**

The inability to void is a symptom of urethral injury, bladder injury, and postrenal ARF. Sphincter damage may have occurred from trauma to the urethra. Extravasation of urine occurs in bladder rupture. The outflow of urine is obstructed in postrenal ARF.

49 Correct answer—**A**

Trauma to the ureters is best treated by surgical repair. Ureteral trauma results in disruption of the structural integrity of the ureters, usually as a result of penetrating abdominal trauma. Surgical anastomosis is required.

50 Correct answer—**C**

Fracture of the penis, usually associated with straddle injuries or violent sexual intercourse, is usually treated by splinting and ice packs. Surgical evacuation of a hematoma may be required if extravasation occurs.

51 Correct answer—**D**

Hematuria, whether frank or microscopic, is a common, nonspecific sign of genitourinary trauma. However, it may not be present in all cases. Menstruation, overdose of anticoagulants, and bleeding disorders must also be ruled out in the patient with hematuria.

52 Correct answer—**A**

Epididymitis and testicular torsion may frequently be confused with one another. Similar signs and symptoms include unilateral testicular pain, swelling, and fever. Differentiation occurs upon elevation of the scrotum, which relieves the pain of epididymitis, but increases the pain of testicular torsion.

53 Correct answer—**C**

Decompressing the urinary tract above the level of the obstruction is essential. That will allow urine to flow out of the kidney and relieve hydronephrosis, which occurs as a result of obstruction. When an obstruction is present, urine flow backs up and stagnates in the kidney. The degree of damage will depend on the duration and completeness of the blockage and presence or absence of infection. The treatment then is to drain the genitourinary tract of urine above the level of the obstruction to prevent damage to the kidney. The type of procedure (cystostomy or nephrostomy) will also depend on the location of the obstruction. This intervention will then prevent ARF by relieving hydronephrosis. These interventions are temporary and are used to improve the general health of the patient until more definitive procedures, such as surgery, can be performed.

54 Correct answer—**A**

When one kidney is obstructed, the urinalysis will remain normal because the unobstructed kidney functions normally, releasing urine of normal composition into the bladder. The obstructed kidney will not be able to release urine. Hematuria may be present, because trauma from the obstruction will cause some bleeding. Sediment is not usually found in the urine.

55 Correct answer—**B**

Before any definitive diagnosis can be made as to any worsening of the patient's condition, the Foley catheter must be assessed. Urine flow can stop when the catheter becomes obstructed from blood clots or kinks. Changing the patient's position is not a therapeutic measure.

56 Correct answer—**B**

A percutaneous nephrostomy is the insertion of a catheter tube above the level of the obstruction, which allows urine to flow from the collecting system of the kidney out through the nephrostomy tube into a drainage bag. When the flow of urine is obstructed, it backs up into the kidney. Over a period of time, this hydronephrosis causes damage to the tubules, which allows greater reabsorption of tubular fluid, especially sodium and water. When obstruction is chronic, tubular function is progressively lost, with concentrating ability the first to cease. The more severe and prolonged the obstruction, the worse the damage. Urinary diversion, such as nephrostomy, is then essential to halt the retrograde flow of urine, which, if allowed to continue, will cause complete failure of that kidney.

Rarely is nephrostomy a cure; rather, it is a temporary measure used to alleviate symptoms, such as pain or acidosis, and promote a better state of health before more permanent and definitive procedures, such as surgery, can be performed. The nephrostomy will help to prevent further damage but it does not reverse the damage that has already been done.

57 Correct answer—**A**

When a patient comes to the ED with renal obstruction, the objectives of emergency management are relief of pain and distress, decompression of the urinary tract above the obstruction, and improvement of the patient's condition to permit more definitive treatment.

58 Correct answer—**D**

IVP is the best technique to delineate the urinary tract. IVP will most clearly identify the exact location of obstruction and degree of hydronephrosis. An abdominal X-ray is the easiest and most readily available of these tests. It will show the presence of calcifications or masses, as well as the position of the kidneys. Ultrasonography does not provide information concerning renal function but yields information about the size, shape, and location of the kidneys and the presence or absence of hydronephrosis. That is valuable in guiding the physician during percutaneous nephrostomy. Arteriography shows the condition and distribution of the renal vasculature, which is not the primary problem in obstruction.

59 Correct answer—**C**

Any condition that reduces perfusion of the kidneys, such as fluid shifting from the intravascular space to the interstitial space, hemorrhage, or hypotension, can result in prerenal azotemia. When the blood supply is reduced, the efferent arteriole will constrict in an attempt to maintain filtration. The filtrate will then remain in the glomerulus for a longer period of time. This allows for a backflow of urea into the blood, accounting for a disproportionate rise in BUN levels compared to creatinine levels. As poor oxygenation to the kidneys persists, ischemic changes occur and cellular debris obstructs filtrate flow into the tubules. If perfusion is restored, renal blood flow and oxygenation will improve, thus restoring kidney function. If the cause is not corrected, ischemic changes persist, the patient remains oliguric, and recovery from ARF can take months.

60 Correct answer—**B**

The nurse should immediately assess for a pulsus paradoxus. Pericardial friction rub is a manifestation of pericarditis that results from the accumulation of uremic toxins and fluid in the pericardial sac. Pericarditis is reversible by hemodialysis, although it is the nurse's primary responsibility to assess for a pulsus paradoxus, which would indicate the extent of fluid accumulation in the pericardial sac. When the pericarditis progresses to pericardial effusion, the friction rub is no longer heard.

61 Correct answer—**C**

Telling the patient that hemodialysis will remove fluid and toxins that the kidneys cannot and that he will then breathe easier is the best explanation at this time. Dialysis does not repair kidney function. The nurse must remember that the patient is very ill and short of breath. The simplest explanation that is truthful and offers hope and support is the most appropriate.

62 Correct answer—**D**

Hyperkalemia is a common complication of ARF. The EKG will show tall tented T waves, then a prolonged PR interval. As hyperkalemia progresses, a wide QRS complex will develop and, if untreated, asystole will ensue. Chronic renal failure results in hypocalcemia and hyperphosphatemia. Calcium and phosphorus balance usually do not present problems in the patient with ARF.

63 Correct answer—**A**

Rupture of the bladder occurs equally in both sexes, and is more likely to occur when it is full. It is associated with blunt abdominal trauma and fracture of the pelvis.

64 Correct answer—**C**

In bladder rupture, the patient should also be assessed for rectal injury, which significantly increases morbidity and mortality. Damage to the iliac vessels also may occur.

65 Correct answer—**D**

Hematuria, pelvic discomfort, and difficulty voiding occur when the bladder is ruptured. Hematuria and pelvic discomfort result from trauma to the tissues. The degree of these symptoms will depend on the degree of damage and the presence of other injuries. Difficulty voiding occurs because the muscles responsible for urination are unable to function.

66 Correct answer—**A**

Immobilization and elevation of the testes will help minimize further bleeding. Because of its severity, relief of pain is a priority for this patient. Ice packs reduce swelling and pain. Trauma may result in bleeding into the penis and scrotal sac. This collection of extravasated blood will produce pain. Application of heat packs will contribute to further bleeding.

67 Correct answer—**C**

Urethral bleeding is present when trauma to the urethra occurs. This must be distinguished from hematuria, which occurs from injury to other parts of the genitourinary system. If the posterior urethra is completely transected, urinary extravasation seldom occurs, because the bladder neck remains competent. An incomplete injury can become a complete transection, so catheterization is not recommended. Hematuria is not present because urine cannot travel down the transected urethra.

Selected References

Ansong, K., and Smith, A. "Emergency Management of Obstructive Uropathy," *Urologic Clinics of North America* 10(1):161-73, February 1983.

Bates, B. *A Guide to Physical Examination,* 3rd ed. Philadelphia: J.B. Lippincott Co., 1983.

Brenner, B.M., and Stine, H.J., eds. "Acute Renal Failure," in *Contemporary Issues in Nephrology,* vol. 6. New York: Churchill Livingstone, 1980.

Budassi, S.A., and Barber, J. *Mosby's Manual of Emergency Care Practices and Procedures,* 2nd ed. St. Louis: C.V. Mosby Co., 1984.

Cass, A.S., et al. "Clinical Indications for Radiographic Evaluation of Blunt Renal Trauma," *The Journal of Urology* 136(2):370-71, August 1986.

Eddins, B. "A Review of the Pathophysiologic Basis of End Stage Renal Disease," *The Journal of Nephrology Nursing* 1:95, September/October 1984.

Espinel, C.H., and Gregory, A.W. "Differential Diagnosis of Acute Renal Failure," *Clinical Nephrology* 13(2):73-77, February 1980.

Flood, S. "Pericardial Effusion in the Uremic Patient: Nursing Considerations and Management," *The American Nephrology Nurses Association Journal* 12:294, October 1985.

Fraumon, A. "An Introduction to Physical Assessment for Nephrology Nurses," *The American Nephrology Nurses Association Journal* 12:112, April 1985.

Freeman, S., and Chapman, J. "Urologic Procedures," *Emergency Medical Clinics of North America* 4(3):543-60, August 1986.

Giving Emergency Care Competently, 2nd ed. New Nursing Skillbook Series. Springhouse, Pa.: Springhouse Corp., 1983.

Green, J., et al. "Extreme Unilateral Hydronephrosis with Normal Glomerular Filtration Rate: Physiological Studies in a Case of Obstructive Uropathy," *The Journal of Urology* 136(2):361-65, August 1986.

Guerriero, W.G. "A Little Known Staph in U.T.I.," *Emergency Medicine* 16(17):58-59, October 15, 1984.

Hanno, P.M., and Wein, A.J. "Urologic Trauma," *Emergency Medical Clinics of North America* 2(4):823-41, November 1984.

Johnson, D. "Pathophysiology of Renal Failure," *Critical Care Nurse* 5:18-20, July/August 1985.

Lancaster, L. "Renal Failure: Pathophysiology, Assessment and Intervention," *Critical Care Nurse* 2:40-55, January/February 1982.

Nien, P.T., and Dretler, S.P. "Acute Genitourinary Disorders," in *Emergency Medicine.* Edited by May, L.H. New York: John Wiley & Sons, 1984.

Sheehy, S.B., and Barber, J. *Emergency Nursing—Principles and Practice,* 2nd ed. St. Louis: C.V. Mosby Co., 1985.

Whittaker, A.A. "Acute Renal Dysfunction: Assessment of Patients at Risk," *Focus on Critical Care* 12:12-17, June 1985.

Chapter 8

Musculoskeletal/Skin Emergencies Questions and Answers

You must begin with Question 1 of this chapter and progress in sequence. **Do not skip around.** Subsequent answers build on previous ones.

Alice Belcher, RN, BSN, CCRN
Deborah Reilly, RN, MSN, CEN
John P. Reilly, MD

1 Which assessment data best indicates a fractured hip?

A. The affected leg is shortened and internally rotated
B. The affected leg is shortened and externally rotated
C. The affected leg is shortened but not rotated
D. There is no visible deformity, but the patient has pain on the affected side

SITUATION

An elderly woman comes to the emergency department (ED) walking with a limp. Two days ago, the patient slipped and fell, landing on her right side. She complains of right groin pain. On physical assessment, no gross deformity is noted.

Questions 2 to 5 refer to the above situation.

2 Which diagnosis should the nurse suspect?

A. Impacted femoral neck fracture
B. Displaced femoral neck fracture
C. Intertrochanteric fracture
D. Subtrochanteric fracture

3 In a patient with a fracture of the femoral shaft, all of the following are late complications *except:*

A. Delayed union
B. Nonunion
C. Fat embolism
D. Infection

4 The most serious complication of femoral shaft fracture in children is:

A. Posttraumatic avascular necrosis
B. Volkmann's ischemia of nerves and muscles
C. Nonunion
D. Progressive coxa vara

5 Children between ages 2 and 9 with uncomplicated femoral shaft fractures can be expected to receive which primary treatment?

A. Bryant's skin traction
B. Fixed skeletal traction
C. A double-hip spica cast
D. Intramedullary nailing

SITUATION

A patient arrives in the ED on a stretcher via ambulance after a head-on automobile accident. The mechanism of injury was a force to the flexed knee with the hip in flexion. The patient reports that his knee struck the dashboard. During assessment, the nurse notes the affected leg is shortened, internally rotated, and adducted. The patient complains of severe hip pain on the affected side.

Questions 6 to 8 refer to the above situation.

6 These findings indicate:

A. Posterior hip dislocation
B. Anterior hip dislocation
C. Central acetabular fracture-dislocation
D. Pelvic fracture

7 The prognosis for a patient with a dislocated hip, without fracture of the acetabulum, will be good if the injury is reduced within the first:

A. 6 hours
B. 12 hours
C. 18 hours
D. 24 hours

8 Which nerve commonly sustains injury in a patient with traumatic hip dislocation?

A. Obturator
B. Sciatic
C. Pudendal
D. Femoral

SITUATION

A 24-year-old man, wearing a football uniform, enters the ED. He is holding his right arm by his side and appears to be quite uncomfortable. He was injured during a game and developed sudden, severe right shoulder pain. The patient resists any passive movement and has a loss of shoulder symmetry.

Questions 9 and 10 refer to the above situation.

9 The nurse should suspect:

A. Anterior dislocation of the shoulder
B. Posterior dislocation of the shoulder
C. Fracture of the clavicle
D. Acute tear of the rotator cuff

10 The nurse understands that this injury results from a combination of:

A. Adduction, extension, and internal rotation of the shoulder
B. Adduction, extension, and external rotation of the shoulder
C. Abduction, extension, and external rotation of the shoulder
D. Abduction, extension, and internal rotation of the shoulder

11 Which pelvic fracture is considered to be a stable or minor fracture?

A. Straddle fracture
B. Malgaigne's hemipelvis fracture-dislocation
C. Combined hemipelvis fracture
D. Fracture of ipsilateral rami

12 The nurse should anticipate direct surgical management for all of the following pelvic fractures *except*:

A. Bilateral pelvic fracture
B. Open pelvic fracture
C. Major vessel injury
D. Patient in extremis

13 Which is an *unacceptable* technique for stabilizing a severely displaced pelvic fracture?

A. External fixation
B. Internal fixation
C. Medical antishock trousers (MAST)
D. Skeletal traction

14 In the patient with a pelvic fracture, blood at the urethral meatus indicates:

A. Foley catheterization is necessary
B. Foley catheterization is contraindicated
C. The bladder has been traumatized
D. There is a retroperitoneal hematoma

15 The principle clinical effects of the MAST for the patient with multiple injuries, including a pelvic fracture, include all of the following *except*:

A. Hemostasis or tamponade
B. Autotransfusion
C. Decreased venous return
D. Increased peripheral vascular resistance

16 Monitoring the patient's blood pressure, while gradually deflating the MAST, is essential. Further deflation is contraindicated when the patient's blood pressure reveals a decrease of:

A. 0 to 5 mm Hg in systolic pressure
B. 5 to 10 mm Hg in systolic pressure
C. 0 to 5 mm Hg in diastolic pressure
D. 5 to 10 mm Hg in diastolic pressure

17 After amputation of major parts, the prognosis for reattachment is poor when warm muscle ischemia time has exceeded:

A. 1 hour
B. 2 hours
C. 4 hours
D. 6 hours

18 Reattachment of an amputated body part has the best prognosis in a patient who sustained a:

A. Guillotine injury
B. Localized crush injury
C. Diffuse crush or explosion injury
D. Avulsion injury

19 When caring for the patient with an amputation, the ED nurse should know that the *least* desirable early treatment of the amputation site is:

A. Application of dry sterile dressing
B. Application of povidone-iodine (Betadine) dressing
C. Irrigation with lactated Ringer's solution
D. Irrigation with normal saline solution

20 All of the following are correct principles of care for the amputated part *except*:

A. Debris should be washed away with irrigation using cool sterile water, normal saline solution, or lactated Ringer's solution
B. The part should be handled with sterile technique
C. The part should be wrapped in sterile gauze and placed directly on ice
D. An X-ray of the part should be obtained

21 A patient with a serious or contaminated amputation, who has no known or previous vaccination, should receive tetanus immunization. To complete the full series of tetanus immunization, how soon after the first dose should the second dose of tetanus toxoid be given?

A. 2 to 4 weeks
B. 4 to 6 weeks
C. 6 to 8 weeks
D. 8 to 10 weeks

22 A 25-year-old man is transported to the ED after the motorcycle he was driving struck a lamppost. His vital signs are stable, and he is alert and oriented. His right leg is splinted. Examination of this leg reveals gross deformity, as 2″ (5 cm) of tibia is exposed, along with an open wound with dirt and denim in it. His foot is warm and has a strong dorsalis pedis and posterior tibial pulse. Sensations are intact. X-rays reveal a comminuted fracture of the mid-shaft tibia and fibula. This type of open tibia fracture is classified as:

A. Grade I
B. Grade II
C. Grade III
D. Grade IV

23 A 45-year-old woman slipped off an icy curb and sustained a left thigh injury when run over by a bus. When evaluated on the scene, her condition is stable, and she is transported to the nearest ED. Though no open wounds are present, her thigh is markedly swollen and tense. Her distal pulses are strong. Distal sensory and motor examination is normal. No pain is present with passive stretch of her foot. X-rays reveal no fractures. Which one of the following is consistent with these findings?

A. Arterial injury
B. Degloving injury
C. Occult fracture
D. Compartment syndrome

24 In the triage setting, all of the following are indicated for a severe soft tissue injury *except*:

A. Wound culture
B. Traction
C. Sterile dressing
D. X-rays

25 A 31-year-old man was cutting logs with a chain saw. When the saw struck a knot, it kicked back and struck him on the right side of his face. Damage sustained from this injury would be *least* likely to involve the:

A. Lacrimal duct
B. Facial nerve
C. Trigeminal nerve
D. Acoustic nerve

SITUATION

A male machinist is seen in the ED, having injured his left hand when his ring and ring finger were caught in a baling machine. He sustained multiple lacerations about the wrist and hand as well as significant loss of soft tissue overlying the hypothenar area. The skin that was torn from his left ring finger was brought to the ED in a plastic bag. The patient is right-hand dominant.

Questions 26 and 27 refer to the above situation.

26 Nursing actions during the initial management of this injury would *not* include:

A. Wrapping the injured finger in sterile gauze
B. Mechanical removal of large pieces of debris from the wound
C. Soaking the injured finger in povidone-iodine (Betadine) solution
D. Assessment of distal neurovascular status

27 What is the most likely outcome of this patient's finger injury?

A. Replacement of avulsed skin; normal sensation
B. Replacement of avulsed skin; decreased sensation and cold intolerance
C. Skin graft for coverage; limited motion
D. Amputation

SITUATION

A 32-year-old man is admitted to the ED with a crush injury to both lower legs. He has been pinned under a bucket-loader for 4 hours. On admission, his vital signs are stable; he is alert and oriented and complaining of extreme pain in his legs. Popliteal pulses are strong; pedal and posterior tibial pulses are weak. The ankles and feet appear dusky; the skin is tense, but the skin envelope is not broken. X-rays show no broken bones.

Questions 28 to 34 refer to the above situation.

28 During assessment, the patient becomes semiconscious and continues moaning with pain. His blood pressure has dropped, and his pulse has increased. The most immediate life-threatening problem for this patient is:

A. Dysrhythmias
B. Hypovolemia
C. Respiratory depression from pain medication
D. Fat embolus to the lung

29 You would anticipate his arterial blood gas measurements to reveal which acid-base imbalance?

A. Metabolic acidosis
B. Respiratory acidosis
C. Metabolic alkalosis
D. Respiratory alkalosis

30 Which symptom is considered to be the classic sign of compartment syndrome?

A. Tenseness of the compartment envelope
B. Weakness of the leg muscles
C. Pain that is out of proportion to the injury
D. Pain on passive stretch of the muscles of the compartment

31 Factors contributing to compartment syndrome include all of the following *except:*

A. Direct soft tissue trauma, causing increased interstitial space pressure and edema
B. Tissue pressure within a fascial compartment that falls below the capillary hydrostatic pressure, preventing arterial inflow
C. Venous outflow obstruction
D. Superficial decubitus formation

32 When perfusion is compromised by compartment syndrome, it is restored by:

A. Elevation of the limb
B. Application of cold packs
C. Application of warm packs
D. Fasciotomy

33 An early major complication of crush injuries is:

A. Adult respiratory distress syndrome
B. Acute renal failure
C. Hepatic failure
D. Paralytic ileus

34 The ED nurse should assess those patients admitted with a crush injury for possible:

A. Substance abuse
B. Gunshot wound
C. Stab injury
D. Infection

SITUATION

A 38-year-old man who spent the night in a snowbank after becoming drunk is brought to the ED. He is conscious and protesting. The fingers of both hands, toes of both feet, and both ears are whitish-yellow, cold, and solid to touch. His rectal temperature is 92° F. (33.3° C.).

Questions 35 to 37 refer to the above situation.

35 Frostbite is a traumatic condition caused by ice crystals forming and expanding in the:

A. Extracellular space
B. Intracellular space
C. Intravascular space
D. Subcutaneous tissues

36 The burned appearance of frostbitten tissue is a direct result of:

A. Tissue destruction by the ice crystals
B. Histamine release with decreased capillary permeability
C. Red blood cell (RBC) aggregation and microvascular occlusion
D. Rewarming

37 Which is the best method to rewarm frostbitten digits?

A. Give the patient alcohol to promote vasodilation
B. Rub the affected areas with crushed ice to promote circulation
C. Allow to thaw indoors, spontaneously and gradually
D. Rewarm rapidly in a water bath at 100° to 105° F. (38° to 40.5° C.)

38 A patient is brought to the ED complaining of burning, tingling, and numbness of the fingers of both hands. On examination, the nurse notes that the tissue is soft and the fingers fail to "pink up" after blanching. This assessment indicates which condition?

A. Raynaud's phenomenon
B. Superficial frostbite
C. Deep frostbite
D. Chilblains

39 What should be included in discharge teaching for a patient with frostbite?

A. Smoking is permissible
B. Children and elderly people are less at risk for frostbite
C. Any insulating effect is diminished when clothing is wet
D. The new insulating fabrics, such as those in a down jacket, are better than multiple clothing layers

40 The major areas of heat loss from the body are the:

A. Hands and feet
B. Head and back of neck
C. Head and chest
D. Exposed chest and abdomen

SITUATION

A woman is burned when a pot of boiling water and spaghetti spills down the front of her body.

Questions 41 to 50 refer to the above situation.

41 When the paramedics arrive at the scene, which action is inappropriate?

A. Removing all jewelry
B. Removing the wet clothing and covering with sterile towels
C. Flushing the burned areas with cool water
D. Applying ice to the burned areas

42 After ensuring airway patency, obtaining baseline vital signs, and establishing an I.V. of lactated Ringer's solution, the paramedics bring the patient to the ED. Because airway obstruction may still occur, approximately how long after injury should frequent airway assessments be made?

A. 12 hours
B. 24 hours
C. 36 hours
D. 48 hours

43 Admission assessment of this patient shows first- and second-degree (partial thickness) and third-degree (full thickness) burns over the anterior chest and abdomen, anterior perineal area, and anterior aspect of both legs and feet. The closest estimate of the total body surface area (BSA) involved would be:

A. 18%
B. 28%
C. 40%
D. 50%

44 Which solution is *most* commonly used during the first 24 hours to prevent hypovolemic shock in the severely burned patient?

A. Dextrose 5% in water
B. Colloids
C. Lactated Ringer's
D. Normal saline

45 The patient weighs 120 pounds (54.54 kg). Based on the standard fluid replacement formula, approximately how much fluid should she receive over the first 24 hours?

A. 2,460 ml
B. 6,100 ml
C. 13,400 ml
D. 61,000 ml

46 What is the cardinal guideline of adequate fluid resuscitation?

A. Half the fluid should be given in the first 8 hours
B. Airway should be patent after 24 hours
C. Urine output should be between 30 and 50 ml/hour
D. Pulse should be less than 100 beats/minute

47 After the shock phase of a burn injury, the capillaries seal and electrolytes remobilize with the fluid. The nurse should monitor the laboratory results for:

A. Elevated hematocrit (hemoconcentration)
B. Elevated RBC count and hypokalemia
C. Hypernatremia and hypokalemia
D. Hyponatremia and hyperkalemia

48 Which statement best describes the rationale for keeping this patient from ingesting food or liquids while in the ED?

A. A danger of esophageal edema exists because of the burn injury
B. It will prevent aspiration from nausea and vomiting
C. Burn patients are prone to develop paralytic ileus
D. It will prevent bowel infarction

49 Before admission to the burn unit, the patient complains of a deep aching pain in both lower legs. Doppler studies reveal no posterior tibial or dorsalis pedis pulses; there is no movement of the lower legs. These findings are consistent with:

A. Normal pain and appearance for this type of injury
B. Tight dressing over affected areas
C. Fluid shifting from interstitial to intravascular spaces
D. Development of compartment syndrome

50 Cold, pain, apprehension, and septic episodes potentiate a catabolic state in the burn patient. Appropriate nutritional support requires large amounts of:

A. Sodium
B. Lipids
C. Protein
D. Glucose

Answer Sheet

	A	B	C	D		A	B	C	D
1	○	○	○	○	31	○	○	○	○
2	○	○	○	○	32	○	○	○	○
3	○	○	○	○	33	○	○	○	○
4	○	○	○	○	34	○	○	○	○
5	○	○	○	○	35	○	○	○	○
6	○	○	○	○	36	○	○	○	○
7	○	○	○	○	37	○	○	○	○
8	○	○	○	○	38	○	○	○	○
9	○	○	○	○	39	○	○	○	○
10	○	○	○	○	40	○	○	○	○
11	○	○	○	○	41	○	○	○	○
12	○	○	○	○	42	○	○	○	○
13	○	○	○	○	43	○	○	○	○
14	○	○	○	○	44	○	○	○	○
15	○	○	○	○	45	○	○	○	○
16	○	○	○	○	46	○	○	○	○
17	○	○	○	○	47	○	○	○	○
18	○	○	○	○	48	○	○	○	○
19	○	○	○	○	49	○	○	○	○
20	○	○	○	○	50	○	○	○	○
21	○	○	○	○					
22	○	○	○	○					
23	○	○	○	○					
24	○	○	○	○					
25	○	○	○	○					
26	○	○	○	○					
27	○	○	○	○					
28	○	○	○	○					
29	○	○	○	○					
30	○	○	○	○					

Answer Sheet

	A	B	C	D		A	B	C	D
1	○	○	○	○	31	○	○	○	○
2	○	○	○	○	32	○	○	○	○
3	○	○	○	○	33	○	○	○	○
4	○	○	○	○	34	○	○	○	○
5	○	○	○	○	35	○	○	○	○
6	○	○	○	○	36	○	○	○	○
7	○	○	○	○	37	○	○	○	○
8	○	○	○	○	38	○	○	○	○
9	○	○	○	○	39	○	○	○	○
10	○	○	○	○	40	○	○	○	○
11	○	○	○	○	41	○	○	○	○
12	○	○	○	○	42	○	○	○	○
13	○	○	○	○	43	○	○	○	○
14	○	○	○	○	44	○	○	○	○
15	○	○	○	○	45	○	○	○	○
16	○	○	○	○	46	○	○	○	○
17	○	○	○	○	47	○	○	○	○
18	○	○	○	○	48	○	○	○	○
19	○	○	○	○	49	○	○	○	○
20	○	○	○	○	50	○	○	○	○
21	○	○	○	○					
22	○	○	○	○					
23	○	○	○	○					
24	○	○	○	○					
25	○	○	○	○					
26	○	○	○	○					
27	○	○	○	○					
28	○	○	○	○					
29	○	○	○	○					
30	○	○	○	○					

1 Correct answer—**B**

The patient with a fractured hip will usually have a shortened leg, external rotation, and painful range of motion. Hip fractures are a common injury, especially in women between ages 70 and 80. Swelling is a guide to the amount of blood loss. Assessment of circulation, sensation, and motor function is important. The major categories of hip fractures are femoral neck and intertrochanteric. The femoral neck fracture is intracapsular and does not usually lead to major blood loss, because the hematoma is contained within the joint capsule. Intertrochanteric fractures are more common among elderly people. These fractures will cause more deformity and a blood loss of approximately 500 to 750 ml in the first few hours. A hip fracture should be splinted. Sandbags to the affected leg and 5 pounds (2.25 kg) of Buck's traction should be applied. The weights may be suspended over the end of the stretcher. The patient should not go to the radiology department without immobilization or traction.

2 Correct answer—**A**

This is probably an impacted femoral neck fracture. Patients with a stress fracture, or a true impacted fracture, usually complain of pain in the groin or medial knee. The patient can be ambulating with a painless limp. Examination reveals no shortening or rotation of the limb. Discomfort with active or passive range of motion may be minor; however, the range of motion will decrease because of muscle spasm. Fractures of the femoral neck are rare in men under age 60. If the fracture is displaced, the patient will not be able to get up because of instability of the fracture and pain. Examination reveals shortening and external rotation of the affected limb. Because the bleeding will be into the joint rather than the soft tissue, swelling is not usually noted. Intertrochanteric fractures usually occur as a result of a fall. The leg will be shortened and externally rotated. The thigh will appear swollen from extracapsular bleeding into the soft tissues. Subtrochanteric fractures are seen in a younger age group. The mechanism is direct trauma with significant force. Hypovolemic shock may occur; this is related to significant blood loss from hemorrhage into the thigh.

3 Correct answer—**C**

Early complications of femoral shaft fractures are shock and fat embolism. The femur is the largest bone in the body, and the shaft is extremely strong. It takes a violent direct injury to fracture the femoral shaft. Internal hemorrhage with shock must be treated expeditiously. During the emergency treatment phase, the limb should be immobilized, because it is a completely unstable fracture. Splinting will help to relieve pain and prevent additional injury to the soft tissue. The patient will have a markedly swollen thigh with deformity. Considerable soft tissue damage and blood loss of up to 1,000 ml is common. A good possibility of associated injuries exists in the same extremity. The patient must be splinted with a Thomas' splint before X-ray, and films must include the joints above and below the injury. A troublesome late complication is persistent knee stiffness. The quadriceps muscle or patella may adhere to the distal femur and require surgical release. Nonunion without infection is rare. Delayed union is an indication for bone grafting.

4 Correct answer—**B**

In children, the most serious complication of femoral shaft fractures is Volkmann's ischemia of nerves and muscles. That results from femoral arterial spasm, which may be secondary to a tear of the intima. Signs and symptoms are pain, pallor, puffiness, pulselessness, paresthesia, and paralysis. Analgesics are dangerous because they mask these signs. The nurse should observe the child for severe and constant pain, especially in the calf. This pain may be worsened by excessive traction. If Volkmann's ischemia is suspected, encircling bandages are removed, thereby restoring circulation. Femoral neck fractures in children may be complicated by nonunion and progressive coxa vara, if internal skeletal traction was either inadequately used or not used. At the time of injury, blood supply to the femoral head may be disrupted, resulting in a posttraumatic avascular necrosis, which occurs in about 30% of the children with this injury.

5 Correct answer—**C**

After stabilization of the patient for 24 hours in Buck's traction, femoral shaft fractures in children under age 9 are treated with a double-hip spica cast. Fixed (balanced-suspension) skeletal traction is used for children over age 9, or for patients in which a hip spica cast is not practical. Only after the child is skeletally mature would intramedullary nailing be considered. Children under age 2 may be treated with Bryant's skin traction, an overhead traction applied to both limbs. That is not used in older children because of the serious risk of femoral arterial spasm and consequent Volkmann's ischemia of nerves and muscles.

6 Correct answer—**A**

A posterior hip dislocation may occur when a force is applied against the flexed knee with the hip in flexion, as when the knee strikes the dashboard during an automobile accident. The higher the degree of hip flexion, the greater the chance of a simple dislocation. Assessment will reveal a shortened, internally rotated, and adducted leg. Associated knee and femur injuries are common. Major complications are sciatic nerve injury and avascular necrosis of the femoral head. An anterior hip dislocation occurs with forced abduction and may result from a fall, an automobile accident, or a blow to the back while squatting. Shortening of the extremity is rare. Assessment will reveal abduction, external rotation, and either flexion or extension, depending on the type of anterior dislocation. Early reduction is essential. Central acetabular fracture-dislocations occur from a blow to the lateral side of the trochanter and pelvis with the force through the femoral head. Assessment will reveal slight shortening and muscle spasm; range of motion will be limited. That type of injury is associated with other serious injuries, such as pelvic and abdominal trauma. Pelvic X-rays are recommended. (Pelvic fractures are the second most common cause of traumatic death.) The mechanism of injury for pelvic, sacral, and coccygeal fractures is direct trauma through the femur. A pelvic fracture should be suspected if there is pain, crepitus, or tenderness over the symphysis pubis, anterior spine, iliac crest, sacrum, or coccyx. The patient must be observed for signs of shock and hemorrhage.

7 Correct answer—**A**

To achieve a good prognosis, a dislocated hip without fracture of the acetabulum must be reduced within the first 6 hours. The prognosis is very poor if the hip is out of the acetabulum for more than 24 hours. If sciatic nerve injury occurs, partial resolution usually occurs after reduction; sensation to the bottom of the feet returns, but footdrop does not resolve.

8 Correct answer—**B**

Assessment of sciatic nerve function and distal pulses must be done in the patient with a hip dislocation, because a high incidence of sciatic palsy exists with these injuries. Trauma to the knee forces the femoral head out of the acetabulum posteriorly. Other injuries, such as patellar fracture, femoral fracture, and injuries to organs, may be present and relate to the level of trauma sustained.

9 Correct answer—**A**

Approximately 50% of all major joint dislocations occur at the shoulder; 95% are anterior dislocations. An anterior dislocation occurs with abduction, extension, and external rotation of the shoulder. The patient will resist passive and active abduction of the arm. Loss of symmetry of the shoulder will be noted. The humeral head can be palpated anteriorly. A neurovascular check before reduction is important. Posterior shoulder dislocations occur with violent internal rotation, and are commonly seen after a convulsion. The patient complains of pain in the shoulder and an inability to lift the arm. Examination shows limited abduction and external rotation. The deformity is less noticeable than with an anterior dislocation. Neurovascular assessment must be done before reduction. A common problem is failure to diagnose. Clavicular fractures may occur with a fall onto the shoulder or outstretched hand, or after a direct blow to the clavicle. Diagnosis is based on history, pain location, and deformity noted by inspection and palpation. Acute tears of the rotator cuff usually occur from a fall on the shoulder, from throwing, or from heavy lifting. Abduction of the shoulder may not be possible, and tenderness is present over the insertion of the rotator cuff into the tuberosities. Passive range of motion should be unrestricted. X-ray findings are normal in most cases.

10 Correct answer—**C**

The anterior shoulder dislocation usually occurs from a combination of abduction, extension, and external rotation of the shoulder. The posterior shoulder dislocation will occur as a result of internal rotation; in many cases, no history of direct injury to the shoulder will exist.

11 Correct answer—**D**

Minor fractures of the pelvis are either fractures of individual bones without a break in the continuity of the pelvic ring, such as avulsion fractures, fracture of the pubic bone, ischium, wing of the ilium, sacrum, and coccyx, and fractures with a single break in the pelvic ring, including fracture of two ipsilateral rami and fracture near or subluxation of the sacroiliac joint. These stable fractures are uncommon in the patient with multiple trauma. Most result from low-energy or well-localized injury to the pelvis. Unstable or major pelvic fractures are more common in multiple trauma, and result in a double break of the pelvic ring. Types of unstable or major pelvic fractures include Malgaigne's hemipelvis fracture-dislocation, straddle fractures, and combined hemipelvis fractures. Malgaigne's hemipelvis fracture-dislocation involves double vertical breaks in the pelvic ring. Straddle fractures include a break of the bilateral superior and inferior rami, and are frequently associated with an increased incidence of complications.

12 Correct answer—**A**

Direct surgical management of pelvic fractures would be indicated for open fractures, major vessel injury, or for the patient in extremis. The open fracture requires debridement, removal of contaminated material, and an external fixation device. Internal fixation may be done at a later time when cardiopulmonary stability has been achieved. Major vessel injury is uncommon with blunt pelvic trauma. Many of these patients will present in extremis and thus will require surgical control. Severe shock after blunt trauma will require intubation, chest tubes, two large-bore intraveneous (I.V.) lines, MAST, blood volume replacement, and surgical intervention. Bleeding sites must be identified, blood loss estimated, and replacement therapy instituted. A bilateral pelvic fracture is usually reduced by skeletal traction on the legs.

13 Correct answer—**B**

Severely disruptive or displaced pelvic fractures should be reduced by either MAST, external skeletal fixation (Hoffman device), or skeletal traction. Massive hemorrhage can be fatal because as much as 5,000 ml of blood loss may result from pelvic or acetabular fractures. MAST immobilizes the fracture and prevents further damage to retroperitoneal tissues from sharp bony fragments. External compression of the pelvic ring impacts the bone fragments against each other and slows bleeding from cancellous bone. MAST may partially reduce the fracture and decrease the intrapelvic volume. Thus, tamponade of the retroperitoneal space occurs. (External fixation is considered by many to be the optimal method to treat pelvic ring fractures.) A decrease in posttraumatic bleeding has been shown when an external device is applied in the initial management of the patient. The frame relieves fracture pain and provides adequate immobilization of stable disruptions. Pelvic ring fractures may also be treated with bed rest, pelvic sling, hip spica cast, or skeletal traction. These devices involve prolonged bed rest, so late pulmonary, urologic, and soft tissue complications are possible. Open reduction and internal fixation should be carried out within the first week, after the patient is hemodynamically stable. It is not done during the early resuscitative period because of the procedure's complexity and significant associated blood loss.

14 Correct answer—**B**

Blood at the tip of the urethral meatus in men indicates urethral injury and contraindicates catheterization until the continuity of the urethra has been confirmed. Blood at the urethral meatus or vagina in women indicates an occult open fracture of the pelvis. Pelvic fractures have been associated with injuries to the rectum, bladder, or male urethra. Trauma to the bladder will cause hematuria that seldom is associated with frank bleeding from the urethral meatus.

15 Correct answer—**C**

The clinical effects of MAST are hemostasis (tamponade), autotransfusion, and increased peripheral vascular resistance. These combined effects produce decreased blood loss, increased venous return, and improved mean arterial pressure. Hemostasis occurs because the external pressure reduces the vessel wall pressure and allows a clot to form. The volume of autotransfusion has been estimated at 250 to 1,000 ml.

16 Correct answer—**B**

The MAST must be removed gradually while monitoring the patient's blood pressure. A decrease in systolic blood pressure greater than 5 to 10 mm Hg contraindicates for further deflation. The abdominal portion is deflated first, then the leg compartments.

17 Correct answer—**D**

Poor reattachment is likely when warm muscle ischemia time has exceeded 6 hours. Because muscle tissue is the most sensitive to anoxia, amputated parts that have not been cooled to decrease metabolism sustain damage. Connective tissue, bone, tendons, nerves, and skin can survive for up to 12 hours. Amputated parts with minimal muscle, such as fingers and thumbs, have been reported to remain viable for up to 30 hours at cold temperatures. Thus, immediate cooling of the amputated part and distal extremity is necessary to increase the success of reattachment.

18 Correct answer—**A**

Sharp guillotine injuries, especially of the area beyond the proximal phalanx, have the best prognosis because minimal debridement is necessary. Such amputations occur as a result of accidents with any objects having a sharp cutting edge, such as knives, glass, meat cleavers, or band saws. Crush and avulsion injuries have poorer prognoses, because extensive debridement and vein grafting are usually required.

19 Correct answer—**B**

The ED nurse must render immediate care to the amputation site. That should include removal of visible foreign bodies and irrigation with 2 liters of lactated Ringer's solution, cool water, or normal saline solution. The area should be covered with sterile gauze, and the extremity should be supported and elevated on a board. Betadine, a desiccant (drying solution) that can dry out subcutaneous tissue, is not appropriate.

20 Correct answer—**C**

The ED nurse should handle the amputated part with sterile technique. Irrigation for foreign body removal may be done with lactated Ringer's solution, cool sterile water, or normal saline solution, but prolonged irrigation should be avoided. An X-ray of the injured extremity and the amputated part should be done. The amputated part should be wrapped in sterile gauze, put into a sterile container, and then placed on top of ice in a large container. Another acceptable method would include wrapping the amputated part in a sterile sponge that has been moistened in a physiologic solution, placing it in a plastic bag or cup, and inserting it into an ice bath at 35° to 39° F. (2° to 4° C.). Direct placement on ice will not provide homogeneous cooling as does the ice bath. The specimen container must be labeled with the patient's name.

21 Correct answer—**B**

A full tetanus immunization series includes three doses of adult tetanus toxoid I.M. The second dose is given 4 to 6 weeks after the first, and the final dose is given 6 months to 1 year later. It is important to obtain a tetanus immunization history and to adhere to the established dosage schedule. In the ED, the nurse will administer 0.5 ml adsorbed tetanus toxoid I.M. and 250 units of tetanus immune globulin I.M. That is appropriate for any serious, old, or contaminated wound, as well as for wounds with destruction of tissue, patients with uncertain or no vaccination history, and patients with major wounds who received fewer than three doses of tetanus toxoid.

22 Correct answer—**C**

This type of open tibial fracture is classified as a Grade III fracture. Open fractures are more serious than closed fractures because of the increased amount of soft tissue damage and increased potential for infection. (For these reasons, open fractures must be treated as an emergency.) Grade I fractures have puncture wounds, usually caused by the sharp edge of the fracture and frequently described as "in-out" wounds. Grade II fractures have wounds greater than 1 cm but less than 8 cm, and more tissue damage but relatively little contamination. Grade III fractures have larger open wounds with a greater degree of soft tissue damage that may include neurovascular structures, and considerable contamination. Recently, Grade III injuries have been subclassified into A, B, and C. Grade IIIA has adequate soft tissue coverage despite extensive lacerations. Grade IIIB has severe soft tissue injury as well as significant contamination and periosteal stripping. Grade IIIC is an extension of IIIB, with associated vascular injury.

23 Correct answer—**B**

These findings suggest a degloving injury. Extremity avulsion injuries are most frequently caused by large vehicles, such as trucks and buses. The large broad double tires produce a tremendous shearing force over a large area, resulting in partial or circumferential avulsion of the skin and subcutaneous tissue. Usually the patient will have a degloving injury with an open wound. The avulsed area is usually severely crushed. Damage to the underlying structures (muscles, nerves, blood vessels, and bone) is variable. Fractures occur in about 80% of these injuries. In this case, the patient will have an atypical degloving injury; the skin and subcutaneous tissue will have a small traction-type wound, along with extensive disruption of the skin and subcutaneous tissue from the underlying structures. Most of the leg will appear normal, except for possible tire tread marks and a region of ecchymosis. A significant hematoma will probably occur in this area. The extent of avulsion at the fascial level is deceptive and can extend the entire length and circumference of the leg. The sequelae of such an injury are insidious because the extent is grossly underestimated. Major skin loss or sepsis from extensive tissue necrosis may occur beneath the intact skin.

Compartment syndrome is an emergency condition that usually occurs 12 to 72 hours after initial injury. It is defined as the progressive vascular compromise of a portion of an extremity, which, if left untreated, results in permanent death of muscle groups and nerves. The most commonly involved area is the lower leg beneath the knee.

24 Correct answer—**B**

Information should be collected with regard to the mechanism of injury, contamination at the scene, and tetanus immunization status. A thorough examination of the wound area must be undertaken with an emphasis on the underlying neurovascular structures. The wound should be cultured and bandaged with sterile dressings, and appropriate X-rays obtained. All patients should receive I.V. antibiotics. Surgical consultation should be obtained for surgical debridement and possibly for reconstruction of associated nerves, blood vessels, or bones. (Inappropriate management of severe soft tissue injuries can have lasting consequences.)

25 Correct answer—**D**

In the facial area, typical kickback injuries may injure the eye, nose, or mouth. The lacrimal duct and branches of the facial or trigeminal nerves are at risk. The acoustic nerve exits from the cranial vault through the internal acoustic meatus and is not located in a particularly hazardous position. (Over the last 10 years, chain saw use has increased dramatically, along with a corresponding rise of associated injuries.) Treatment of these devastating injuries should include neurovascular assessment based on anatomic location, debridement, antibiotics, and tetanus prophylaxis.

26 Correct answer—**C**

Appropriate nursing actions during the initial management of this patient would include wrapping the injured finger in sterile gauze after removing pieces of debris and assessing distal neurovascular status. After the patient is stabilized, the wound should not be soaked in Betadine, which is a desiccant that can dry out subcutaneous tissue.

27 Correct answer—**D**

Amputation is the most likely outcome when the skin is completely detached and the finger is completely denuded. Skin replacement or graft usually results in unacceptable hand function.

Industrial accidents frequently involve the hands or fingers being caught in moving machinery. These injuries can range from crushing, to degloving, to amputation. Parts of the hand may be torn or ground off and may not be suitable for salvage. Full-thickness injury to the palm is frequently seen with falls from motorcycles or bicycles. A degloving injury is characterized by avulsion of skin, frequently leaving underlying tendons and bones intact. The primary problem in this injury is the viability of the skin. When skin is still attached distally, vascularity is difficult to assess, and replacement of the skin may be possible.

28 Correct answer—**B**

Extravasation of fluid into the ischemic, crushed limbs produces hypovolemia, the most urgent problem in this patient. As much as 8 liters may extravasate into each limb. Dysrhythmias are possible, and the patient should be monitored. The pain medication has probably not yet been given. Fat embolus, although a possibility, is not consistent with these signs and symptoms.

29 Correct answer—**A**

The nurse would anticipate this trauma patient's arterial blood gas measurements to reveal metabolic acidosis. That acid-base imbalance occurs as decreased tissue perfusion releases metabolic ischemic by-products from crushed tissues and increases lactic acid production.

30 Correct answer—**C**

The complaint of pain that seems out of proportion to the injury is a classic symptom of compartment syndrome. Tenseness, muscle weakness, and pain on passive stretch are other symptoms.

31 Correct answer—**B**

Direct soft tissue injury, causing increased interstitial pressure, may contribute to compartment syndrome. When tissue pressure in a fascial compartment rises above the capillary hydrostatic pressure or mean arterial pressure, arterial inflow and venous outflow are obstructed. The prolonged inflow occlusion produces cellular ischemia, muscle necrosis, and decubitus formation. These allow bacterial invasion, infection, and rapid deterioration.

32 Correct answer—**D**

To minimize deficits to neurologic function, local blood flow must be promptly restored. In this patient, fasciotomy would probably be the treatment of choice. If direct manometry of intramuscular pressures is available, fasciotomy is indicated when pressures exceed 45 cmH_2O. Elevation of the limb would not help quickly enough for this urgent situation. Cold packs are an early measure and of little help at this time. Warm packs intensify the problem.

33 Correct answer—**B**

Acute renal failure is a major complication. The initial hypovolemic insult causes peripheral and renal vasoconstriction. Compensating mechanisms of circulating catecholamines, aldosterone, antidiuretic hormone, and renin further decrease renal blood flow and glomerular filtration rate. Lastly, circulating myoglobins from rhabdomyolysis produce rapid rises of serum potassium, phosphate, and uric acid levels. Paralytic ileus may develop 3 to 5 days after injury as a result of the hypokalemia that follows crush injuries.

34 Correct answer—**A**

Alcohol, heroin, analgesic, tranquilizer, sleeping pill, or antidepressant drug abuse all circumvent the protective effect of pain. During the excessive sedation period, the addicted patient can sleep deeply with one or more limbs compressed by the full body weight for a prolonged period of time.

35 Correct answer—**A**

The ice crystals enlarge in the extracellular space, compressing the cells and resulting in cell membrane rupture.

36 Correct answer—**C**

As ice crystals enlarge, cells rupture, interrupting enzymatic and metabolic activity. That causes histamine release and increased capillary permeability with resultant RBC aggregation and microvascular occlusion, causing the burned appearance.

37 Correct answer—**D**

The treatment of choice is rapid rewarming in a water bath, no warmer than 106° F. (41° C.). No mechanical friction, such as rubbing, should be used, nor should the affected part touch the bottom of the basin. Analgesics may be used to control pain. Use sterile technique, provide tetanus prophylaxis, and use a bed cradle to prevent pressure and friction, because thawed tissue is extremely sensitive to trauma and infection. The other answer choices, used before 1955, have been found ineffective in preserving tissue.

38 Correct answer—**B**

These are typical signs and symptoms of superficial frostbite. Deep frostbite exhibits whitish tissue, which is cold and solid to the touch and turns pink or purplish-blue, with pain. Blisters form after thawing. Raynaud's phenomenon is characterized by intermittent attacks of pallor and cyanosis after exposure to cold or emotional stimuli. Chilblains are the result of intermittent exposure to temperatures ranging from 33° to 60° F. (10° to 15° C.). Tissue appears edematous, with reddish-blue patches that itch and burn.

39 Correct answer—**C**

Cold conduction is enhanced by wet clothing. Therefore, extra garments should be taken along when people expect to be in the cold for an extended period. Multiple layers of clothing still offer more effective insulation than a single garment. Smoking causes peripheral vasoconstriction, resulting in decreased blood flow. Children, with a smaller body mass, and elderly persons with peripheral vascular disease are at increased risk.

40 Correct answer—**B**

The large amount of blood flowing near the surface area of the head and neck makes these the major areas of heat loss.

41 Correct answer—**D**

Applying ice to already compromised tissue could cause frostbite. All jewelry should be removed from burn victims as soon as possible. Covering with sterile towels or sheets helps to conserve heat that the victim paradoxically loses from the damaged microcirculation. It also protects exposed nerves and minimizes the risk of wound infection.

42 Correct answer—**D**

Frequent airway assessments should be done within 48 hours after injury. Mechanical airway obstruction may not occur as a result of the burn; however, edema occurs as fluid shifts from plasma to the interstitial space. That happens because of endothelial cellular swelling and disruption of the capillaries, which allows escape of colloidal and isotonic fluid. Fluids must be replaced during the first 24 to 48 hours to prevent hypovolemic shock. That fluid replacement can add to the edema, thereby decreasing lung compliance. After about 48 hours, patients enter the diuretic phase, and the danger of airway obstruction decreases. If burn injuries occur in an enclosed space, the toxic products of combustion can cause deterioration of pulmonary function.

43 Correct answer—**B**

Using the Rule of Nines, the anterior chest and abdominal area is 18% (so one-half is 9%). The perineal area is 1%. The anterior aspect of one full leg is 9%, so two legs equal 18%. The total indicates damage to 28% of the BSA.

44 Correct answer—**C**

Lactated Ringer's solution, which contains no dextrose and closely approximates the composition of the extracellular fluid, should be infused. In the severely burned patient, dextrose significantly increases the blood glucose level and produces osmotic diuresis. Normal saline solution may be selectively used in patients with electrolyte imbalances. Colloids are not used at this stage except in small children or in patients with burns covering 50% of BSA, because the albumin will leak into the tissue.

45 Correct answer—**B**

The standard formula is 4 ml of lactated Ringer's solution x body weight in kg x % burn area = amount of fluid given in 24 hours: 4 ml x 54.54 kg x 28 = 6,108 or 6,100 ml.

46 Correct answer—**C**

Because evaporative losses from wounds are difficult to estimate, fluid replacement is titrated to achieve a serum sodium level of 135 to 145 mEq/liter, a urine output of 30 to 50 ml/hour, a pulse between 60 and 140 beats/minute, systolic pressure between 100 and 140 mm Hg, and a clear sensorium. The goal is to perfuse vital organs as fully as possible without overloading the circulatory system and causing cardiac and respiratory complications.

47 Correct answer—**C**

Hypernatremia can result because interstitial fluid, with its high sodium content, now shifts back into the cell, and there are evaporative losses at the wound site. Hypokalemia occurs because of the potassium loss from damaged tissue and destroyed RBCs along with the selective renal excretion of potassium that occurs with high aldosterone levels. Hemoconcentration and sludging of RBCs occur with the early fluid shift to interstitial tissues, resulting in decreased intravascular volume and slowed blood flow.

48 Correct answer—**C**

Patients with massive burns frequently develop gastric distention and paralytic ileus from the stress of the injury. A nasogastric tube should be inserted, and gastric output should be measured and recorded. The aspirate should be checked for occult blood, and pH should be measured every 2 hours. Cimetidine (Tagamet) or ranitidine (Zantac) may be ordered. A sliding scale antacid coverage may be ordered for a gastric pH less than 5.0. If the pH is 3.0, then 60 ml of an antacid is given; if pH is 4.0, then 30 ml of an antacid is given.

49 Correct answer—**D**

Pain disproportionate to the injury and the loss of distal pulses are typical signs of compartment syndrome, which is the result of fluid shifting from intravascular to interstitial spaces. Pain would be expected, but not necessarily deep, aching pain. In this situation, an appropriate nursing action upon assessment of altered peripheral perfusion would be to notify the physician and prepare for an escharotomy.

50 Correct answer—**C**

Nutritional support requires large amounts of protein. Extensive burns produce a hypermetabolic response, which increases caloric and protein requirements to 2½ times the patient's preburn state. A positive nitrogen balance is maintained by a caloric intake of 6,000 to 10,000 per day.

Selected References

Bayley, E.W., and Smith, G.A. "The Three Degrees of Burn Care," *Nursing87* 17:33-41, March 1987.

Braunholer, W. "The Critical Process of Rewarming Frozen Tissue," *Consultant* 25:50-54, January 30, 1985.

Cooke, S.S. "Major Thermal Injury—The First 48 Hours," *Critical Care Nurse* 6:55-62, January/February 1986.

Dunham, C.M., and Cowley, R.A., eds. *Shock Trauma/Critical Care Manual: Initial Assessment and Management.* Baltimore: Aspen Systems Corp., 1986.

Freeman, J.A. "Nursing Care of the Patient with a Burn Injury," *Critical Care Nurse* 4:52-68, November/December 1984.

Iversen, L.D., and Clawson, D.K. *Manual of Acute Orthopaedic Therapeutics,* 2nd ed. Boston: Little, Brown & Co., 1982.

Lanros, N.E. *Assessment: Intervention Emergency Nursing,* 2nd ed. Bowie, Md.: Robert J. Brady Co., 1983.

Lucas, C.E. "Answers to Questions of Crush Injury," *Hospital Medicine* 21:101-12, May 1985.

May, H.L., ed. *Emergency Medicine.* New York: John Wiley & Sons, 1984.

McMurtry, R.Y. "Multiple Trauma and Pelvic Bleeding: Diagnosis and Treatment," in *Techniques in Orthopaedics: Topics in Orthopaedic Trauma.* Edited by P.G. Spiegel Baltimore: University Park Press, 1984.

Meyers, M.H. *The Multiple Injured Patient with Complex Fractures.* Philadelphia: Lea & Febiger, 1984.

Orthopaedic Knowledge Update I: Home Study Syllabus. Chicago: American Academy of Orthopaedic Surgeons, 1984.

Salter, R.B. *Textbook of Disorders and Injuries of the Musculoskeletal System.* Baltimore: Williams & Wilkins, 1970.

Sheehy, S.B., and Barber, J.M. *Emergency Nursing: Principles and Practice,* 2nd ed. St. Louis: C.V. Mosby Co., 1985.

Stroud, S.D., et al. "Chainsaw Injuries," *Journal of Emergency Nursing* 11:242-45, September/October 1985.

Tile, M. *Fractures of the Pelvis and Acetabulum.* Baltimore: Williams & Wilkins, 1984.

Chapter 9

Obstetric/Gynecologic Emergencies Questions and Answers

You must begin with Question 1 of this chapter and progress in sequence. **Do not skip around.** Subsequent answers build on previous ones.

Consultant: Vincent J. Ferragano, MD
Joanne Lapidus-Graham, RN, MA
Lisa Mayercik, RN, BSN
Theresa Nauta, RN, MSN

SITUATION

A woman in the 38th week of pregnancy comes to the emergency department (ED) complaining of painless vaginal bleeding that occurred, without warning, when she got out of bed this morning. Her abdomen is soft, and the uterus is nontender. The fetal heart rate is assessed at the umbilicus at 120 beats/minute.

Questions 1 and 2 refer to the above situation.

1 Based upon the patient's history and physical presentation, the nurse should suspect which of the following conditions?

A. Abruptio placentae
B. Antepartal hemorrhage
C. Spontaneous miscarriage
D. Placenta previa

2 The highest priority in caring for this patient is:

A. Preparing for a potential cesarean section
B. Maintaining strict bed rest and observing for further bleeding
C. Assessing for signs of shock caused by blood loss
D. Avoiding pelvic examinations or the insertion of any foreign objects into the vagina

3 The bleeding associated with abruptio placentae is accompanied by:

A. Premature labor
B. Severe abdominal pain
C. Hemorrhagic shock
D. A rapid decrease in blood pressure

4 Any third-trimester vaginal bleeding calls for close fetal monitoring. An ominous fetal heart rate pattern is:

A. Late decelerations below normal baseline
B. Accelerations, to 160 beats/minute, lasting 15 seconds
C. Heart rate stable at 120 beats/minute
D. All of the above

5 If impending shock is suspected in a woman with vaginal bleeding during pregnancy, the initial nursing action is to stay with the patient and alert other staff. The next action is to:

A. Start intravenous (I.V.) infusion of dextrose 5% in water (D_5W)
B. Monitor fetal heart rate
C. Position patient on left side
D. Massage the fundus

SITUATION

A woman comes to the ED in labor. Her membranes ruptured earlier, and uterine contractions are occurring every 2 to 3 minutes, lasting approximately 60 to 90 seconds. With the next contraction, the patient experiences the urge to bear down. Pelvic examination indicates the cervix is fully dilated and 100% effaced, the fetal station is +2, and the presenting part is the head.

Questions 6 to 10 refer to the above situation.

6 Which of the following equipment should be available for the delivery?

A. Sterile gloves and scissors, two sterile Kelly clamps, warm blankets, Ambu bag, and bulb syringe
B. Sterile gloves and basin, sterile Kelly clamp, and DeLee suction apparatus
C. Sterile gloves and scissors, sterile Kelly clamp, and 1% lidocaine
D. Sterile gloves and scissors, and two sterile Kelly clamps

7 Which of the following signs indicates imminent delivery?

A. Bulging of the perineum
B. Crowning of the fetal head on the perineum
C. Receding of the fetal head between contractions
D. Involuntary movement of bowels

8 The nurse instructs the client to pant or breathe through contractions during the delivery. The rationale for this intervention is to:

A. Assist the mother in coping with the pain of the contractions
B. Avoid fetal hypoxia or distress
C. Avoid a too-rapid or uncontrolled delivery of the head during bearing-down efforts
D. Assist the physician in a more efficient and safe delivery

9 The patient gives birth to a girl. Initial assessment of the neonate's condition and necessary steps to support respiration and cardiac function are completed:

A. By the delivering physician
B. Immediately after delivery
C. After the neonate has made the transition to extrauterine life
D. With clamping and cutting of the umbilical cord

10 The first sign indicating placental separation is:

A. Lengthening of the umbilical cord
B. A gush of blood from the vagina
C. Rising of the fundus as it contracts and separates from the placenta
D. "Shakes and chills" experienced by the patient

SITUATION

A woman in the 36th week of pregnancy comes to the ED. She complains of persistent headache and a feeling of indigestion. Her blood pressure (BP) is 150/100 mm Hg. Her ankles show 2+ pitting edema. Urinalysis reveals 3+ proteinuria. She is placed in a quiet, private ED evaluating room, and the physician is notified.

Questions 11 to 13 refer to the above situation.

11 Eclampsia is diagnosed when:

A. BP reaches 160/110 mm Hg
B. Generalized edema is present
C. Seizures occur
D. 4+ proteinuria is present

12 The physician orders magnesium sulfate at 1 gram/hour via continuous infusion. Which of the following symptoms should immediately be reported to the physician?

A. BP less than 120/80 mm Hg
B. Urine output of 50 ml/hour
C. Respirations less than 16 breaths/minute
D. Patient appears to be resting more comfortably

13 The primary rationale for placing this patient in a quiet, private room is to:

A. Prevent onset of early labor
B. Reduce external stimuli
C. Protect her from the emotional upset of seeing other patients
D. Protect her from infection

14 Which is the initial nursing action for a patient with eclampsia?

A. Turn the patient on her side to prevent aspiration
B. Insert an I.V. line for medication administration
C. Monitor vital signs continuously
D. Maintain a patent airway and administer supplemental oxygen

15 In an antepartal patient, the first change in BP that indicates the onset of mild preeclampsia is:

A. Increase in systolic pressure of 30 mm Hg or greater
B. BP of 140/90 mm Hg or greater
C. Any increase in the diastolic pressure above 90 mm Hg
D. A minimum of three consecutive BP measurements above the patient's baseline

SITUATION

A woman is brought to the ED via ambulance after giving birth at home, 1 hour ago, to a normal, healthy girl. Since her arrival, she has bled through four or five perineal pads. Her BP is 100/70 mm Hg; pulse, 82 beats/minute and regular; respirations, 18 breaths/minute. The patient does not complain of syncope or light-headedness, and has not lost consciousness. Blood is sent to the laboratory for complete blood count (CBC) with differential, electrolyte levels, and type and cross match. Two units of packed red blood cells (RBC) will be available.

Questions 16 to 20 refer to the above situation.

16 The nurse palpates the fundus and assesses it to be soft. What is most appropriate to do next?

A. Recheck the vital signs
B. Massage the fundus gently until firm
C. Request an order for oxytocin (Pitocin)
D. Assess the amount of bleeding

17 A slow rate of continuous postpartum vaginal bleeding is usually indicative of:

A. Cervical laceration
B. Clots in the uterus
C. Retained placental fragments
D. Vigorous massage of the uterus

18 The physician orders ergonovine (Ergotrate), 0.2 mg I.M. stat and every 4 hours for two doses. The nurse would withhold this medication and notify the physician if the patient was found to have:

A. Tachycardia of 102 beats/minute
B. Urticaria
C. Ataxia
D. BP greater than 130/90 mm Hg

19 Two hours later, the bleeding has lessened but continues to be heavier than normal. The fundus is soft and located above and to the right of the umbilicus. The most appropriate initial nursing intervention is to:

A. Notify the physician and prepare the patient for a D & C
B. Record the findings on the patient's chart
C. Assist the patient in using a bedpan and encourage voiding
D. Assist the patient in getting out of bed and encourage ambulation

20 The patient's BP is now 90/60 mm Hg; pulse, 92 beats/minute; respirations, 16 breaths/minute. She complains of some light-headedness and appears restless. The fundus is firm with a moderate amount of lochia rubra. The initial nursing action is to stay with the patient, alert other staff, and:

A. Place the patient in Trendelenburg's position
B. Increase I.V. fluids to 150 ml/hour
C. Recheck CBC with differential
D. Massage fundus to remove clots

SITUATION

A 26-year-old female is admitted to the ED. She complains of severe right lower quadrant abdominal pain and moderate, bright-red vaginal bleeding that started this morning as spotting. The patient has not menstruated for 2 months. She has had five or six episodes of nausea without vomiting in the morning. She states she has swelling of her breasts and an occasional feeling of fatigue. She thinks she is pregnant but has not yet had it confirmed. Medical history includes an episode of pelvic inflammatory disease (PID) 3 years ago, which was treated with a course of antibiotic therapy. Patient's vital signs taken every 15 minutes remain stable at BP, 110/70 mm Hg; pulse, 100 beats/minute; respirations, 24 breaths/minute; and temperature, 100.6° F. (38.1° C.). She is pale, but alert and responsive. The physician orders a CBC, type and cross match for 2 units of blood, a radioimmunoassay, and ultrasound. I.V. administration of 1,000 ml lactated Ringer's solution is initiated. Within 2 hours, the laboratory data and ultrasound confirm an ectopic pregnancy.

Questions 21 to 26 refer to the above situation.

21 Over 90% of ectopic pregnancies are located at which site?

A. Fallopian tube
B. Cervix
C. Abdominal cavity
D. Retroperitoneal area

22 Which assessment factors indicate the potential for development of an ectopic pregnancy?

A. Amenorrhea for 8 weeks
B. Nausea without vomiting
C. History of PID
D. Radioimmunoassay of human chorionic gonadotropin (HCG)

23 Clinical symptoms of ectopic pregnancy may also include:

A. Back pain
B. Shoulder and neck pain
C. Leg cramping
D. Intestinal cramping

24 For ultrasound of the uterus to be done correctly, the nurse should:

A. Monitor the patient's vital signs every 15 minutes
B. Increase fluids to fill the patient's bladder
C. Obtain consent for the procedure
D. Encourage the patient to ask questions about the procedure

25 Discharge planning for this patient includes knowledge of:

A. The importance of physician follow-up
B. The signs and symptoms of pregnancy
C. The signs and symptoms of PID
D. All of the above

SITUATION

A 29-year-old female is admitted to the ED to rule out PID. The patient is complaining of bilateral lower abdominal pain and a slight, whitish-yellow, odorless vaginal discharge. BP is 100/70 mm Hg; pulse, 96 beats/minute; respirations, 24 breaths/minute; temperature, 100.6° F. (38.1° C.). She states she has had the discharge for 3 days; the lower abdominal pain began 2 days ago and has become increasingly worse. Fever has persisted since the day before admission. She has an intrauterine device (IUD) in place. The physician orders CBC, blood cultures, cervical culture, urinalysis, and ultrasound.

Questions 26 to 31 refer to the above situation.

26 Causative organisms for PID include which of the following?

A. *Neisseria gonorrhoeae*
B. *Mycobacterium tuberculosis*
C. *Chlamydia trachomatis*
D. All of the above

27 Signs and symptoms of PID may be confused with:

A. Pregnancy
B. Gallbladder disease
C. Acute pancreatitis
D. Appendicitis

28 Which of the following are potential complications of PID?

A. Infertility
B. Ectopic pregnancy
C. Peritonitis
D. All of the above

29 What would increase a patient's risk of developing PID?

A. Overwhelming infection
B. Stress
C. IUD
D. Continued use of antibiotics

30 When antibiotic therapy is to be continued after discharge, the nurse should be primarily concerned with the patient's understanding of:

A. The need for bed rest
B. The need to complete the medication regimen
C. The need for follow-up with the physician
D. The signs and symptoms of recurrence

31 Discharge planning should include:

A. Genetic counseling for future pregnancies
B. Education and treatment of sexual contacts
C. Education for stress reduction
D. Follow-up ultrasound studies every 6 months

SITUATION

A 33-year-old female, para 6006, is admitted to the ED via stretcher. She arrived by ambulance approximately 1 hour after an extramural delivery at home of a 6-pound, 5-ounce (2.9-kg) healthy girl. During transfer from the ambulance stretcher to the ED stretcher, it is noted that the sheets under the patient are saturated with bright-red blood. The patient is pale and restless. Her BP is 90/60 mm Hg; pulse, 108 beats/minute; respirations, 28 breaths/minute; and temperature, 99.6° F. (37.5° C.). The fundus is firm at the level of the umbilicus; lochia rubra completely saturates the perineal pads. Blood loss is estimated at greater than 500 ml. After examination by the physician, the diagnosis is postpartum hemorrhage caused by a vaginal laceration.

Questions 32 to 35 refer to the above situation.

32 Which assessment data indicates that this patient is at risk for postpartum hemorrhage?

A. Vital signs
B. Vaginal laceration
C. High parity
D. Weight of the infant

33 Which signs suggest postpartum hemorrhage related to a vaginal laceration?

A. Extramural delivery with infant weighing 6 pounds, 5 ounces (2.9 kg)
B. Vital signs, restlessness, and pallor
C. Blood loss of greater than 500 ml
D. Firm fundus with bright-red bleeding

34 The nursing action that has the highest priority for this patient is to monitor the:

A. Vital signs for indications of shock
B. Response to oxytocin (Pitocin) therapy
C. Response to fundal massage
D. Response to verbal stimuli

35 Patient education is begun as part of discharge planning. Which observation would provide the basis for an objective evaluation of teaching effectiveness?

A. Patient understands the crisis she has just experienced
B. Patient verbalizes her understanding of the need to notify her physician of any change in physical status
C. Patient understands need for frequent rest periods during the day
D. Patient understands the need for medical follow-up

SITUATION

A 27-year-old woman is admitted to the ED after losing consciousness at home. Now fully alert, she complains of achiness, nausea, vomiting, and fever, which began yesterday morning. The patient has no medical or gynecologic history. She is 3 days into her menstrual period. When questioned, she states she uses super-absorbant tampons and, occasionally, contraceptive sponges. The patient's vital signs are as follows: BP, 86/48 mm Hg; temperature, 103° F. (39.4° C.); pulse, 124 beats/minute; respirations, 28 breaths/minute.

Questions 36 to 41 refer to the above situation.

36 Given the above findings, the nurse would interpret the patient's symptoms as:

A. Salmonella poisoning
B. Appendicitis
C. Toxic shock syndrome
D. Rocky Mountain spotted fever

37 The patient with the above condition exhibits other symptoms, which include:

A. Cutaneous petechiae over trunk
B. Diffuse macular erythroderma
C. Mucous membrane lesions
D. Vesicular rash over palms of hands and soles of feet

38 The causative agent of this patient's condition is:

A. *Staphylococcus aureus*
B. *Chlamydia trachomatis*
C. *Escherichia coli*
D. *Treponema pallidum*

39 Which high-risk factors are associated with toxic shock syndrome?

A. Poor personal hygiene, use of deodorant tampons, use of IUD
B. Prolonged use of super-absorbant tampons, contraceptive sponges, or the diaphragm
C. Prolonged use of tampons and frequent use of commercial douche preparations
D. Prolonged oral antibiotic therapy, alternating use of tampons and vaginal pads during menses

40 The main priority in management of this patient would be:

A. Rapid I.V. fluid infusion; close monitoring of vital signs and urine output
B. Administering antipyretic medications and tepid sponge bath to reduce fever
C. Drawing blood for cultures; monitoring vital signs
D. Preparing for a spinal tap; monitoring temperature

41 The nurse should observe this patient for which condition associated with untreated toxic shock syndrome?

A. Adult respiratory distress syndrome (ARDS)
B. Disseminated intravascular coagulation (DIC)
C. Severe metabolic acidosis
D. All of the above

Answer Sheet

	A	B	C	D		A	B	C	D
1	○	○	○	○	31	○	○	○	○
2	○	○	○	○	32	○	○	○	○
3	○	○	○	○	33	○	○	○	○
4	○	○	○	○	34	○	○	○	○
5	○	○	○	○	35	○	○	○	○
6	○	○	○	○	36	○	○	○	○
7	○	○	○	○	37	○	○	○	○
8	○	○	○	○	38	○	○	○	○
9	○	○	○	○	39	○	○	○	○
10	○	○	○	○	40	○	○	○	○
11	○	○	○	○	41	○	○	○	○
12	○	○	○	○					
13	○	○	○	○					
14	○	○	○	○					
15	○	○	○	○					
16	○	○	○	○					
17	○	○	○	○					
18	○	○	○	○					
19	○	○	○	○					
20	○	○	○	○					
21	○	○	○	○					
22	○	○	○	○					
23	○	○	○	○					
24	○	○	○	○					
25	○	○	○	○					
26	○	○	○	○					
27	○	○	○	○					
28	○	○	○	○					
29	○	○	○	○					
30	○	○	○	○					

Answer Sheet

	A	B	C	D
1	○	○	○	○
2	○	○	○	○
3	○	○	○	○
4	○	○	○	○
5	○	○	○	○
6	○	○	○	○
7	○	○	○	○
8	○	○	○	○
9	○	○	○	○
10	○	○	○	○
11	○	○	○	○
12	○	○	○	○
13	○	○	○	○
14	○	○	○	○
15	○	○	○	○
16	○	○	○	○
17	○	○	○	○
18	○	○	○	○
19	○	○	○	○
20	○	○	○	○
21	○	○	○	○
22	○	○	○	○
23	○	○	○	○
24	○	○	○	○
25	○	○	○	○
26	○	○	○	○
27	○	○	○	○
28	○	○	○	○
29	○	○	○	○
30	○	○	○	○
31	○	○	○	○
32	○	○	○	○
33	○	○	○	○
34	○	○	○	○
35	○	○	○	○
36	○	○	○	○
37	○	○	○	○
38	○	○	○	○
39	○	○	○	○
40	○	○	○	○
41	○	○	○	○

1 Correct answer—**D**

In women carrying pregnancies until midterm or later, the cardinal sign of placenta previa is painless vaginal bleeding. The degree of placental placement over the internal cervical os determines the bleeding's severity and the onset of the initial episode. Bleeding associated with spontaneous miscarriage occurs earlier in a pregnancy, usually before the 20th week.

2 Correct answer—**C**

Essential nursing interventions that assist in assessment of blood loss include monitoring vital signs. A blood specimen should also be obtained for a CBC and type and cross match. Two units of blood should be available in case of bleeding or if hemoglobin and hematocrit values are lowered. I.V. fluids, such as lactated Ringer's or normal saline solution, are started to replace lost fluids and to prepare an access site for blood transfusion if it becomes necessary. When the patient is stabilized, strict bed rest is maintained and vaginal pads are counted to assess further blood loss. A cesarean section may not be necessary if bleeding is not severe and fetal well-being is maintained. If no emergency exists, maturity of the fetus should be assessed by the physician before delivery is performed. Pelvic examinations are contraindicated in the ED because manipulation of the cervix, without knowing the cause of the problem, may cause tearing of the placenta. Any pelvic examination of a patient with suspected placenta previa should be performed in the labor and delivery suite under a "double set-up"; that is, the patient is prepared and draped for a cesarean section and all personnel are ready to operate should hemorrhage occur.

3 Correct answer—**B**

The bleeding in abruptio placentae is accompanied by severe abdominal pain related to changes in the uterus as the placenta separates from the myometrium. This is described as a Couvelaire uterus, and a boardlike abdomen accompanies the pain. An extremely tense and painful abdomen indicates placental bleeding into the myometrium; an enlarging uterus may indicate blood is accumulating behind the placenta.

4 Correct answer—**A**

Any significant changes in the baseline fetal heart rate, which is normally 120 to 160 beats/minute, are important, particularly late decelerations of any degree. Periodic late decelerations are indicative of fetal hypoxia or anoxia. Accelerations to 160 beats/minute that last 15 seconds, or a fetal heart rate stable at 120 beats/minute are normal. Periodic baseline accelerations are indicative of an adequate fetal-placental circulation. Any situation that disturbs maternal hemodynamics or the uteroplacental blood flow will eventually affect fetal well-being. Continuous or frequent monitoring with a Doppler ultrasound stethoscope or bell stethoscope is necessary.

5 Correct answer—**B**

The fetal heart rate is monitored closely for any significant changes in the normal baseline rate and for any late decelerations that may indicate dysfunction in uteroplacental blood flow.

Placing the patient on the left side minimizes compression of the ascending vena cava by the gravid uterus. Such compression can impede blood return to the right atrium, resulting in a drop in cardiac output and hypotension. The patient can also be placed in a supine position with the right hip elevated. Supplemental oxygen should be provided. The I.V. infusion is then started to administer fluids and have an available access for administration of medications. Massage or stimulation of the fundus, the top of the uterus, is always contraindicated to avoid pressure on the presenting part, particularly if it is the placenta.

6 Correct answer—**A**

The nurse's priorities in an imminent or emergency delivery include establishing effective respirations in the neonate, maintaining asepsis, and preventing hypothermia. Two sterile Kelly clamps and a pair of scissors are preferable to maintain asepsis, and to clamp and cut the umbilical cord. Warm, dry blankets are used to dry the neonate's face, nose, and mouth and to wrap the neonate's head and body for warmth. If the fetal head is delivered slowly while the thorax is still being squeezed in the birth canal, seepage of fluid into the neonate's nose and mouth can occur. A bulb syringe is used to first suction the mouth and then the nose. Suctioning the nose first may elicit a reflex inhalation of amniotic fluids into the respiratory tract before the mouth has been cleared. If no respirations are present, an Ambu bag is used for resuscitation.

7 Correct answer—**B**

Crowning refers to the process by which the vaginal opening completely encircles the head. It is a sign of imminent delivery, especially in the multiparous patient. In the nulliparous patient, delivery may occur up to 30 minutes after crowning occurs. If the amniotic sac is still intact at this point, the nurse will tear it to prevent the neonate from aspirating amniotic fluid with its first respiration.

8 Correct answer—**C**

The mother is instructed to continue to pant or breathe through her contractions and to bear down only when asked to do so, to avoid a too-rapid or uncontrolled delivery. The nurse applies gentle pressure on the advancing head to control the delivery and prevent too-rapid delivery. The other hand supports the perineum and prepares to receive the head as it emerges. Depending on the patient, one or more contractions may be necessary to distend maternal tissues and allow passage of the head through the introitus. The nurse should be sure to maintain a supportive and calm attitude at this time. The head is usually delivered between contractions.

9 Correct answer—**B**

The Apgar score measures the neonate's transition into extrauterine life. The overall physiologic status of the neonate must be observed at the exact time of delivery and again after 5 minutes. The Apgar score assesses the heart rate and respirations, muscle tone, reflexes, and color. A heart rate below 100 beats/minute indicates neonatal asphyxia, for which resuscitative measures may be necessary. Respirations are observed with heart rate; crying is a good indicator. Muscle tone refers to the degree of flexion and resistance in the neonate. The neonate should not appear flaccid or floppy, and normal handling of the neonate will permit this determination. Reflex irritability is assessed through the first suctioning efforts that elicit a cough or gag. Also the soles of the feet may be tickled or the startle reflex elicited. Most neonates will not appear pink immediately after delivery. The extremities may be blue, and the torso pink (acrocyanosis). This condition is frequently reversed by providing warmth to the neonate.

10 Correct answer—**B**

A gush of blood from the vagina is the first sign of placental separation. The umbilical cord will then lengthen and, finally, the fundus will rise as the uterus contracts and separates from the placenta. Pushing on the fundus or pulling on the umbilical cord is contraindicated before delivery of the placenta. A patient may feel an uncomfortable contraction as the placenta passes through the cervix. After the placenta is delivered, it must be examined for completeness and the presence of all cotyledons.

11 Correct answer—**C**

Eclampsia refers to the development of seizures secondary to the hyperreflexive state associated with preeclampsia. The cause of preeclampsia is unknown. This patient is experiencing signs of severe preeclampsia; however, the severity of symptoms is not always indicative of the potential for seizures. Although the seizures are not life-threatening to the mother, fetal hypoxia may occur during a seizure. Efforts towards delivery of the fetus are made after a seizure occurs.

12 Correct answer—**C**

Respiratory depression, less than 16 breaths/minute, may indicate that the patient is receiving too much of the medication. Magnesium sulfate, a central nervous system (CNS) depressant, reduces the activity at the neuromuscular junction and helps prevent convulsions. Assessment parameters include respirations, reflexes, and urine output. An absent or sluggish patellar reflex also suggests overdose. The blood magnesium levels should be checked every 4 to 6 hours to maintain therapeutic levels of 4 to 7 mg/dl. Serum magnesium levels above 10 mg/dl produce CNS and respiratory depression, and levels above 20 mg/dl can result in cardiac arrest. Magnesium sulfate can be administered intravenously or intramuscularly. The loading dosage of I.V. magnesium sulfate is 4 to 6 grams administered over 10 minutes, followed by a continuous infusion of 1 to 2 grams/hour. Intramuscular (I.M.) dosage is 4 grams every 4 hours. Calcium gluconate should be available at the bedside to reverse the effects of magnesium sulfate, if necessary.

13 Correct answer—**B**

Reduction of stimuli in the environment plays an important role in limiting stimulation to the CNS and preventing seizures.

14 Correct answer—**D**

The priority action in managing an eclamptic patient is to establish a patent airway and provide supplemental oxygen. The patient should be positioned on her left side to reduce compression of the inferior vena cava by the enlarged uterus, thus increasing the blood supply to the fetus.

15 Correct answer—**A**

Mild preeclampsia is indicated by a rise in systolic pressure of 30 mm Hg or more and a rise in diastolic pressure of 15 mm Hg or more on two occasions, at least 6 hours apart. The patient should be maintained on bed rest in the left lateral position during these 6 hours. A prepregnancy or first-trimester blood pressure reading is necessary as a baseline to assess any blood pressure changes in the second or third trimester. Blood pressure normally decreases in the second trimester as a result of blood volume expansion.

16 Correct answer—**B**

Bleeding soon after delivery is usually caused by uterine atony. Fundal massage, administration of oxytocin, and nipple stimulation from breast-feeding all help to promote uterine tone and hemostasis. When the fundus is massaged, it stimulates the myometrium to contract, promoting hemostasis and expulsion of any existing clots. When massaging the fundus, two hands are always used. One hand anchors the lower uterine segment just above the symphysis pubis, and the other hand gently massages the fundus. Anchoring the lower segment of the uterus provides support, because the uterus may be relaxed after delivery. Massage should be gentle to avoid a partial or complete uterine prolapse. If massage is ineffective, oxytocin may be ordered, because overmassage may cause muscle fatigue and relaxation. Some physicians routinely use I.M. or I.V. oxytocin (Pitocin) after delivery to aid in uterine contraction.

17 Correct answer—**A**

A slow rate of continuous postpartum vaginal bleeding usually indicates a cervical laceration. Lacerations of the vagina, perineum, and labia also can occur. Continued bleeding will be observed despite efficient postpartum uterine contractions. This requires immediate inspection of the birth canal. Continuous bleeding is potentially dangerous, because it can lead to hemorrhagic shock. In this situation, the potential for lacerations is increased because the delivery was spontaneous and unattended at home. Retained placental fragments usually result in vaginal bleeding at a fast rate.

18 Correct answer—**D**

Elevated BP may occur with Ergotrate administration; therefore, Ergotrate should not be administered to a patient with a BP of 130/90 mm Hg or greater. Ergotrate is used after delivery of the placenta to produce firm uterine contractions and to decrease any uterine bleeding. Ergotrate can be administered orally or intramuscularly. Adverse effects include nausea and vomiting, dizziness, headache, cramps, dyspnea, and chest pain.

19 Correct answer—**C**

When the uterus is located to the right of the umbilicus, it is a sign of bladder distention. That increases pressure on the uterus and may increase vaginal bleeding. If the patient cannot urinate on the bedpan, catheterization may be necessary to empty the bladder and control the bleeding. The amount of urine obtained, the status of the uterus, the presence of bleeding, and the comfort level of the patient should then be recorded.

20 Correct answer—**A**

Trendelenburg's position places the legs higher than the head, thereby increasing circulation back to the heart. Increasing I.V. fluids with the physician's order and obtaining a second CBC are appropriate subsequent interventions. Remember that this CBC may not be indicative of immediate blood loss.

21 Correct answer—**A**

Although ectopic pregnancies can also develop at the cervix, ovary, peritoneal surface, and abdominal cavity, at least 90% develop in the fallopian tube. Tubal ectopic pregnancies may be the result of any condition that causes a narrowing or constriction within the fallopian tube. Under such circumstances, the lumen of the fallopian tube is large enough to permit spermatozoa to ascend but not large enough to permit the fertilized ovum to pass downward.

22 Correct answer—**C**

Kinking of the fallopian tube, segmental narrowing of the tube, and partial agglutination of the opposing surfaces of the tube can be caused by endometriosis, developmental defects, or inflammatory processes, such as PID. Patients with a confirmed diagnosis of PID, such as the patient in this situation, are at increased risk for ectopic pregnancy.

23 Correct answer—**B**

Patients with ectopic pregnancy complain of shoulder and neck pain, which radiates as sharp lower abdominal pain. Although not always present, it is frequently precipitated by activities that increase abdominal pressure, such as defecation.

24 Correct answer—**B**

Filling the bladder lifts the uterus and allows for better visualization of the uterus and other structures during ultrasonography.

25 Correct answer—**D**

The patient must be seen by her physician before returning to activities of daily living. Knowledge of the signs and symptoms of pregnancy and PID will alert the patient to any recurrence.

26 Correct answer—**D**

Pathogens carrying sexually transmitted disease, such as *N. gonorrhoeae* and *C. trachomatis*, enter the body from the outside via the cervical canal and travel to the uterus and pelvis via lymphatic channels, uterine veins, or the fallopian tubes. *M. tuberculosis* enter through the lungs and are transported via the bloodstream.

27 Correct answer—**D**

Signs and symptoms of PID can also be seen in patients with ectopic pregnancy or appendicitis. Ultrasound and cultures will assist in making the correct diagnosis.

28 Correct answer—**D**

As with any infection in the lower abdominal region, peritonitis can be a potential complication if appropriate treatment is not prescribed and maintained. Because of the inflammatory process affecting the reproductive organs, patients with PID are at a higher risk for tubal ectopic pregnancies and subsequent fertility problems.

29 Correct answer—**C**

The risk of PID is 4 to 8 times greater in women who use an IUD. During an episode of PID, many physicians recommend removal of the device once antibiotic therapy has been initiated.

30 Correct answer—**B**

The patient must verbalize her understanding of antibiotic therapy and the need to continue the medication until the regimen is completed, and not just when the signs and symptoms have disappeared or she is feeling better.

31 Correct answer—**B**

Depending upon the infecting organism, sexual contacts should be treated and educated to prevent reinfection.

32 Correct answer—**C**

High parity is considered a predictive assessment factor associated with potential postpartum bleeding; other factors include rapid labor, overdistention of the uterus, and an overly large infant. Any relaxation of the uterine muscle fibers gives rise to a continuous oozing of blood, one of the forms of postpartum hemorrhage. Assessing the patient before delivery helps define the patient's risk of postpartum hemorrhage. In the obstetric designation para 6006, the first number is the number of pregnancies, the second is the number of induced or spontaneous abortions, the third is the number of premature deliveries, and the fourth is the number of full-term deliveries.

33 Correct answer—**D**

Lacerations of the birth canal are particularly likely to cause serious bleeding. Bright-red arterial blood and a firm, contracted uterus suggest hemorrhage from the birth canal. The physician must inspect the birth canal to make the diagnosis. The cervix and vagina should also be examined before repairing the episiotomy, if performed.

34 Correct answer—**A**

When hemorrhaging occurs, the body activates certain compensatory mechanisms to delay the onset of shock. The condition and size of the patient determine the amount of blood loss that can be tolerated. However, when hemorrhaging has been profuse, the mechanisms of compensation can fail and shock ensues. As shock deepens, restlessness, diaphoresis, cool and clammy skin, tachypnea, unconsciousness, and death may follow.

35 Correct answer—**B**

The best basis for an objective evaluation is the patient's verbalization of her understanding. Anytime the nurse gives the patient information about care or treats the patient, she is performing a professional nursing responsibility. It is also a potential source of liability, because to state that a patient understands care or treatment is only the nurse's perception. The nurse is the health professional who spends the most time with the patient and can evaluate the patient's understanding of what is being taught. The nurse must document that the patient can verbalize an understanding of what is taught or, if it is a specific skill, demonstrate what has been taught.

36 Correct answer—**C**

Characteristically, toxic shock syndrome has a rapid onset of nausea and vomiting followed by profuse diarrhea. Severe abdominal pain or rebound tenderness may occur. Fever in excess of 102° F. (39.9° C.) is early and nearly always present. Volume loss with postural dizziness and hypotension develops quickly. Disorientation or alteration in consciousness without focal neurologic signs is sometimes prominent. Other symptoms may include photophobia, headache, diffuse muscle aches, joint stiffness, and sore throat. Toxic shock syndrome primarily affects previously healthy young women during their menstrual periods, although it may occur in women not menstruating and in children.

37 Correct answer—**B**

The symptoms of toxic shock syndrome are accompanied by diffuse macular erythroderma that desquamates and progresses to marked peeling of the palms of the hands and soles of the feet about 10 days after onset.

38 Correct answer—**A**

The toxic shock syndrome toxin is secreted by group I, *Staphylococcus aureus*, and causes the toxic shock syndrome.

39 Correct answer—**B**

The vagina is a favorable environment for the growth of *S. aureus* and its toxins, and it is believed that insertion of a tampon, contraceptive sponge, or diaphragm may traumatize the vaginal mucosa, thereby facilitating infection and absorption of the toxin. Extra-absorbant tampons seem to cause increased incidence because of increased absorbancy and fewer tampon changes. The absorbancy may cause occlusion of the flow and less frequent changes, permitting a contaminated environment for a longer time. The latter holds true also for contraceptive sponges and a diaphragm that is left in the vagina for 6 to 24 hours.

40 Correct answer—**A**

The hypotension of toxic shock syndrome is frequently difficult to control, and immediate supportive care for shock should be initiated. Immediate volume repletion is imperative, or refractory hypotension with resulting vascular, cardiac, and renal abnormalities may result. Systolic pressure should be maintained at 90 mm Hg.

41 Correct answer—**D**

ARDS, severe metabolic acidosis, and DIC have developed in patients in response to vascular depletion, which causes decreased peripheral perfusion.

Selected References

Beisher, N., and Mackay, E. *Obstetrics and the Newborn.* Philadelphia: W.B. Saunders Co., 1986.

Bobak, I.M., and Jensen, M. *Essentials of Maternity Nursing.* St. Louis: C.V. Mosby Co., 1984.

Emergencies. Nurse's Reference Library. Springhouse, Pa.: Springhouse Corp., 1985.

Hahn, A. *Pharmacology in Nursing.* St. Louis: C.V. Mosby Co., 1982.

Howe, C.L. "Dealing with Third Trimester Bleeding," *RN* 48:29-31, February 1985.

Lee, G. "Eclampsia: Toxemia of Pregnancy," *Journal of Emergency Nursing* 11:225-26, 1985.

Neeson, J.L., and May, K.A. *Comprehensive Maternity Nursing.* Philadelphia: J.B. Lippincott Co., 1986.

Quilligan, E., et al. *Current Therapy in Obstetrics and Gynecology 2.* Philadelphia: W.B. Saunders Co., 1983.

Reeder, S., et al. *Maternity Nursing.* Philadelphia: J.B. Lippincott Co., 1983.

Roberts, J. "Emergency Birth," *Journal of Emergency Nursing* 11:125-31, May/June 1985.

Chapter 10

Eye/Ear/Nose/Throat Emergencies Questions and Answers

You must begin with Question 1 of this chapter and progress in sequence. **Do not skip around.** Subsequent answers build on previous ones.

Laura Gasparis, RN, MA, CCRN, CEN
Patricia Murphy, MD
Neil Nepola, MD

SITUATION

A 22-year-old woman who has a recent history of an upper respiratory tract infection is seen in the emergency department (ED). She complains of hoarseness that has lasted 3 days, along with pain on speaking, nasal congestion, and dysphagia. Assessment findings reveal a purulent nasal discharge, erythematous posterior oropharynx, and a temperature of 101° F. (38° C.).

Questions 1 to 3 refer to the above situation.

1 These assessment findings indicate what condition?

A. Acute laryngitis
B. Chronic laryngitis
C. Laryngeal carcinoma
D. Vocal cord polyps

2 The nurse would anticipate treatment for this patient to include:

A. Voice rest, with whispering permitted
B. Complete voice rest
C. Swish and gargle with alcohol-based astringent
D. Gargle with aspirin and salt water

3 Which nursing action is most effective in providing patient comfort?

A. Administer metaproterenol (Alupent)
B. Apply an icebag to the patient's throat
C. Instruct the patient to gargle with an antiseptic solution
D. Instruct the patient to swish and swallow a topical anesthetic solution of lidocaine (Xylocaine) before eating

SITUATION

An 18-year-old man, who was sleeping and awoke suddenly with complaints of "something moving" in his ear, comes to the ED. On physical examination a large, live cockroach is noted in his external auditory canal.

Questions 4 and 5 refer to the above situation.

4 The nurse would anticipate the initial treatment to be:

A. Removing the insect with forceps
B. Spraying lidocaine (Xylocaine) 10% in the auditory canal
C. Irrigating the ear with warm water
D. Instilling warm mineral oil into the ear

5 After efforts to remove the insect are successful, subsequent management should include:

A. Administering ampicillin (Amcill) 500 mg P.O. to prevent infection
B. Irrigating the ear canal with peroxide and applying a dry sterile dressing
C. Packing the ear canal with iodoform gauze
D. Applying antibacterial drops into the ear and packing the ear canal with ¼-inch gauze strips

SITUATION

A 65-year-old man with a known history of chronic obstructive pulmonary disease (COPD) and laryngeal carcinoma is seen in the ED. He is currently undergoing radiation therapy and presents symptoms of acute respiratory distress. Assessment reveals inspiratory stridor, dyspnea, increasing apprehension, and facial flushing.

Questions 6 and 7 refer to the above situation.

6 Immediate action should include:

A. Arterial blood gas evaluation (ABGs) and 100% oxygen via mask
B. Tracheotomy
C. Intubation
D. Chest X-ray

7 If an attempt to intubate this patient is unsuccessful, the nurse would anticipate priority action to include:

A. Obtaining a smaller endotracheal (ET) tube
B. Assembling equipment necessary for a tracheotomy
C. Obtaining a cricothyroidotomy tray
D. Ordering an X-ray of the lateral neck

SITUATION

A 40-year-old man is brought to the ED after being mugged. Blood is coming from his left ear, and the physician diagnoses a ruptured tympanic membrane.

Questions 8 and 9 refer to the above situation.

8 The initial treatment for this patient should include:

A. Remove clots and pack canal
B. Administer antibacterial otic drops
C. Administer ampicillin (Amcill) 500 mg P.O. t.i.d.
D. Administer tetanus toxoid

9 During discharge teaching, the nurse would stress the importance of:

A. Gentle nose-blowing
B. Avoiding heavy lifting
C. Rinsing the ear canal with warm water daily
D. Retaining packing in the ear canal for 1 week

SITUATION

A 6-year-old child is seen in the ED with complaints of ear pain and a 2-day history of itchiness, diminished hearing, and fever. The child had been swimming in a public pool last week.

Questions 10 to 15 refer to the above situation.

10 The above manifestations indicate which possible condition?

A. Acute otitis externa
B. Acute otitis media
C. Ruptured tympanic membrane
D. Ear canal cellulitis

11 Treatment for this patient includes all of the following *except*:

A. Acetaminophen (Tylenol) administration
B. Oral antibiotic administration
C. Otic antibiotic administration
D. Ice packs to the ear

12 The patient with acute otitis externa commonly demonstrates:

A. Otalgia
B. Upper respiratory tract infection
C. Temperature above 102° F. (38.9° C.)
D. Periauricular lymphadenopathy

13 The otic emergency more common in children than adults is:

A. Acute otitis externa
B. Acute otitis media
C. Meniere's disease
D. Bullous myringitis

14 If otitis media is not treated aggressively, serious complications include all of the following *except*:

A. Meningitis
B. Ototoxicity
C. Mastoiditis
D. Permanent hearing loss

15 Which diagnostic procedure is *not* warranted for the patient with acute otitis media?

A. Myringotomy
B. Tympanocentesis
C. Caloric test
D. Blood cultures

SITUATION

A 54-year-old man with a history of alcohol abuse is seen in the triage area. He complains of difficulty breathing through his nose since last night, after an alleged fall. His symptoms include a lacerated bridge of the nose, periorbital edema, and dried blood in his nares.

Questions 16 to 19 refer to the above situation.

16 The most serious cause of this patient's breathing difficulty can be attributed to:

A. Blood clots in nares
B. Edema of the nose
C. Deviated septum
D. Septal hematoma

17 In caring for this patient, which intervention is appropriate?

A. Ask patient to blow his nose in order to remove clot
B. Insert intranasal packing
C. Examine nasal bone for mobility
D. Administer tetanus toxoid

18 Treatment for a linear fracture with nasal bleeding may include:

A. Nasal packing and establishment of an intravenous (I.V.) line
B. Administration of a decongestant and vasoconstrictor
C. Application of a cold pack to bridge of nose
D. All of the above

19 Which nursing action is *not* appropriate for the patient with epistaxis?

A. Alleviating patient apprehension
B. Pinching nose for 4 to 5 minutes
C. Placing patient in semirecumbent position with head tilted forward
D. Beginning administration of I.V. fluids

20 A 5-year-old child who recently underwent adenotonsillectomy is brought to the ED because of profuse bleeding from the nose and mouth. The child is weak, pale, tachycardic, and hypotensive. A priority nursing action is to:

A. Clear clots from nose and mouth
B. Place packing into the nose
C. Draw blood sample for hemoglobin and hematocrit testing, type and cross-match
D. Administer I.V. lactated Ringer's solution

SITUATION

A 19-year-old man is brought to the hospital by emergency medical service (EMS) after an automobile accident. He has multiple facial lacerations, nasal deformity, and cheek flattening, as well as diplopia and difficulty in opening his mouth.

Questions 21 to 25 refer to the above situation.

21 Patient assessment findings most likely indicate which of the following?

A. Mandibular fracture
B. Maxillary fracture
C. Zygomatic fracture
D. Temporomandibular joint (TMJ) dislocation

22 An *inappropriate* nursing action during the immediate care of this patient is to:

A. Prepare for definitive treatment of fracture by physician
B. Assess the patient's level of consciousness
C. Evaluate patient for cervical or spinal trauma
D. Observe for potential airway obstruction

23 Which nursing action is considered *unsafe* when assisting the patient with optimal airway clearance?

A. Positioning patient on his side
B. Inserting a nasopharyngeal airway
C. Positioning patient in a semi-Fowler's position
D. Having tracheotomy equipment available

24 During the assessment of this patient, which diagnostic procedure should be included?

A. Water's view
B. Submental-vertex view
C. Cervical spine films
D. All of the above

25 The patient's condition is stable. Cervical or spinal injury has been ruled out, and no neurologic deficit exists. Continued pain is best relieved by:

A. Administering narcotics or analgesics as physician orders
B. Positioning patient with head elevated
C. Applying cold compresses to the fracture site
D. All of the above

SITUATION

A 35-year-old man is seen in the ED with complaints of ear pain and inability to close his mouth completely. He has pain on attempting to clench his teeth, and a click is noted on full opening of his mouth. The patient states that he recently stopped smoking and admits to frequent gum chewing as a substitute.

Questions 26 to 28 refer to the above situation.

26 Patient assessment data most likely indicate:

A. Acute odontalgia
B. TMJ dislocation
C. Bilateral malocclusion
D. Dental abscess of wisdom tooth

27 A manual reduction of the patient's jaw is indicated. Which of the following interventions would facilitate this procedure?

A. Administration of I.V. diazepam (Valium)
B. Application of topical anesthetic spray to mucous membranes of mouth cavity
C. Giving atropine sulfate I.M. to reduce oral secretions
D. Holding hot compresses to each side of face

28 Discharge planning for this patient should include the importance of:

A. Frequent mouth exercises to strengthen muscles
B. Wearing a jaw brace while sleeping
C. A soft diet for 3 to 4 days
D. Daily compliance with muscle relaxant therapy

SITUATION

A 40-year-old woman comes to the ED with unilateral flaccid facial paralysis of acute onset. Physical examination reveals lag on the affected side when closing eyes, decreased lacrimation, and drooping of mouth. A diagnosis of Bell's palsy is made.

Questions 29 and 30 refer to the above situation.

29 To avoid development of corneal abrasions, the nurse should:

A. Administer 1% methylcellulose to affected eye
B. Place a Steri-Strip to maintain closure of the affected eye
C. Rinse eye with an antibiotic irrigating solution
D. Apply eye patches bilaterally until treatment is instituted

30 Discharge teaching for this patient should include instructions regarding:

A. Facial massage, exercises, and application of moist heat to face
B. Techniques for corneal protection
C. Therapy with analgesics and steroids
D. All of the above

SITUATION

A 50-year-old woman comes to the hospital because of intermittent episodes of excruciating right-sided facial pain.

Questions 31 and 32 refer to the above situation.

31 In caring for this patient with trigeminal neuralgia, the nurse would anticipate pharmacologic management to include which medication?

A. Oxycodone with acetaminophen (Percocet)
B. Carbamazepine (Tegretol)
C. Diazepam (Valium)
D. Steroids

32 Which statement is *true* regarding trigeminal neuralgia?

A. The majority of patients respond to drug therapy in 4 hours
B. Eventually all patients fail to respond to drug therapy and will require surgical intervention
C. Diagnosis is made on the basis of history and physical examination alone
D. Painful paroxysm is precipitated by touching of trigger zone on contralateral (opposite side) anterior face

SITUATION

A 25-year-old male carpenter is seen by the triage nurse. He complains of severe right eye pain with a gritty sensation and sensitivity to light. This began suddenly while he was hammering a nail. Patient appears very angry and states he is going to sue his boss.

Questions 33 and 34 refer to the above situation.

33 When obtaining a history from the patient, which question has the *least* priority?

A. Describe your visual acuity before this accident; did you have any previous eye disease?
B. Were goggles or glasses worn and did damage occur to them?
C. What was the mechanism of injury; suspected object, its pathway, direction, and distance to your head?
D. Are you seeing halos around the lights at present?

34 Which nursing action would be *least* effective for pain relief?

A. Instilling a fluorescein stain
B. Application of topical analgesics
C. Covering eye with an occlusive patch
D. Irrigating eye with normal saline solution

SITUATION

A 60-year-old woman comes to the triage nurse after having sustained blunt trauma to her right eye during a fall. Her only complaint is that of blurred vision in the right eye. A diagnosis of hyphema is made.

Questions 35 to 37 refer to the above situation.

35 All of the following information is important to obtain during initial data collection from the patient. Which holds the *highest* priority?

A. Mechanism of injury
B. Previous history of ocular disorders
C. Symptoms before arrival at hospital
D. Prior use of any medications, especially aspirin

36 Which nursing action should be included in the plan of care for this patient?

A. Maintain the patient in a supine position
B. Patch eyes during the acute phase
C. Irrigate eye frequently with normal saline solution during the acute phase
D. Massage the eye gently with fingers

37 Which instruction should *not* be included in patient teaching before discharge?

A. Avoid coughing and Valsalva's maneuver
B. Remain on bed rest for 2 weeks
C. Elevate head of bed to 30 degrees
D. Reduce stress and physical strain

SITUATION

A 29-year-old man is brought to the hospital via ambulance after sustaining a chemical burn of his eyes. The patient was involved in a fight during which lye was thrown in his face.

Questions 38 to 40 refer to the above situation.

38 Which nursing action has the *highest* priority for this patient?

A. Check pH of eyes with litmus paper
B. Instill antibiotic optic drops
C. Flush eyes with a sodium bicarbonate solution
D. Continuously irrigate the eye with copious amount of normal saline solution

39 All of the following statements regarding chemical burns of the eye are true *except*:

A. Alkaline burns are the most destructive
B. Acid burns are extremely irritating
C. An acid substance continues to dissolve soft tissue in the eye until it is removed
D. The principles of management are similar for alkaline and acid burns

40 What is the best indication that treatment has been effective for this patient?

A. Slight evidence of corneal whitening
B. A pH value of 7.0 on litmus paper reading
C. Extraocular movements
D. Visual acuity limited to light perception

Answer Sheet

	A	B	C	D		A	B	C	D
1	○	○	○	○	31	○	○	○	○
2	○	○	○	○	32	○	○	○	○
3	○	○	○	○	33	○	○	○	○
4	○	○	○	○	34	○	○	○	○
5	○	○	○	○	35	○	○	○	○
6	○	○	○	○	36	○	○	○	○
7	○	○	○	○	37	○	○	○	○
8	○	○	○	○	38	○	○	○	○
9	○	○	○	○	39	○	○	○	○
10	○	○	○	○	40	○	○	○	○
11	○	○	○	○					
12	○	○	○	○					
13	○	○	○	○					
14	○	○	○	○					
15	○	○	○	○					
16	○	○	○	○					
17	○	○	○	○					
18	○	○	○	○					
19	○	○	○	○					
20	○	○	○	○					
21	○	○	○	○					
22	○	○	○	○					
23	○	○	○	○					
24	○	○	○	○					
25	○	○	○	○					
26	○	○	○	○					
27	○	○	○	○					
28	○	○	○	○					
29	○	○	○	○					
30	○	○	○	○					

Answer Sheet

	A	B	C	D
1	○	○	○	○
2	○	○	○	○
3	○	○	○	○
4	○	○	○	○
5	○	○	○	○
6	○	○	○	○
7	○	○	○	○
8	○	○	○	○
9	○	○	○	○
10	○	○	○	○
11	○	○	○	○
12	○	○	○	○
13	○	○	○	○
14	○	○	○	○
15	○	○	○	○
16	○	○	○	○
17	○	○	○	○
18	○	○	○	○
19	○	○	○	○
20	○	○	○	○
21	○	○	○	○
22	○	○	○	○
23	○	○	○	○
24	○	○	○	○
25	○	○	○	○
26	○	○	○	○
27	○	○	○	○
28	○	○	○	○
29	○	○	○	○
30	○	○	○	○

	A	B	C	D
31	○	○	○	○
32	○	○	○	○
33	○	○	○	○
34	○	○	○	○
35	○	○	○	○
36	○	○	○	○
37	○	○	○	○
38	○	○	○	○
39	○	○	○	○
40	○	○	○	○

1 Correct answer—**A**

A patient with a recent history of an upper respiratory tract infection, hoarseness, fever, and erythematous oropharynx has acute laryngitis. Patients with vocal cord polyps have hoarseness but no upper respiratory tract infection, whereas those with laryngeal cancer may have hoarseness and difficulty breathing only if the lesion is large. Laryngeal cancer usually occurs in older men with a long history of smoking and alcohol abuse.

2 Correct answer—**B**

Treatment for acute laryngitis is complete voice rest. No whispering is permitted. Smoking, alcohol, and aspirin may cause further irritation, inflammation, edema, and pain. Saline solution gargles and topical anesthetics may be helpful.

3 Correct answer—**B**

The most effective nursing action for the patient with acute laryngitis is the application of an icebag to the throat. Alupent treatments and antiseptic gargles are inappropriate. To swish and swallow with an anesthetic solution before eating is unsafe, because aspiration may occur.

4 Correct answer—**B**

Recent studies reveal that insects may be removed from the ear by spraying a topical neurostimulant, such as lidocaine, into the external auditory canal. If this is unavailable, the insect should be immobilized and drowned in mineral oil, then removed with minute forceps. Irrigation with water may cause the insect's body to swell or may push the insect closer to the tympanic membrane.

5 Correct answer—**D**

Attempts to remove foreign objects from the ear produce trauma, which may cause more swelling and even bleeding of the ear canal walls. Bleeding may be controlled by using ¼-inch gauze strips as a light packing. Insects are potential disease carriers; thus, if trauma caused by bites or scratchings occurs, a topical otic antibiotic is used for prophylaxis. Oral antibiotics and iodoform gauze are not necessary.

6 Correct answer—**C**

Immediate establishment of airway is required, and intubation is appropriate. Patients undergoing radiation therapy to the head and neck are subject to complications, including edema of the upper airway, severe dryness of the oral cavity, and burns of the skin. Tracheotomy should not be performed in a patient with laryngeal cancer, because this may lead to stomal carcinoma by direct extension of the tumor. A patient with COPD should not receive 100% oxygen; ABG studies are not an immediate need.

7 Correct answer—**C**

The next step for such a patient is an immediate cricothyroidotomy. The edema or tumor may be so great that an ET tube cannot be passed; further attempts produce greater edema.

8 Correct answer—**A**

When a patient has a ruptured tympanic membrane and basal skull fracture has been ruled out, bleeding from the ear may be controlled by evacuating the clot and packing the ear canal. The packing may be removed when bleeding has stopped. Tympanic membrane rupture does not require antibiotics; a healthy exposed middle ear mucosa is especially vulnerable to ototoxicity from ear drops. The tympanic membrane should heal in 1 to 2 weeks.

9 Correct answer—**B**

During discharge teaching, the patient must be encouraged to avoid heavy lifting, or straining from Valsalva's manuever, for 1 to 2 weeks. Other activities to be avoided are swimming, or any other situation that would involve water getting into the ear canal, and blowing the nose.

10 Correct answer—**A**

Swimming in a public pool is a common source of contamination, especially for the ears, producing an inflammatory disorder of the auricle and external auditory canal known as acute otitis externa. It is most often caused by bacterial or fungal infections, particularly *Pseudomonas*. Predisposing factors include moisture in the ear canal, which may occur in a warm, moist climate or as a result of swimming, and trauma resulting from attempts to clean or scratch an itchy ear.

11 Correct answer—**D**

Appropriate treatment includes medications such as analgesics, antibiotics (oral, otic, or topical), antipyretics, and application of hot, moist compresses to the affected ear.

12 Correct answer—**D**

Periauricular lymphadenopathy is present in acute otitis externa. History of an upper respiratory tract infection, a temperature of 102° F. (38.8° C.) or higher, and otalgia that increases with prone position are manifestations of acute otitis media.

13 Correct answer—**B**

Otitis media is more common in children than adults because of children's narrower eustachian tubes, which can occlude easily. The condition is commonly preceded by an upper respiratory tract infection or childhood disease, such as measles or scarlet fever. This is because of the proximity and connection of the eustachian tube to the upper respiratory tract.

14 Correct answer—**B**

If otitis media is not treated aggressively, complications include meningitis, mastoiditis, intracranial abscess, and permanent hearing loss. Ototoxicity is an adverse reaction to salicylates or antibiotics, such as kanamycin (Kantrex) and streptomycin.

15 Correct answer—**C**

The diagnostic procedures usually performed when a patient has acute otitis media include pneumatic otoscopy, hearing test, and blood cultures if the patient's temperature is 102.2° F. (39° C.) or higher. Tympanocentesis, aspiration of the middle ear, may be required for effusion, and myringotomy may be needed if the tympanic membrane is bulging. The caloric test is used in neurologic examinations to assess cranial nerve function.

16 Correct answer—**D**

In nasal trauma, a collection of blood develops under the septal mucosa, forming a septal hematoma. This bulging mass then causes breathing difficulties in both nares. Blood clots in the nares, edema of the nose, and a deviated septum also may cause breathing difficulty, but are less serious.

17 Correct answer—**D**

This patient sustained a nasal laceration, which requires cleansing with povidone-iodine (Betadine) and peroxide, followed by irrigation with normal saline solution. Tetanus toxoid should be given for an open wound. Before applying intranasal packing or blowing the nose, cerebrospinal fluid (CSF) rhinorrhea must be ruled out by observing for drainage from the nose and testing this drainage for glucose. CSF contains 60% of serum glucose content.

18 Correct answer—**D**

Treatment for a linear nasal fracture with nasal bleeding includes establishing an I.V. line, packing the nasal cavity, administering decongestants and vasoconstrictors, and applying cold packs to the bridge of the nose.

19 Correct answer—**D**

Active bleeding can be controlled temporarily by pinching the nose for 4 to 5 minutes. If bleeding persists, cauterization with silver nitrate sticks or electrocautery should be attempted. If bleeding still is not controlled, the physician will anesthetize the nasal chamber and insert nasal packing. Whenever nasal packing of any sort is used, the patient should be placed on broad-spectrum antibiotics until packs are removed. Alleviating the patient's apprehension and placing the patient in a semirecumbent position with head tilted forward are appropriate.

20 Correct answer—**A**

Bleeding after adenotonsillectomy must be treated with utmost urgency. Priority action always includes clearing the airway of blood and clots. I.V. fluids should be started promptly because children become hypovolemic much faster than adults, and the patient must be ready to go to the operating room immediately. Tonsillar sponges may be used to apply pressure to the tonsils, but a physician must place postnasal packing to control adenoidal bleeding.

21 Correct answer—**C**

Patient assessment findings of nasal deformity, cheek flattening, difficulty in opening the mouth, and diplopia most likely indicate a zygomatic fracture. This type of facial fracture is associated with asymmetry of the face, pain with jaw movement, limited movement of lower jaw, and visual disturbances. Zygomatic fractures are most commonly caused by automobile accidents and fights. They are commonly associated with orbital floor fractures, also referred to as "blow-out fractures."

22 Correct answer—**A**

The immediate management of a patient who sustained a zygomatic fracture would not include preparation for definitive treatment of the fracture by a physician. Definitive treatment may require semi-open reduction, open reduction, or internal wire fixation. Appropriate nursing actions aim to maintain a patent airway by examining for potential obstruction from blood clots, saliva, and loose teeth. Level of consciousness should be assessed, thereby establishing a baseline by which deterioration in neurologic status from associated head trauma can be recognized. The patient also should be evaluated for possible cervical or spinal trauma. Subsequent actions include controlling bleeding from facial lacerations and applying cold compresses to prevent facial edema. Prompt application of compresses will permit fractures to be tended sooner.

23 Correct answer—**B**

Nursing interventions to ensure a patent airway hold the highest priority. The patient must be in a side-lying or semi-Fowler's position for optimal airway clearance. Suction equipment must be readily available. Aspiration of teeth, bony fragments, blood clots, and vomitus must be prevented. Emergency intubation or tracheotomy equipment should be accessible quickly to ensure the immediate establishment of an airway, if necessary. The insertion of a nasopharyngeal airway is inappropriate and unsafe in the patient with a zygomatic fracture, because more trauma and bleeding may result.

24 Correct answer—**D**

Diagnostic procedures are essential for determining the extent of injuries and formulating a plan of care based on individual needs of the patient. Water's view X-rays permit evaluation of malar or zygoma eminence, and submental-vertex view permits evaluation of the zygomatic arch. Cervical spine X-rays, which are in many cases neglected because the facial deformities are most striking, must be obtained to evaluate fractures or dislocations that may result from the trauma.

25 Correct answer—**D**

Appropriate interventions that facilitate patient comfort include administering narcotics or analgesics as the physician orders, positioning the patient for comfort by elevating his head, and applying cold compresses to the fracture site to decrease edema.

26 Correct answer—**B**

Patient assessment data most likely indicate TMJ dislocation. This condition results in jaw displacement in which spasms of jaw muscles prevent the condyles from returning to their normal position. TMJ dislocation may be unilateral or bilateral, caused by trauma or simply by opening one's mouth too widely. It may also occur in individuals in high-stress occupations or constant chewers. On assessment, the patient cannot close his mouth completely and has referred pain to his teeth, temples, or ears.

27 Correct answer—**A**

The administration of I.V. diazepam (Valium) facilitates manual reduction of the jaw by alleviating tension and anxiety, relaxing facial muscles, and increasing patient cooperation during the procedure. After the procedure, postreduction X-rays are necessary.

28 Correct answer—**C**

Discharge planning for a patient with TMJ dislocation should include the importance of remaining on a soft diet for 3 to 4 days. This will avoid adding stress to the TMJ dislocation from excessive chewing or opening the mouth widely. Medication instructions regarding analgesics, if prescribed p.r.n., should be reviewed. Frequent mouth exercises could precipitate a TMJ dislocation.

29 Correct answer—**A**

Nursing interventions that help to prevent corneal abrasions include administering a 1% methylcellulose (artificial tears) solution to the affected eye, gentle periodic manual closure of the eyelid, sunglasses, and applying an eye patch to the affected eye.

30 Correct answer—**D**

The nurse prepares the patient with Bell's palsy for discharge by providing instructions for patient participation in recovery by encouraging facial massage, facial muscle exercises, and the application of moist heat to the face. Medication instructions regarding analgesics and steroids are essential to foster patient compliance. Techniques that promote corneal protection should be stressed.

31 Correct answer—**B**

Carbamazepine is the initial treatment of choice for trigeminal neuralgia. Trigeminal neuralgia is a disorder of unknown etiology that appears to result from sudden, episodic discharges along the distribution of the trigeminal nerve (fifth cranial nerve). It occurs predominantly in women age 40 or older; exacerbations tend to occur in the spring and fall. The right side of the face is affected more commonly than the left. Other medications used to treat trigeminal neuralgia include phenytoin and baclofen. Narcotics and analgesics are minimally effective.

32 Correct answer—**C**

The diagnosis of trigeminal neuralgia is commonly made on the basis of patient history and physical examination alone. Diagnostic tests are not required unless evidence of intracranial lesion exists, or if neurologic disorders are suspected. Painful paroxysms can be precipitated by touching the trigger zone on the ipsilateral (same side) anterior face. Pain is partially or completely eliminated within 48 hours after pharmacologic therapy begins. Twenty percent to fifty percent of patients will eventually fail to respond to drug therapy and will require surgical intervention, such as percutaneous rhizotomy or microsurgical decompression of the trigeminal nerve root.

33 Correct answer—**D**

Asking the patient if he sees halos around lights has the least priority. This symptom is usually associated with glaucoma, not extraocular foreign body emergencies. Because this type of trauma may be associated with future compensation, be sure to conduct a comprehensive interview. Information obtained must include time since occurrence, circumstances of the injury, safety apparatus worn, treatment before arrival, medical history including present medications, last tetanus immunization, allergies, visual status before accident, and time since fluid or food was last taken by mouth.

34 Correct answer—**A**

Instilling a fluorescein stain into the eye is a diagnostic procedure and does not contribute to pain relief. Effective interventions for helping the patient achieve pain relief include irrigating the eye gently with a normal saline solution and applying topical analgesics. Photosensitivity is common in ocular injuries; therefore, the eye should be covered with an occlusive patch.

35 Correct answer—**D**

Initial interview of the patient with an ocular emergency must elicit information regarding injury, the mechanism, time elapsed since occurrence, treatment before arrival, changes in clinical status, description of pain, visual changes, and medical history. Of particular importance is the patient's current medication history. Hyphema is a condition in which the blood vessels in the iris bleed into the anterior chamber of the eye. Prior use of any medications that may increase bleeding and decrease clotting time must be known; if bleeding is not minimized, severe ocular problems and loss of vision may ensue.

36 Correct answer—**B**

During the initial phase of treatment, the patient's eyes are patched. To minimize recurrent bleeding, patient activities are restricted. The patient is put on bed rest in a semi-Fowler's position, with bathroom privileges only. Sedation may be given judiciously. Hyphema usually clears in 5 to 6 days.

37 Correct answer—**B**

Discharge teaching for the patient with hyphema includes instructions to avoid coughing and Valsalva's maneuver, because they increase intraocular pressure; maintain head of bed at a 30-degree angle to decrease intraocular pressure; and try to reduce stress and physical strain during the recovery period. Remaining on bed rest for an extended time of 2 weeks has no therapeutic importance.

38 Correct answer—**D**

Do not delay in instituting eye irrigation with copious amounts of normal saline solution, preferably a continuous irrigation setup. Flushing the eyes with sodium bicarbonate is inappropriate because it is an alkaline substance. Checking the pH of the eye with litmus paper and instilling antibiotic drops are appropriate after complete eye irrigation. Steroids are also applied after irrigation, to reduce local inflammation.

39 Correct answer—**C**

Alkaline burns are an absolute ocular emergency. The most destructive chemicals to enter the eye are alkaline substances, which include lye, ammonia, and plaster. Alkaline chemicals cause necrosis of the conjunctiva and cornea, which will continue to react with ocular tissues, producing severe damage. All traces of the chemical must be removed to halt its corrosive action. Acid burns are usually not as devastating to the eye as are alkaline burns. Acid chemicals cause a coagulation necrosis of the cornea. The extent of damage to the eye is limited by the coagulation formed in the process. Similar principles of management apply to alkaline and acid burns of the eye.

40 Correct answer—**C**

A pH value of 7.0 on a litmus paper reading best indicates that treatment has been effective for the patient. This finding verifies adequate irrigation and absence of chemical in the eye. Whitening of cornea and visual acuity limited to light perception result from ocular tissue damage, which produces varied degrees of vision loss.

Selected References

Ausband, J.R. *Ear, Nose and Throat Disorders,* 2nd ed. New Hyde Park, N.Y.: Medical Examination Pub. Co., 1982.

Boies, R.L., et al. *Fundamentals of Otolaryngology.* Philadelphia: W.B. Saunders Co., 1983.

Cosgriff, J.A., and Andersen, D.L. *The Practice of Emergency Care,* 2nd ed. Philadelphia: J.B. Lippincott Co., 1984.

Mathog, R.H. *Maxillofacial Trauma.* Baltimore: Williams & Wilkins Co., 1984.

Rosen, P., et al. *Emergency Medicine: Concepts and Clinical Practice.* St. Louis: C.V. Mosby Co., 1983.

Sheehy, S.A., and Barber, J. *Emergency Nursing: Principles and Practice*, 2nd ed. St. Louis: C.V. Mosby Co., 1985.

Tintinalli, J.E., et al. *Emergency Medicine—A Comprehensive Study Guide.* New York: McGraw-Hill Book Co., 1985.

Warner, C.B. *Emergency Care: Assessment and Intervention,* 3rd ed. St. Louis: C.V. Mosby Co., 1983.

Chapter 11

Systemic Emergencies Questions and Answers

You must begin with Question 1 of this chapter and progress in sequence. **Do not skip around.** Subsequent answers build on previous ones.

Alice Belcher, RN, BSN, CCRN
Kathleen McMahon, RN, MSN, CEN
Joanne Scotto, RN, BSN

SITUATION

A 75-year-old woman with a long history of rheumatoid arthritis is brought to the emergency department (ED) in convulsions. About 4 hours earlier, she complained that her arthritis had been very painful. Methyl salicylate (wintergreen oil) was ordered topically by her primary physician, but the patient's son believes she may have taken it orally (1 tsp = 21 adult aspirin tablets).

Questions 1 to 5 refer to the above situation.

1 The absorption of aspirin tablets is nearly complete in how many hours?

A. 2
B. 3
C. 4
D. 6

2 Symptoms of acute salicylate intoxication may occur from single doses greater than which amount of mg/kg?

A. 50
B. 100
C. 150
D. 200

3 Symptoms of salicylate poisoning (salicylism) include:

A. Tetany
B. Seizures
C. Hypernatremia
D. Hypothermia

4 Emergency treatment for this patient would *not* include:

A. Gastric lavage with activated charcoal
B. Ipecac syrup
C. Parenteral calcium gluconate
D. Hemodialysis

5 Which is true regarding salicylate intoxication after ingestion of enteric-coated aspirin?

A. Because of the coating, symptoms will not be as severe
B. Hospitalization probably will not be required
C. Toxic effects will be delayed because absorption is delayed
D. Early blood levels are a reliable guide to prognosis

SITUATION

A 3-year-old girl who weighs 35 pounds (15 kg) is brought to the ED. She is alert but has been nauseated, vomiting, and diaphoretic since this morning. Last night an open bottle of pediatric acetaminophen (children's Tylenol) was found in a bathroom at the patient's home.

Questions 6 to 10 refer to the above situation.

6 Symptoms of acetaminophen overdose usually occur within how many hours after ingestion?

A. 1 to 3
B. 4 to 6
C. 12 to 24
D. 24 to 48

7 Toxic effects of acetaminophen include all of the following *except:*

A. Liver necrosis
B. Liver failure
C. Impaired renal function
D. Mucous membrane inflammation

8 Which laboratory value should be abnormal with acetaminophen toxicity?

A. Creatinine phosphokinase (CPK) level
B. Alkaline phosphatase level
C. Prothrombin time (PT)
D. Direct Coombs' test

9 The appropriate treatment for this patient is administration of:

A. Activated charcoal
B. Oxygen
C. Acetylcysteine (Mucomyst)
D. Dialysis (peritoneal or hemodialysis)

10 Acetaminophen affects which of the following systems?

A. Cardiovascular
B. Respiratory
C. Hepatic
D. Central nervous system (CNS)

SITUATION

A mother brings her 5-year-old son to the pediatric clinic because she thinks that he swallowed 5 to 10 iron supplement tablets. He is vomiting and complaining of severe abdominal pain.

Questions 11 to 15 refer to the above situation.

11 Which statement regarding iron poisoning is true?

A. It makes no difference whether the child swallowed ferrous fumarate, ferrous sulfate, or ferrous gluconate
B. Death can occur after ingestion of 50 to 100 ferrous sulfate tablets
C. Acute iron poisoning occurs primarily in elderly people
D. Shock is the most common cause of death in iron poisoning

12 Iron ingestion may be confirmed by:

A. Gastric fluid analysis
B. Serum triiodothyronine (T_3) and thyroxine (T_4) levels
C. Serum hemoglobin levels
D. Abdominal X-rays 72 hours after ingestion

13 If a potentially toxic ingestion is suspected, which procedure should be done first?

A. Administer a saline cathartic
B. Administer ipecac syrup or gastric lavage
C. Obtain abdominal X-rays
D. Measure serum iron levels

14 Which may indicate iron toxicity?

A. Metabolic alkalosis
B. Abdominal pain and hemorrhagic gastroenteritis
C. Seizures
D. Renal failure

15 Supportive care for this patient should consist of which procedure?

A. Maintenance of body temperature
B. Administration of antihypertensives
C. Administration of diuretics
D. Dialysis

SITUATION

A 12-year-old boy arrives by ambulance to the ED. On a playmate's dare, the patient drank 2 ounces (60 ml) of liquid bleach (an alkaline substance).

Questions 16 to 20 refer to the above situation.

16 Which statement is true concerning caustic substances?

A. Acidic substances have the same effect as alkaline substances
B. The severity of an alkaline burn depends on the pH of the substance and the duration of contact with the mucosa
C. Oropharyngeal and esophageal damage is more common with liquids than with solids
D. The absence of oral burns excludes the possibility of esophageal burns

17 Which is a symptom of caustic ingestion?

A. Tinnitus
B. Hyperthermia
C. Drooling
D. Dyspnea

18 Treatment of caustic ingestion would include:

A. Dilution with 8 ounces (240 ml) of milk or water
B. Administration of activated charcoal
C. Administration of a cathartic
D. Induction of emesis or gastric lavage

19 In adults, the lethal dose of concentrated acids or alkalis is (in milliliters):

A. 5
B. 10
C. 15
D. 30

20 Which statement is true concerning management of caustic ingestion?

A. Dermal and ocular decontamination should be carried out
B. Antibiotics may be administered prophylactically
C. Steroids should never be administered
D. Barium swallow is contraindicated

SITUATION

A 21-year-old woman comes to the ED complaining of blurred vision, sore throat, dizziness, and nausea. The patient reports that her sister has similar symptoms. Both women ate the same type of food at a restaurant yesterday.

Questions 21 to 24 refer to the above situation.

21 Which statement about botulism is true?

A. Ingestion of improperly home-processed vegetables, fruits, and meats causes the majority of cases
B. Botulism is not caused by fresh vegetables that have been grown in the ground
C. Danger arises when cooked foods remain at room temperature for more than 2 hours
D. The spores of *Clostridium botulinum* cannot withstand boiling temperatures for more than 30 minutes

22 Botulism is caused by a neurotoxin that blocks release of acetylcholine at peripheral nerve endings. The differential diagnosis of botulism includes which entity?

A. Guillain-Barré syndrome
B. Brown-Séquard syndrome
C. Salmonella poisoning
D. Acetaminophen overdose

23 Eight serologically different toxins of *C. botulinum* exist, but types A, B, and E most commonly affect human beings. Which statement is true?

A. Identification of the type of toxin requires serum or stool analysis
B. The incubation period for Type A is longer than that for Types B and E
C. Patient care is unchanged, regardless of toxin type
D. Respiratory insufficiency occurs with the same frequency, regardless of toxin type

24 Treatment of botulism includes which therapy?

A. Magnesium citrate (Milk of Magnesia)
B. Acetylcysteine (Mucomyst)
C. Exchange transfusion
D. Hemofiltration

SITUATION

A 51-year-old woman was admitted to the ED about 2 hours ago. She has a history of asthma, and her admitting diagnosis is pneumonia. She is complaining of breathing difficulty, and an audible wheeze is present. An erythematous rash, not seen on admission, is noted over her entire body. She received an initial dose of penicillin by intravenous piggyback 1 hour ago but has no history of allergies to antibiotics.

Questions 25 to 27 refer to the above situation.

25 Signs and symptoms of anaphylaxis may include:

A. Bradydysrhythmias
B. Cheyne-Stokes respiration
C. Acute pulmonary hyperinflation
D. Hypertension

26 Which statement concerning drug reactions is true?

A. The eruption begins as macules that spread in a symmetrical pattern, first on the head and proximal extremities
B. First episodes of hypersensitivity drug reactions of the exanthematous type always occur within 1 week after the drug is started
C. When a patient has received a drug many times without a reaction, it is safe to say that a reaction will never develop
D. The morphology of the eruption provides clues to the causative agent

27 Immediate treatment of a severe allergic reaction to a drug includes:

A. Oxygen therapy
B. Norepinephrine (Levophed)
C. Furosemide (Lasix)
D. Prednisone (Deltasone)

SITUATION

A 72-year-old man is admitted to the ED after an automobile accident. He was trapped in the wreckage for 3 hours. The air temperature was 30° F. (−1° C.). Although his fingers and toes were not frostbitten, he is stuporous. His pulse is 52 beats/minute, and his respiratory rate is 8 breaths/minute. His core temperature is 81° F. (27.2° C.).

Questions 28 to 33 refer to the above situation.

28 Elderly people are at risk for hypothermia because of:

A. Impaired hypothalamic function
B. Impaired thyroid function
C. Impaired circulation
D. Higher use of vasoactive medications

29 Which statement regarding hypothermia is false?

A. The myocardium is depressed and irritable, which may cause dysrhythmias
B. Decreased retention of water and sodium causes generalized dehydration (cold diuresis)
C. Insulin release is increased
D. Hepatic function (for example, handling of substrates or drugs) is altered

30 Which group of nursing interventions is *unsafe* for this patient?

A. Electrocardiographic (EKG) monitoring, core temperature and urine output measurements, neurologic check
B. Warmed I.V. fluids, frequent blood pressure checks, arterial blood gas (ABG) measurements
C. Serum electrolyte and glucose measurements
D. Frequent positioning of the patient to enhance rewarming

31 The extreme range of temperature compatible with life is:

A. 77° to 113° F. (25° to 45° C.)
B. 78.8° to 108° F. (26° to 42.2° C.)
C. 87.8° to 104° F. (31° to 40° C.)
D. 89.6° to 105.8° F. (32° to 41° C.)

32 Afterdrop or afterfall in the hypothermic patient refers to:

A. Drooping of the fingers or toes after rewarming
B. Impaired gait for several days after rewarming of lower extremities
C. Continued drop of core temperature by 4 to 6 F. degrees (2 to 3 C. degrees) as cold blood is returned from peripheral to core circulation
D. Microcirculatory sludging, which may result in renal or hepatic failure

33 Which method of rewarming is preferred for the hypothermic patient?

A. Hyperthermia blankets to the whole body
B. Warm-water immersion at temperatures of 100° to 105° F. (37.8° to 40.6° C.)
C. Warm enemas, warm I.V. infusions, peritoneal dialysis
D. Inhalation of warm saturated oxygen

SITUATION

The ED has just received word that the rescue team is bringing a victim of radiation exposure with associated injuries.

Questions 34 to 39 refer to the above situation.

34 In preparation for the patient's arrival, which of the following should be done?

A. Probably no procedure has been established at your hospital because of the rarity of radiation exposure. Protect other patients and personnel from exposure as best as possible
B. Prepare any available treatment room to isolate the patient and cover the floor with newspaper or nonskid plastic
C. Notify maintenance to shut off the air circulation system to any one available treatment area and to cover the floor in that room with nonskid plastic
D. Notify maintenance to shut off the air circulation system; use only a room with a lead-lined shield or an X-ray room; gather necessary equipment: Geiger counter, water, scrub brushes, soap, lead-lined containers for disposal, dosimeters, and protective garb for personnel who will care for the patient

35 Upon patient arrival, which should be done after breathing and circulation have been stabilized?

A. Remove all clothing and jewelry, disposing of them properly; wash patient with soap and water scrub
B. Assess amount of external radiation with Geiger counter; if detected, cover patient with plastic sheet and move to treatment room
C. Assess and treat serious associated injuries
D. Debride open wounds or radiation burns

36 Which patient is *least* likely to have been exposed to radiation?

A. A cancer patient complaining of fatigue, vomiting, and diarrhea
B. A firefighter who suffered smoke inhalation 2 days ago during a warehouse fire and now complains of vomiting
C. A nuclear plant worker who complains of weakness and epistaxis but who was not involved in a plant accident
D. A 55-year-old female bank employee with fever, chills, nausea, and vomiting

37 Clinical manifestations of radiation exposure (100 to 2,000 rads) include:

A. Tremors
B. Nausea and vomiting
C. Convulsions
D. Death

38 After the decontamination process, the Geiger counter readings do not show a reduction in the amount of external radiation. These findings indicate that:

A. The patient may have internal contamination
B. Convulsions and death will soon follow
C. You have no need for concern because this is common
D. The patient should receive additional body scrubs

39 After radiation exposure, leukopenia and thrombocytopenia usually are seen:

A. Immediately
B. Anywhere from 1 to 5 weeks after exposure, depending on amount of exposure
C. 2 months after exposure
D. None of the above

SITUATION

A 15-year-old boy is brought to the ED by his father for evaluation of a painful, erythemic lesion on his right leg. He had been walking through a wooded area earlier in the day and thinks that he may have been stung or bitten.

Questions 40 to 44 refer to the above situation.

40 Which precaution is appropriate when dealing with insect bites or stings?

A. Careful use of tourniquet proximal to sting or bite
B. Emergency equipment available in the event of respiratory failure
C. Antivenom available for I.V. administration
D. No precautions necessary because serious complications do not usually result

41 In all types of bites, which therapy is most likely to be administered?

A. Antibiotic
B. Antipruritic
C. Calcium gluconate
D. Tetanus toxoid

42 In most cases, to reduce the risk of future bites or stings, the patient should be instructed to:

A. Spray infested areas with creosote at least every 2 months; use protective clothing when hiking or working outdoors near sheds or woodpiles; and check protective clothing before use
B. Spray repellent in yard, on self, and on clothing
C. Nothing can be done to prevent bites
D. None of the above

43 Before discharge, instructions given to the patient who experienced an insect-related allergic reaction would include all of the following *except*:

A. The necessity of wearing a Medic Alert bracelet indicating allergy
B. If allergic to bee stings, the importance of carrying an anaphylaxis kit and knowing its proper use
C. Avoiding the use of perfumes, sprays, and brightly colored clothing, because these attract insects
D. Providing information that serum sickness may occur 2 to 3 days after the sting

44 Unlike other bites, that of the brown recluse spider:

A. Can occur any time of the year, but usually between September and March
B. Can occur any time of the year, but usually between April and October
C. Can be the most disfiguring, sometimes requiring skin grafting to close the wound
D. Has no particular differentiating characteristic

SITUATION

A 23-year-old man who had been hiking is brought to the ED, having sustained a snake bite to his lower left leg 20 minutes ago.

Question 45 refers to the above situation.

45 Prompt treatment should begin with:

A. Accurate identification of snake type
B. Immobilization and elevation of involved limb
C. Immobilization of limb below heart level and application of a lightly constrictive tourniquet
D. Application of ice to the skin over the snake bite wound

In most cases, to reduce the [illegible] the patient should be instructed to:

A. [illegible] infested area with [illegible] clothing when [illegible] wooded [illegible]
B. [illegible] repellents [illegible]
C. [illegible]
D. None of the above.

After desensitization, instructions given to the patient who experienced an anaphylactic reaction would include all of the following, except:

A. The necessity of [illegible]
B. [illegible] and [illegible] the proper use
C. Avoiding the use of perfumes, sprays, and brightly colored clothing [illegible]
D. [illegible]

[illegible]

A. [illegible]
B. [illegible]
C. [illegible]
D. [illegible]

EDUCATION

[illegible]

[illegible] of the above [illegible]

[illegible]

A. [illegible]
B. Immobilize [illegible]
C. Immobilize [illegible] below heart level [illegible] application of a tight [illegible]
D. Application of ice to the [illegible]

Answer Sheet

	A	B	C	D		A	B	C	D
1	○	○	○	○	31	○	○	○	○
2	○	○	○	○	32	○	○	○	○
3	○	○	○	○	33	○	○	○	○
4	○	○	○	○	34	○	○	○	○
5	○	○	○	○	35	○	○	○	○
6	○	○	○	○	36	○	○	○	○
7	○	○	○	○	37	○	○	○	○
8	○	○	○	○	38	○	○	○	○
9	○	○	○	○	39	○	○	○	○
10	○	○	○	○	40	○	○	○	○
11	○	○	○	○	41	○	○	○	○
12	○	○	○	○	42	○	○	○	○
13	○	○	○	○	43	○	○	○	○
14	○	○	○	○	44	○	○	○	○
15	○	○	○	○	45	○	○	○	○
16	○	○	○	○					
17	○	○	○	○					
18	○	○	○	○					
19	○	○	○	○					
20	○	○	○	○					
21	○	○	○	○					
22	○	○	○	○					
23	○	○	○	○					
24	○	○	○	○					
25	○	○	○	○					
26	○	○	○	○					
27	○	○	○	○					
28	○	○	○	○					
29	○	○	○	○					
30	○	○	○	○					

Answer Sheet

	A	B	C	D		A	B	C	D
1	○	○	○	○	31	○	○	○	○
2	○	○	○	○	32	○	○	○	○
3	○	○	○	○	33	○	○	○	○
4	○	○	○	○	34	○	○	○	○
5	○	○	○	○	35	○	○	○	○
6	○	○	○	○	36	○	○	○	○
7	○	○	○	○	37	○	○	○	○
8	○	○	○	○	38	○	○	○	○
9	○	○	○	○	39	○	○	○	○
10	○	○	○	○	40	○	○	○	○
11	○	○	○	○	41	○	○	○	○
12	○	○	○	○	42	○	○	○	○
13	○	○	○	○	43	○	○	○	○
14	○	○	○	○	44	○	○	○	○
15	○	○	○	○	45	○	○	○	○
16	○	○	○	○					
17	○	○	○	○					
18	○	○	○	○					
19	○	○	○	○					
20	○	○	○	○					
21	○	○	○	○					
22	○	○	○	○					
23	○	○	○	○					
24	○	○	○	○					
25	○	○	○	○					
26	○	○	○	○					
27	○	○	○	○					
28	○	○	○	○					
29	○	○	○	○					
30	○	○	○	○					

1 Correct answer—**A**

The absorption of regular aspirin tablets is nearly complete within 2 hours. If patients ingest methyl salicylate or enteric forms of aspirin, absorption may not be complete for 4 to 6 hours. Absorption will also be delayed in the presence of food.

2 Correct answer—**C**

Symptoms of salicylate intoxication occur when more than 150 mg/kg is ingested.

3 Correct answer—**B**

Seizures that result from CNS excitement are a sign of acute salicylism. A variable degree of CNS depression may occur, producing lethargy and coma. Dehydration, hyponatremia, and hypokalemia are other symptoms of acute salicylism, along with the hallmark symptoms of tinnitus, vomiting, hyperthermia, and hyperpnea.

4 Correct answer—**C**

Emergency treatment for this patient does not include parenteral calcium gluconate. Emesis should be induced with ipecac syrup or gastric lavage if the patient is alert; however, it is contraindicated in the patient with convulsions or an altered state of consciousness. Activated charcoal will bind salicylates and prevent further absorption, and may be given via a Levin tube, if necessary. Parenteral sodium bicarbonate will correct metabolic acidosis and shift salicylates from the tissues into the plasma. Indications for hemodialysis include a potentially lethal salicylate blood level (greater than 100 mg/dl), a deteriorating condition despite conservative therapy, or an inability to effect alkaline diuresis.

5 Correct answer—**C**

If the aspirin or salicylate product ingested had an enteric coating, the toxic effects could be delayed, because absorption of these products occurs more slowly. The patient must be kept under observation for at least 24 hours, because enteric-coated salicylates may not reach their highest concentration until 24 hours or more after the overdose. Since absorption occurs more slowly, early levels may be unreliable as a guide to prognosis.

6 Correct answer—**C**

Initial symptoms of nausea, vomiting, lethargy, and diaphoresis occur within 12 to 24 hours after ingestion. Elevated serum glutamic-oxaloacetic transaminase (SGOT), serum glutamic-pyruvic transaminase (SGPT), and serum bilirubin levels, as well as prolonged prothrombin time (PT) and tenderness in the right upper abdominal quadrant over the liver, occur after 24 to 48 hours. Three to five days after ingestion, jaundice, hepatic coma, hypoglycemia, oliguria, and severely prolonged PT may occur.

7 Correct answer—**D**

The hepatotoxicity of acetaminophen is related to depleted glutathione stores and the accumulation of a toxic metabolite of acetaminophen. Renal failure is less common and is usually mild, although severe tubular necrosis may ensue. Acetaminophen is not irritating to mucous membranes.

8 Correct answer—**C**

The hepatotoxic effects of acetaminophen result in elevation of SGOT, SGPT, and bilirubin levels, and in prolonged PT.

9 Correct answer—**C**

Within the first 12 hours, initial treatment begins with the clearing of residual acetaminophen from the GI tract by the use of emesis, or lavage and saline cathartics. If a high probability of developing hepatic damage exists, then the currently recommended treatment is acetylcysteine (Mucomyst) within 12 to 16 hours of ingestion. Activated charcoal binds acetylcysteine and should not be given. Oxygen is not indicated as an emergency treatment; peritoneal dialysis or hemodialysis is indicated in severe cases when early treatment is not administered.

10 Correct answer—**C**

Acetaminophen can be toxic to the liver when therapeutic doses are exceeded. It has no effect on the cardiovascular or respiratory systems or on the CNS.

11 Correct answer—**D**

Shock is the most common cause of death in iron poisoning. Toxicity is based on the amount of elemental iron ingested, not on the amount of iron salt ingested. Ferrous fumarate has 33% elemental iron, ferrous sulfate has 20%, and ferrous gluconate has 11.5%. The ingestion of fewer than 10 tablets of ferrous sulfate can be fatal. Acute iron poisoning is seen most commonly in young children as a result of accidental ingestion.

12 Correct answer—**A**

Iron ingestion may be confirmed in several ways. Gastric fluid may be analyzed qualitatively by the deferoxamine color test. Plain X-rays of the abdomen may demonstrate radiopaque particles; however, iron tablets may dissolve after 4 hours and iron solutions are not radiopaque. The provocative chelaton test, which uses 50 mg/kg of I.M. deferoxamine, requires significant iron absorption before the urine appears pinkish red. Serum iron levels and iron-binding capacity should be determined in any patient who has ingested an unknown or potentially toxic amount of iron.

13 Correct answer—**B**

If a potentially toxic ingestion of elemental iron is suspected, the stomach should be emptied as soon as possible. The method of choice is induction of emesis using ipecac syrup. If the patient has an altered sensorium or if hematemesis has occurred, gastric lavage is indicated.

14 Correct answer—**B**

GI symptoms resulting from direct irritation of the GI mucosa occur within 1 to 6 hours of ingestion. Severity ranges from mild epigastric distress and vomiting to marked abdominal pain and hemorrhagic gastroenteritis. In patients who have taken a severe overdose, the serum iron level exceeds the iron-binding capacity and results in free-circulating iron. Free iron causes the systemic symptoms that develop over 24 to 48 hours. Metabolic acidosis and shock are common early features of severe overdose. Coagulation defects and hepatic damage are variable and inconsistent.

15 Correct answer—**A**

Supportive care consists of maintaining body temperature, administering parenteral fluids to maintain hydration, and correcting hypotension with vascular expanders and vasopressors, if necessary. Hypoxia may be treated with oxygen therapy; metabolic acidosis may be treated with sodium bicarbonate.

16 Correct answer—**B**

Strong alkaline products produce a liquefactive necrosis, penetrate deeply and rapidly, and result in esophageal stricture. Acidic substances cause a coagulation necrosis and thus do not penetrate as deeply as alkalis. Damage to the oropharynx and esophagus is more common by solids than by liquids. In 10% to 15% of cases, esophageal burns are present despite the absence of oral burns.

17 Correct answer—**C**

Drooling occurs as a result of dysphagia combined with an outpouring of saliva. Although local pain or burning is almost always present, severe burns may damage nerve endings, resulting in anesthesia. Dysphagia is common. A physical examination may reveal mucosal burns, appearing as whitish grey or red patches.

18 Correct answer—**A**

If tolerated, dilution of the ingested acid or alkaline substance with 6 to 8 oz (180 to 240 ml) of milk or water is beneficial. After that, the patient should take nothing by mouth. Induced emesis, gastric lavage, and administration of activated charcoal and cathartics are inappropriate. Airway management, adequate fluid replacement, and careful monitoring for perforation and hemorrhage are essential.

19 Correct answer—**A**

In adults, the lethal dose of concentrated acids or alkalis is 5 ml.

20 Correct answer—**A**

Dermal and ocular decontamination should be carried out when appropriate. Antibiotics are not useful prophylactically. Barium swallow at 10 days to 3 weeks may assess severity of damage. Steroids are controversial but may be recommended if burns are found or esophagoscopy is not performed.

21 Correct answer—**A**

The majority of botulism cases occur from improperly home-processed vegetables, fruits, and meats. The spores of *C. botulinum* can withstand boiling temperatures for several hours; after cooling to room temperature, they can germinate and begin to produce toxin. Danger arises when cooked food remains at room temperature for more than 16 hours. Fresh vegetables grown in the ground also can produce botulism.

22 Correct answer—**A**

The differential diagnosis of botulism includes Guillain-Barré syndrome, basilar artery stroke, chemical intoxication, tick-borne paralysis, trichinosis, and various neuropsychiatric syndromes.

23 Correct answer—**A**

Identification of specific types of *C. botulinum* requires serum or stool analysis. Type A toxin is more dangerous than Types B and E because of its prolonged morbidity and increased mortality. The incubation period is shorter in Type A, with the onset of symptoms ranging from 12 hours to 8 days after ingestion of the toxin. Acute onset of respiratory insufficiency, requiring prolonged mechanical ventilation, occurs more commonly in Type A.

24 Correct answer—**A**

Medical therapy for botulism can include magnesium citrate, saline solution enemas, equine antitoxin, and plasmapheresis. Medical therapy is aimed first at preventing progression of the toxic effects and complications by eliminating any nonabsorbed toxin and neutralizing unfixed toxin. Subsequent supportive care is directed toward maintaining body functions to allow for metabolism of the fixed toxin.

25 Correct answer—**C**

The anatomic findings associated with fatal systemic anaphylaxis include acute pulmonary hyperinflation caused by airway obstruction or laryngeal edema, urticaria, or vascular collapse.

26 Correct answer—**A**

An anaphylactic drug reaction usually begins as a macular eruption on the head and proximal extremities, then spreads in a symmetrical pattern. First episodes of exanthematous-type reactions occur most commonly within 1 week after the patient has started taking the drug. Occasionally, however, the rash appears as long as 14 days after the drug has been discontinued. A patient may be treated with a drug many times before developing a reaction. The morphology of the eruption gives no clue to the specific causative agent; therefore, a careful history of all medications and other substances that have entered any body orifice is essential in making the proper diagnosis.

27 Correct answer—**A**

Immediate treatment includes oxygen therapy. This patient has signs of systemic anaphylaxis. Since she is a known asthmatic, she has a greater risk of anaphylaxis than a nonasthmatic person. Anaphylaxis is a life-threatening condition that must be treated quickly. Treatment is directed toward impairing absorption of the antigen, enhancing oxygenation, and treating or preventing hypotension. Emergency treatment includes oxygen therapy, epinephrine (Adrenalin), aminophylline (Phyllocontin), and hydrocortisone (Cortef). Prednisone may take 4 to 6 hours to start working.

28 Correct answer—**A**

Elderly people have impaired hypothalamic function, presumably because of atherosclerotic changes. They are at risk even without any predisposing causes, such as impaired thyroid function or circulation, or the use of vasoactive medications.

29 Correct answer—**C**

Insulin release is suppressed in hypothermia; as a result, the serum glucose level may be elevated to 500 to 600 mg/dl. However, glucose uptake and insulin secretion return to normal during rewarming.

30 Correct answer—**D**

To prevent ventricular fibrillation, extreme caution must be used when moving, transporting, manipulating, and intubating these patients, because defibrillation is ineffective below 86° to 87° F. (30° to 30.6° C.). At 85° F. (29.4° C.), the heart will not respond to drug therapy. Appropriate nursing interventions would include EKG monitoring, recording of core temperature, neurologic checks, and monitoring of urine output, serum electrolyte levels, vital signs, and ABG measurements. Warming the I.V. fluids is also therapeutic.

31 Correct answer—**A**

The extreme temperature range compatible with life is 77° to 113° F. (25° to 45° C.). Hypothermia, a core temperature of 95° F. or below (35° C.), is categorized as follows: *mild* hypothermia, 95° F., shivering, sluggish and decreased coordination; *moderate* hypothermia, 89.6° F. (32° C.), muscular rigidity, stupor, dilated pupils; *severe* hypothermia, 78.8° to 82.4° F. (26° to 28° C.), pulse and respiration undetectable, ventricular fibrillation likely, electroencephalogram likely to be flat; death imminent.

32 Correct answer—**C**

Afterdrop is a familiar phenomenon in postoperative patients in whom the core temperature continues to drop 2 to 3 C. degrees after the cause of hypothermia is removed. Vasodilation and increased muscular activity return peripherally sequestered blood to the central circulation. Microcirculatory sludging does occur but is not referred to as afterdrop.

33 Correct answer—**D**

Inhalation of warm saturated oxygen (active internal warmth) has a greater benefit for the heart and body core; peripheral heating and vasodilation occur more slowly. External warming with hyperthermia blankets, warm-water enemas, warm I.V. fluids, and warm peritoneal dialysis must occur concurrently to prevent afterdrop and ventricular fibrillation.

34 Correct answer—**D**

Notify maintenance to shut off the air circulation system. Use only a room with a lead-lined shield or an X-ray room. Gather the necessary equipment: Geiger counter, water scrub, brushes and soap, lead-lined containers for disposal, and protective garb for personnel who will care for the patient. Cover the floor with newspaper or nonskid plastic.

35 Correct answer—**B**

The amount of external radiation should be assessed first, thereby providing a baseline of the extent of exposure. The other procedures are part of the decontamination process. After decontamination, reassessment with a Geiger counter will be necessary.

36 Correct answer—**D**

The bank employee with fever, chills, nausea, and vomiting is least likely to be suffering from radiation exposure. All of the other patients should be ruled out carefully, since they show signs of radiation exposure and have a likely source of contamination.

37 Correct answer—**B**

Mild to severe nausea and vomiting are seen in most cases of radiation exposure, regardless of the amount of exposure. Tremors, convulsions, and death are seen in severe contamination (exposure over 2,000 rads).

38 Correct answer—**A**

If the Geiger counter readings do not show a reduction in the amount of external radiation after the decontamination process, this patient probably has internal contamination. Additional body scrubs will not help. Body fluids (saliva, blood, and waste) must be tested. Gastric lavage, cathartics, or emetics may be administered, as well as chelating or blocking agents, which prevent uptake of radioactive iodine by the thyroid gland. Convulsions and death can still be avoided if appropriate treatment is instituted promptly.

39 Correct answer—**B**

Leukopenia and thrombocytopenia always occur in these patients. In mild exposure (100 rads), they will be manifested 4 to 5 weeks later. They are seen in 3 weeks with an exposure of 300 to 600 rads. In exposures over 600 rads, hematologic abnormalities are seen in 1 to 3 weeks.

40 Correct answer—**B**

Respiratory failure is always a possibility after insect stings and bites. Emergency equipment must be readily available for a severe allergic reaction or anaphylaxis. Antivenom I.V. is recommended for scorpion and black widow spider bites. Tourniquet application is used for scorpion and snake bites.

41 Correct answer—**D**

Tetanus toxoid should be administered in all cases, unless the patient has received a tetanus toxoid booster within 5 years. Prophylactic antibiotics may be prescribed. Calcium gluconate controls muscle spasms associated with black widow spider and scorpion bites. Antipruritics reduce itching associated with tick bites.

42 Correct answer—**A**

Spraying infested areas with creosote, wearing protective clothing when hiking or working outdoors or near sheds or woodpiles, and checking protective clothing before use are recommended to reduce infestation and to prevent bites. Insect repellents are useful only against bees.

43 Correct answer—**D**

Before discharge from the ED, the patient admitted with an insect-related allergic reaction should be informed that he may experience serum sickness 10 to 14 days after the sting. The necessity of wearing a Medic Alert bracelet must be stressed. The patient should be instructed to obtain and to familiarize himself with an emergency insect bite kit. Inform the patient to avoid using perfumes, sprays, and brightly colored clothing because these attract insects.

44 Correct answer—**C**

Brown recluse spider bites are quite disfiguring and can require skin grafting. Ulcers form and, with a graft, can take 6 to 8 weeks to heal.

45 Correct answer—**C**

If less than 30 minutes has elapsed since the snake bite, prompt treatment must begin with immobilization of the affected limb below heart level and the immediate application of a lightly constrictive tourniquet. The skin should be washed, but ice should not be applied to the bite. Snake bites involving the head or trunk are the most dangerous, but most snake bites occur below the elbow or knee. Remember never to elevate the affected extremity because this action increases envenomation. In the United States, rattlesnakes, water moccasins, copperheads, and coral snakes are poisonous to human beings. Identifying the type of snake that inflicted the bite is helpful, although valuable treatment time must not be wasted in doing so.

Selected References

Barber, J.M., and Budassi, S. *Mosby's Manual of Emergency Care, Practices and Procedures.* St. Louis: C.V. Mosby Co., 1979.

Biddle, C. "Hypothermia: Implications for the Critical Care Nurse," *Critical Care Nurse* 5:34-38, March/April 1985.

Braunohler, W. "The Critical Process of Rewarming Frozen Tissue," *Consultant* 25:50, January 30, 1985.

Clark, D., and Scovill, N. "Botulism: Coping With an Epidemic," *Critical Care Nurse* 7, January/February 1987.

Conn, J. *Conn's Current Therapy.* Philadelphia: W.B. Saunders Co., 1987.

Curtis, R., et al. "Efficacy of Ipecac and Activated Charcoal/Cathartic: Prevention of Salicylate Absorption in a Simulated Overdose," *Archives of Internal Medicine* 144(1):48-52, January 1984.

DeLapp, T.D. "Accidental Hypothermia," *American Journal of Nursing* 83:62-67, January 1983.

Drucker, J. *Infections: Recognition, Understanding, Treatment.* Philadelphia: Lea & Febiger, 1984.

Finch, R.G. *Textbook of Infectious Diseases.* New Hyde Park, N.Y.: Medical Examination Pub. Co., 1984.

Gilman, A.G., et al., eds. *Goodman and Gilman's The Pharmacological Basis of Therapeutics,* 7th ed. New York: Macmillan Publishing Co., 1985.

Joubert, D. "Use of Emetic, Adsorbent, and Cathartic Agents in Acute Drug Overdose," *Journal of Emergency Nursing* 13:49-51, January/February 1987.

Lanros, N.E. *Assessment and Intervention Emergency Nursing,* 2nd ed. Bowie, Md.: Robert J. Brady Co., 1983.

Linden, C., and Rumack, B. "Acetaminophen Overdose," *Emergency Medicine Clinics of North America* 2(1):103-19, February 1984.

MacDonald, K., et al. "Type A Botulism from Sauteed Onions: Clinical and Epidemiological Observations," *Journal of the American Medical Association* 253(9):1275-78, March 1985.

Maroncelli, R. "Action Stat: Accidental Poisoning," *Nursing86* 16:25, July 1986.

May, H., ed. *Emergency Medicine.* New York: John Wiley & Sons, 1984.

Newton, M., et al. "General Treatments of Household Poisonings," *Journal of Emergency Nursing* 13:12-15, January/February 1987.

Ruthman, J.C., and Hendricksen, D.K. "Emergency Department Presentation of Type A Botulism," *American Journal of Emergency Medicine* 3(3):203-05, May 1985.

Smith, D.S. "Living Death: Don't Let Hypothermia Fool You into a Fatal Mistake," *RN* 46:48-51, January 1983.

Spyker, D., and Rogol, A. *Current Emergency Therapy '84.* East Norwalk, Conn.: Appleton-Century-Crofts, 1984.

Thurkauf, G. "Acetaminophen Overdose," *Critical Care Nurse* 7:20, January/February 1987.

Chapter 12

Gastrointestinal Emergencies Questions and Answers

You must begin with Question 1 of this chapter and progress in sequence. **Do not skip around.** Subsequent answers build on previous ones.

Stephanie Higie, RN, BSN, CEN
Joanne Noone, RN, MSN, CCRN, CEN
Patricia Tooker, RN, MSN, CCRN

1 A patient arrives in the emergency department (ED) with an ice pick protruding from his left lower abdominal quadrant. An appropriate nursing action is to:

A. Immediately remove the object and apply firm pressure to the wound
B. Leave the object in place until the patient is in the operating room (OR)
C. Establish two large-bore intravenous (I.V.) lines and then remove the object
D. Obtain an abdominal X-ray and then remove the object

2 Which type of penetrating injury would a gunshot wound at the sixth intercostal space be?

A. Chest
B. Abdominal
C. Thoracoabdominal
D. Pelvic

3 A patient arrives to the ED with a gunshot wound to the left lower abdominal quadrant. His vital signs are blood pressure (BP), 110/70 mm Hg; pulse, 96 beats/minute; respirations, 24 breaths/minute. Which intervention is the *most* appropriate treatment?

A. Emergency exploratory laparotomy
B. Abdominal computed tomography (CT) scan
C. Diagnostic peritoneal lavage
D. Close observation in the ED over the next several hours

4 A patient has a penetrating gunshot wound to the abdomen and hematuria. Which diagnostic test is indicated before surgery?

A. Diagnostic peritoneal lavage
B. An abdominal X-ray
C. Intravenous pyelogram (IVP)
D. Abdominal CT scan

5 A gunshot wound to the right upper abdominal quadrant may cause injury to the:

A. Liver
B. Transverse colon
C. Stomach
D. All of the above

6 Before a patient with a penetrating abdominal wound is taken to the OR, which should be inserted?

A. Two large-bore I.V. lines
B. A nasogastric (NG) tube
C. An indwelling (Foley) catheter
D. All of the above

7 A young, healthy adult sustains a penetrating abdominal wound. Clinical signs of shock will occur only after what percentage of blood volume is lost?

A. 15%
B. 25%
C. 30%
D. 50%

8 All of the following are considered penetrating traumas *except*:

A. A stab wound to the right upper abdominal quadrant
B. A severe abdominal laceration caused by a fall
C. A gunshot wound to the left lower abdominal quadrant
D. A BB pellet to the lower abdomen

9 Clinical manifestations of perforated gastric ulcer include all of the following *except*:

A. Paralytic ileus
B. Shock
C. Anxiety, respiratory difficulty
D. Severe upper abdominal pain radiating to the jaw

10 Chemical peritonitis associated with a perforated gastric ulcer is caused by:

A. Overuse of antacids
B. Salicylate ingestion
C. Gastric and intestinal content spillage
D. Sodium and calcium imbalance

SITUATION

A 38-year-old man is admitted to the ED with complaints of severe epigastric pain. His vital signs upon admission are within normal limits. His diagnosis is pancreatitis.

Questions 11 to 20 refer to the above situation.

11 Pancreatitis occurs as a complication of perforated duodenal ulcer when:

A. Serum amylase is elevated to dangerous levels
B. A perforation erodes into the pancreas
C. The patient has a high alcohol intake
D. The pancreatic duct is obstructed

12 Ulcers that perforate most commonly are located in the:

A. Stomach
B. Jejunum
C. Duodenum
D. Ileum

13 Gastrointestinal (GI) emergencies, such as obstruction, perforation, and acute intractable hemorrhage, are usually treated by:

A. Surgical intervention
B. Fluid and blood replacement
C. Antacids, anticholinergics, sedatives, and ataractic drugs
D. Decreased stress and alteration in diet

14 The most common cause of pancreatitis is:

A. Excessive alcohol intake
B. Excessive fat intake
C. Heredity
D. Stress

15 Common symptoms of hemorrhagic pancreatitis include:

A. Jaundice
B. Extreme epigastric or umbilical pain extending to back or flank
C. Shock
D. All of the above

16 The patient with acute pancreatitis should be monitored for an elevated level of serum:

A. Cholesterol
B. Amylase
C. Potassium
D. Calcium

17 The analgesic of choice in the treatment of acute pancreatitis is:

A. Acetaminophen (Tylenol) with codeine
B. Oxycodone with aspirin (Percodan)
C. Meperidine (Demerol)
D. Morphine

18 Treatment of acute hemorrhagic pancreatitis includes which procedure?

A. Administer large volumes of colloid and electrolyte solution
B. Administer calcium gluconate
C. Monitor central venous pressure (CVP) and urine output
D. All of the above

19 A broad-spectrum antibiotic that is metabolized by the liver and excreted into the biliary tract is indicated:

A. Frequently
B. Only if surgery is required
C. Rarely
D. Never

20 As symptoms of pancreatitis resolve, the patient should be placed on which diet?

A. Low-fat, no-alcohol, no-caffeine
B. Low-fat, low-cholesterol
C. Low-salt, low-sugar, no-alcohol
D. No-alcohol, no-caffeine, no-sugar

SITUATION

A 21-year-old man comes to the ED with abdominal pain of sudden onset. A diagnosis of acute appendicitis is made.

Questions 21 and 22 refer to the above situation.

21 Which assessment data indicate acute appendicitis?

A. Rovsing's sign
B. Leukopenia
C. Abdominal distention
D. Audible borborygmi

22 In caring for a patient with sudden abdominal pain, which practice is considered *unsafe?*

A. Infusion of I.V. lactated Ringer's solution
B. Insertion of an NG tube attached to suction
C. Prompt administration of analgesics to decrease discomfort
D. Measurement of rectal temperature

23 When compared with older children and adults, very young children have a higher incidence of perforation of the appendix with resulting peritonitis, because they:

A. Describe their symptoms poorly
B. Have a greater pain tolerance
C. Have a weaker appendiceal wall
D. Have less resistance to infection

24 An 8-year-old boy is sent home from school after complaining of a persistent stomachache. At home, he has an episode of nausea and vomiting. He is afebrile. His mother attributes his symptoms to indigestion or an upset stomach, and decides not to seek medical attention. The decision to treat the child at home is a threat to his health because:

A. Any abdominal pain in school-aged children must be medically evaluated
B. Absence of fever does not necessarily mean absence of illness
C. Vomiting is the primary cause of water and electrolyte loss in pediatric patients
D. Early recognition of appendicitis prevents rupture and complications

SITUATION

A 26-year-old man is brought to the ED via ambulance after an automobile accident. No obvious fractures or injuries are noted. A diagnosis of possible blunt abdominal trauma is made.

Questions 25 to 28 refer to the above situation.

25 Patients with blunt abdominal trauma commonly have injuries to which internal organs?

A. Liver and spleen
B. Kidneys and spleen
C. Pancreas and spleen
D. Pancreas and liver

26 To restore circulatory dynamics in this patient, which type of solution should be included?

A. Hypertonic
B. Hypotonic
C. Isotonic
D. Hypo-osmolar

27 Two diagnostic tools that may be used for detecting intra-abdominal injury are paracentesis and peritoneal lavage. Peritoneal lavage is *contraindicated* in the patient:

A. With a colostomy
B. Who is unconscious
C. With multiple abdominal scars
D. Between ages 2 and 10

28 Which statement regarding suspected splenic injury is *false?*

A. The normal spleen is palpable below the lower left costal margin
B. The spleen is injured more often than any other abdominal organ
C. The high incidence of splenic injury is directly related to the organ's high vascularity
D. A positive Kehr's sign is seen in approximately 50% of patients with splenic bleeding

SITUATION

A 74-year-old man is brought to the hospital by his nephew after complaining of severe abdominal cramping and noticeable swelling of his abdomen. He claims he has had a "stomach virus" for a few days. His symptoms include nausea, anorexia, mild discomfort, and constipation. The pain has increased in intensity in the last 12 hours, and he has experienced several episodes of vomiting small amounts of "greenish" liquid. A diagnosis of possible bowel obstruction is made.

Questions 29 to 32 refer to the above situation.

29 Bowel obstruction is most commonly seen in very young and very old patients. The hallmark signs and sympoms of intestinal obstruction are:

A. Pain, distention, vomiting, and prolonged constipation
B. Absence of pain, nausea and vomiting, and prolonged constipation
C. Loss of bowel sounds, distention, constipation, and nausea
D. Hyperactive bowel sounds, diarrhea, vomiting, and cramping

30 The primary cause of large-bowel obstruction is:

A. Adhesions
B. Volvulus
C. Carcinoma
D. Diverticulitis

31 While the nurse is completing the initial physical assessment and history, the patient becomes increasingly restless and confused. A second set of vital signs is obtained, and the physician on call is notified. Vital signs are BP, 90/58 mm Hg; pulse, 134 beats/minute and weak; temperature, 96.6° F. (35.9° C.), with a cool skin surface; respirations, 16 breaths/minute and shallow. These findings indicate development of:

A. Cerebrovascular accident
B. Congestive heart failure
C. Shock
D. Anxiety

32 The correct sequence for assessment and evaluation of the patient's abdomen is:

A. Auscultation, percussion, inspection, and palpation
B. Auscultation, inspection, percussion, and palpation
C. Inspection, auscultation, percussion, and palpation
D. Inspection, auscultation, palpation, and percussion

SITUATION

A 38-year-old male stockbroker is brought to the ED by a co-worker after experiencing an episode of severe weakness following a business luncheon. Although he denies any medical or surgical history, he takes large amounts of liquid antacids "to help keep his stomach calm." He has had several episodes of bloody vomitus within the past 3 to 4 days. A diagnosis of upper GI bleeding is made.

Questions 33 to 38 refer to the above situation.

33 Which nursing action is most helpful in determining the cause of the patient's bleeding?

A. Inserting an NG tube to measure the pH of gastric fluids
B. Collecting blood specimens for complete blood count (CBC), type and screen, and coagulation profiles
C. Prompt scheduling of an endoscopy
D. Obtaining a thorough history and physical examination

34 In assessing the patient's health status, the nurse should know that hematemesis is most commonly the result of:

A. Malignant tumors
B. Peptic ulcers
C. Blood dyscrasias
D. Esophageal varices

35 Anticholinergic drugs, commonly used to treat peptic ulcer disease, produce which pharmacologic action?

A. Decrease the responsiveness of the patient
B. Increase gastric emptying
C. Interfere with histamine formation
D. Block the effects of vagal nerve impulses on smooth muscles

36 Esophageal varices are:

A. Abnormalities within the circulation of the splenic artery
B. Nearly always caused by portal hypertension
C. The result of frequent use of alcohol, tobacco, or spicy foods
D. Almost always the result of an existing esophageal carcinoma

37 Nursing care of the patient who has a Sengstaken-Blakemore tube includes all of the following *except:*

A. Maintaining constant observation while the balloons are inflated
B. Ensuring that the balloon pressures are kept at the levels required to control bleeding
C. Remaining alert for any complaints of chest pain
D. Placing the patient in a supine position to prevent development of shock

38 The three most common causes of upper GI bleeding are:

A. Neoplasms, gastritis, duodenal ulcer
B. Peptic ulcer, acute mucosal lesions, esophageal varices
C. Esophagitis, gastric ulcer, hematologic disorders
D. Mallory-Weiss tear, peptic ulcer, vascular anomalies

SITUATION

A 72-year-old man is brought to the ED by his daughter after an episode of rectal bleeding. He has been treated in the past for hemorrhoidal discomfort and bleeding.

Questions 39 to 44 refer to the above situation.

39 If clinical findings suggest the lower bowel to be the source of bleeding, which diagnostic test should be performed first?

A. Angiography
B. Abdominal CT scan
C. Esophagogastroduodenoscopy
D. Proctoscopy

40 After initial treatment in the ED, the patient will probably be:

A. Prepared for emergency surgery
B. Admitted to the intensive care unit
C. Admitted to a medical unit
D. Sent home and referred to an outpatient clinic

41 In instances of prolonged bleeding, anemia is a possible complication. The resultant pallor is usually most easily detected in the:

A. Lips
B. Gums
C. Sclera
D. Nail beds

42 Which is the most common cause of lower GI bleeding?

A. Diverticulitis
B. Hemorrhoids
C. Ischemic bowel disease
D. Neoplasms

43 When undergoing emergency endoscopy, the patient should be monitored for which potential complication?

A. Cardiac dysrhythmias
B. Perforation
C. Aspiration
D. All of the above

44 Lower GI bleeding is defined as bleeding from:

A. The colon
B. A source below the ligament of Treitz
C. A source below the appendix
D. Diverticuli

SITUATION

A 28-year-old woman is admitted to the ED after being involved in a high-speed, head-on automobile accident. She is conscious and alert; her skin is cool and dry. Vital signs are BP, 110/70 mm Hg; pulse, 100 beats/minute; respirations, 24 breaths/minute. The emergency medical technicians (EMTs) report severe front-end damage to the car and a broken steering wheel.

Questions 45 to 51 refer to the above situation.

45 After assessment of the patient's airway, breathing, and circulatory status, the next priority is to:

A. Ask the patient when her last meal was
B. Initiate two large-bore I.V. lines
C. Insert a Foley catheter
D. Insert an NG tube

46 The earliest sign of impending shock is:

A. Tachycardia
B. Hypotension
C. Narrowing pulse pressure
D. Cool and clammy skin

47 The patient's BP suddenly drops to 88/60 mm Hg and her pulse increases to 130 beats/minute. After administration of 500 ml of lactated Ringer's solution, BP increases to 100/70 mm Hg and her pulse is 100 beats/minute. Which of the following should be done next?

A. Prepare the patient for an IVP
B. Prepare the patient for a diagnostic peritoneal lavage
C. Prepare the patient for the OR
D. Immediately transfuse with O-positive or O-negative blood, depending on availability

48 A diagnostic peritoneal lavage may yield a false-negative result in:

A. Splenic bleeding
B. Diaphragmatic rupture
C. Bladder tear
D. Retroperitoneal hematoma

49 Diagnostic peritoneal lavage is performed on children:

A. Frequently
B. Rarely
C. Under age 2
D. Never

50 An IVP is indicated if which sign is present?

A. Blood at the meatus
B. High-riding prostate on rectal examination
C. Hematuria
D. All of the above

51 A large mass in the left upper abdominal quadrant, displacement of the stomach, and associated rib fractures in the left lower thorax are consistent with injury to the:

A. Liver
B. Small intestine
C. Spleen
D. Colon

Answer Sheet

	A	B	C	D		A	B	C	D
1	○	○	○	○	31	○	○	○	○
2	○	○	○	○	32	○	○	○	○
3	○	○	○	○	33	○	○	○	○
4	○	○	○	○	34	○	○	○	○
5	○	○	○	○	35	○	○	○	○
6	○	○	○	○	36	○	○	○	○
7	○	○	○	○	37	○	○	○	○
8	○	○	○	○	38	○	○	○	○
9	○	○	○	○	39	○	○	○	○
10	○	○	○	○	40	○	○	○	○
11	○	○	○	○	41	○	○	○	○
12	○	○	○	○	42	○	○	○	○
13	○	○	○	○	43	○	○	○	○
14	○	○	○	○	44	○	○	○	○
15	○	○	○	○	45	○	○	○	○
16	○	○	○	○	46	○	○	○	○
17	○	○	○	○	47	○	○	○	○
18	○	○	○	○	48	○	○	○	○
19	○	○	○	○	49	○	○	○	○
20	○	○	○	○	50	○	○	○	○
21	○	○	○	○	51	○	○	○	○
22	○	○	○	○					
23	○	○	○	○					
24	○	○	○	○					
25	○	○	○	○					
26	○	○	○	○					
27	○	○	○	○					
28	○	○	○	○					
29	○	○	○	○					
30	○	○	○	○					

Answer Sheet

1 ○ ○ ○ ○
2 ○ ○ ○ ○
3 ○ ○ ○ ○
4 ○ ○ ○ ○
5 ○ ○ ○ ○
6 ○ ○ ○ ○
7 ○ ○ ○ ○
8 ○ ○ ○ ○
9 ○ ○ ○ ○
10 ○ ○ ○ ○
11 ○ ○ ○ ○
12 ○ ○ ○ ○
13 ○ ○ ○ ○
14 ○ ○ ○ ○
15 ○ ○ ○ ○
16 ○ ○ ○ ○
17 ○ ○ ○ ○
18 ○ ○ ○ ○
19 ○ ○ ○ ○
20 ○ ○ ○ ○
21 ○ ○ ○ ○
22 ○ ○ ○ ○
23 ○ ○ ○ ○
24 ○ ○ ○ ○
25 ○ ○ ○ ○
26 ○ ○ ○ ○
27 ○ ○ ○ ○
28 ○ ○ ○ ○
29 ○ ○ ○ ○
30 ○ ○ ○ ○
31 ○ ○ ○ ○
32 ○ ○ ○ ○
33 ○ ○ ○ ○
34 ○ ○ ○ ○
35 ○ ○ ○ ○
36 ○ ○ ○ ○
37 ○ ○ ○ ○
38 ○ ○ ○ ○
39 ○ ○ ○ ○
40 ○ ○ ○ ○
41 ○ ○ ○ ○
42 ○ ○ ○ ○
43 ○ ○ ○ ○
44 ○ ○ ○ ○
45 ○ ○ ○ ○
46 ○ ○ ○ ○
47 ○ ○ ○ ○
48 ○ ○ ○ ○
49 ○ ○ ○ ○
50 ○ ○ ○ ○
51 ○ ○ ○ ○

1 Correct answer—**B**

Impaled objects should never be removed until the patient is in the OR, where hemorrhage can be surgically controlled once the object is removed.

2 Correct answer—**C**

The diaphragm, which separates the chest from the abdomen, rises to the level of the sixth intercostal space on respiratory exhalation. Therefore, this injury is considered a thoracoabdominal one, because the bullet may enter both the abdomen and the chest.

3 Correct answer—**A**

An exploratory laparotomy is the most appropriate treatment for the patient with a gunshot wound to the left lower abdominal quadrant. This procedure must be done to determine which structures have been penetrated by the bullet to control hemorrhage. A peritoneal lavage and abdominal CT scan do not assist in identifying the extent of injury to vessels. These procedures take considerable amounts of valuable time to perform, thus predisposing the patient to hemorrhage.

4 Correct answer—**C**

An IVP will ensure that at least one kidney is functioning should a nephrectomy be necessary. An abdominal X-ray, peritoneal lavage, and a CT scan do not provide information on renal function.

5 Correct answer—**D**

Predicting the direction a bullet takes once it enters the abdomen is impossible, so penetration of the liver, transverse colon, or stomach may occur.

6 Correct answer—**D**

The I.V. lines will provide access for administration of fluids and blood products. The NG tube will empty the stomach and relieve distention. The Foley catheter will empty the bladder and provide a means by which to measure hourly urine output; less than 30 ml/hour is an indicator of shock.

7 Correct answer—**A**

Clinical signs of hypovolemic shock, especially tachycardia and orthostatic hypotension, usually develop after blood loss of 15% occurs. Hypotension is significant after loss of 25% of blood volume. Once 40% to 50% of blood volume is lost, irreversible shock occurs.

8 Correct answer—**B**

Injuries that penetrate the surface of the skin, except abrasions or lacerations, and are not caused by blunt trauma are classified as penetrating.

9 Correct answer—**D**

Paralytic ileus, shock, anxiety, respiratory difficulty, and severe upper abdominal pain radiating to the shoulders are clinical manifestations of perforated gastric ulcer. This radiating pain is caused by irritation of the diaphragm and phrenic nerves.

10 Correct answer—**C**

Chemical peritonitis is caused by a rapid escape of gastric and intestinal contents after perforation. Peritonitis is an inflammation of a portion or all of the parietal and visceral surfaces of the abdominal cavity. The primary response of the peritoneum to injury includes edema in the subperitoneal tissues, hypermotility of the bowel, and an outpouring of plasmalike fluid from the extracellular, vascular, and interstitial compartments into the peritoneal space.

11 Correct answer—**B**

Perforation of a duodenal ulcer with ensuing peritonitis erodes the wall of the pancreas, causing pancreatitis.

12 Correct answer—**C**

Duodenal ulcers perforate most commonly. Approximately 80% of ulcers are duodenal and 20% are gastric. Duodenal ulcers usually occur in patients age 30 to 50; gastric ulcers are commonly seen in later years.

13 Correct answer—**A**

Surgical intervention is indicated in life-threatening emergencies, such as perforation, acute obstruction, and acute intractable hemorrhage. The other treatments may be used in less serious illnesses.

14 Correct answer—**A**

The most common cause of pancreatitis is excessive alcohol intake, which has either a direct toxic effect of the pancreas or causes back-up of pancreatic juices into the pancreas. Biliary tract disease, another common cause of pancreatitis, includes disorders such as biliary stones in the ampulla of Vater, which cause pancreatic duct obstruction with build-up of pancreatic juices, and cholecystitis, which results in a reflux of bile components into the pancreatic duct. These irritating, altered substances cause a chemical inflammation.

Decreasing fat intake and reducing stress can help reduce symptoms, but fat intake and stress are not necessarily implicated as causal factors. Heredity is not a causal factor.

15 Correct answer—**D**

Jaundice is caused by common bile duct obstruction as a result of pancreatic edema. Shock develops when trypsin, in the inflammatory fluid that is spilled into the peritoneum, activates kinin, a vasodilator. Hemorrhage occurs when activated elastase dissolves the fibers of surrounding blood vessels. Pain results from distention of the pancreatic capsule, ductal spasm, or increased secretion of enzymes after eating.

16 Correct answer—**B**

Within a few hours after onset of acute pancreatitis, the serum amylase level rises and remains elevated for about 3 days. After 24 hours, the serum lipase level will also rise and remain elevated for up to 10 days.

17 Correct answer—**C**

Demerol is the drug of choice. Morphine and its opiate derivatives increase spasm of Oddi's sphincter. Tylenol with codeine and Percodan are probably not strong enough to relieve the severe pain associated with acute pancreatitis.

18 Correct answer—**D**

Colloids and electrolyte solutions are volume expanders that combat shock. The CVP and urine output should be monitored hourly to assess impending shock and its treatment. Calcium gluconate corrects the hypocalcemia that commonly occurs in acute pancreatitis.

19 Correct answer—**A**

Bacterial organisms readily multiply in necrotic tissue; therefore, a broad-spectrum antibiotic, such as ampicillin (Amcill) or gentamicin (Garamgem), commonly is indicated.

20 Correct answer—**A**

A low-fat, no-alcohol diet will avoid pancreatic stimulation. Avoiding caffeine will prevent stimulation of gastric acid secretion, which activates pancreatic activity.

21 Correct answer—**A**

Rovsing's sign, pain in the right lower abdominal quadrant that is intensified by left lower abdominal quadrant pressure, is present in acute appendicitis. Also, temperature is usually slightly elevated (99° to 101° F. [37.2° to 38.3° C.]) and moderate leukocytosis (elevation in the white blood cell [WBC] count) exists. These symptoms occur in about 60% of patients. The patient may also have anorexia, nausea, and vomiting. Abdominal distention and audible borborygmi are associated with bowel obstruction.

22 Correct answer—**C**

Narcotics, which may mask important signs and symptoms, are not given until the cause of the pain has been determined and a decision regarding surgery has been made. Appropriate nursing interventions include monitoring rectal temperature and WBC count, obtaining blood cultures, administering antipyretics and antibiotics as ordered, administering an I.V. infusion of lactated Ringer's or normal saline solution, and inserting a gastric tube for suction.

23 Correct answer—**A**

Young children have difficulty describing symptoms; therefore, complications occur more commonly than in older children or adults. Also, the abdominal omentum is not well developed in children. If the appendix perforates, peritonitis can easily develop because the infection cannot be walled off as quickly as in adults.

24 Correct answer—**D**

In children age 2 and older, inflammation with infection of the vermiform appendix is one of the most common conditions requiring surgery. It is rare in infants, and boys are affected more commonly than girls. Pain is always present, so any child with persistent abdominal pain should be suspected of having appendicitis and should be evaluated. Diarrhea is the primary cause of dehydration in children.

25 Correct answer—**B**

Some abdominal organs are more likely to be injured than others. The frequency of which organ is involved depends largely on how the injury is produced and its location. The frequency of organ injury in abdominal trauma is as follows: spleen, kidneys, intestines, liver, and then pancreas.

26 Correct answer—**C**

An isotonic solution, such as lactated Ringer's or normal saline solution, is administered intravenously. This solution maintains the same osmotic pressure as blood serum; therefore, cellular constituents remain unchanged. To restore circulatory dynamics, fluid replacement is essential in blunt abdominal injury with suspected trauma to internal organs. Thus, blood volume is maintained until surgery can be performed.

27 Correct answer—**C**

Peritoneal lavage is contraindicated in patients who have a history of many abdominal operations. Adhesions increase the likelihood that the bowel will be penetrated and that the lavage fluid will be trapped, making its return difficult. Peritoneal lavage is also contraindicated in pregnant patients, because of possible damage to the fetus. This procedure is not contraindicated in unconscious patients or in those having a history of a single operative procedure, such as a colostomy.

28 Correct answer—**A**

The spleen is injured more often than any other abdominal organ. It is located in the left upper abdominal quadrant, under the diaphragm, and near the abdominal wall. The spleen is partly protected by the lower left ribs and cannot be palpated until triple its normal size. Kehr's sign, referred pain to the left shoulder from blood irritating the diaphragm, is evident in 50% of patients. The danger of splenic injury is directly related to the fact that the spleen is the most vascular organ in the body. Splenic lacerations and ruptured hematomas are notorious sources of persistent bleeding into the peritoneal cavity.

29 Correct answer—**A**

The hallmarks of intestinal obstruction are abdominal pain, distention, vomiting, and prolonged constipation (obstipation). All four signs and symptoms are not necessarily present in every case, and the severity varies with the level and type of obstruction. When an obstruction is high in the small intestine, copious vomiting appears early, with minimal abdominal distention. When obstruction is low in the colon, distention is marked but vomiting may not occur at all. Constipation may be overlooked because the patient may have two or three bowel movements early in its initial stages, until the bowel, distal to the point of obstruction, is evacuated. On physical examination, bowel sounds typically are high-pitched and occur in rushes. The abdomen is usually distended but is not tender unless the bowel is ischemic.

30 Correct answer—**C**

The primary cause of large-bowel obstruction in an adult is carcinoma. Diverticulitis is the second most common cause, with volvulus the third. Cancer of the colon and rectum accounts for more than 50,000 deaths annually—the second highest death rate in the United States for any type of cancer. Men are affected more commonly than women. The highest incidence occurs in people about age 50. The 5-year survival rate is 40% to 50%, the best of the visceral cancers.

31 Correct answer—**C**

Shock is a condition in which effective circulating blood volume decreases; inadequate organ and tissue perfusion result and lead to derangements of cellular function. Clinical manifestations include decreasing arterial pressure (systolic pressure falls more rapidly than diastolic), tachycardia, cold and clammy skin, circumoral pallor, alterations of mental status, and suppression of kidney function.

32 Correct answer—**C**

Although all four examination techniques are utilized, the order is inspection, auscultation, percussion, and palpation. Auscultation precedes percussion and palpation to prevent distortion of auscultatory findings related to pressure on the abdominal wall. Percussion precedes palpation to screen for an enlarged spleen before deep palpation. The necessary equipment is a stethoscope, flexible tape measure, and wrist watch.

33 Correct answer—**D**

Acute GI bleeding is a potentially life-threatening condition that requires immediate assessment of extent and source. Determining the cause of bleeding relies on physical clues, the patient's history, and the physical examination. Once it has been determined that the patient is not in shock, concise information pertaining to the patient's past and present health history must be collected. A history and subsequent physical examination will help to identify the sequence of events that led the patient to seek aid, the character of bleeding, history of previous bleeding, associated symptoms or diseases, and drug use.

34 Correct answer—**B**

Hematemesis, the vomiting of gross blood, is most commonly caused by peptic ulcers (80%), gastric and duodenal ulcers (20%), bleeding esophageal varices (5% to 10%), and gastric carcinoma (3%).

35 Correct answer—**D**

Anticholinergic agents, such as atropine, methantheline (Banthine), and propantheline (Pro-Banthine), are administered to suppress gastric secretions and to delay gastric emptying by blocking the effects of vagal nerve impulses on smooth muscle. Sedatives are usually administered with anticholinergics to decrease the patient's level of responsiveness. Histamine (H_2)-receptor antagonists, such as cimetidine (Tagamet) and ranitidine (Zantac), inhibit the action of histamine, which causes gastric acid secretion.

36 Correct answer—**B**

Esophageal varices are dilated tortuous veins found in the submucosa of the lower esophagus that may extend throughout the esophagus and into the stomach. These varices are nearly always caused by portal hypertension, which results from obstruction of the portal venous circulation and/or cirrhosis of the liver (from excessive use of alcohol). Abnormalities of the circulation within the splenic vein or superior vena cava are lesser-known causes of esophageal varices. Overuse of alcohol, tobacco, and spicy foods can lead to esophageal carcinoma, but none of these is directly associated with varices.

37 Correct answer—**D**

The Sengstaken-Blakemore tube has gastric and esophageal balloons that can be inflated to control esophageal bleeding. During use, the head of the bed must remain slightly elevated, unless the patient is in shock. Elevation helps to avoid gastric regurgitation and to diminish nausea and a sense of gagging. Another potential complication is airway obstruction from migration of the esophageal balloon into the trachea. If this occurs, the balloons should be deflated immediately by cutting the tube with scissors, and the tube should be removed.

38 Correct answer—**B**

The three most common causes of upper GI bleeding are peptic ulcer, acute mucosal lesions (resulting from gastritis, esophagitis, or Mallory-Weiss tears), and esophageal or gastric varices.

39 Correct answer—**D**

If the clinical findings suggest the lower bowel is the source of bleeding, proctoscopy should be the first diagnostic procedure. Proctoscopy will determine if the bleeding is from the rectosigmoid colon, rectum, or anal canal. Bleeding lesions commonly identified by proctoscopy include diffuse mucosal lesions, such as ulcerative and ischemic colitis; local vascular lesions, such as hemorrhoids; and tumors, such as polyps or cancer.

40 Correct answer—**D**

The treatment for ED patients with lower GI bleeding depends on the extent and type of bleeding. If bleeding is caused by hemorrhoids or fissures, emergency admission is rarely necessary, and the patient may be referred to an outpatient clinic. If the bleeding is overt and from polyps, carcinoma, or ulcerative colitis, blood replacement may be necessary.

41 Correct answer—**D**

Skin color is an unreliable index of the degree of anemia because of wide individual variations in the amount of melanin in the skin. When the amount of hemoglobin has been significantly reduced, the nail beds or palms will reveal anemia, unless the hand has been held in an awkward position or has been exposed to extreme cold or heat.

42 Correct answer—**B**

With hemorrhoids, the most common cause, bleeding usually occurs intermittently and produces small amounts of bright-red blood on the outside of formed stool or on toilet tissue. Massive bleeding rarely occurs. Bleeding from the colon is much less common than from the stomach or duodenum; however, the blood loss may be abrupt. Perirectal diseases, such as hemorrhoids, fissures, diverticulitis, and tumors, usually result in lower GI bleeding.

43 Correct answer—**D**

Although endoscopy is a very useful tool for identifying the specific cause of upper GI bleeding, it is contraindicated in some situations. The risk of perforation or aspiration is greater in patients who are uncooperative or unresponsive, or who have esophageal obstruction. The endoscope increases airway resistance and may cause cardiac dysrhythmias. However, these are relative contraindications; that is, if emergency surgery is being considered to control bleeding, important information that aids the surgeon in the proper approach can be rapidly obtained. Thus, surgical morbidity will be reduced.

44 Correct answer—**B**

The ligament of Treitz at the duodenojejunal junction is considered the dividing point for upper and lower GI bleeding.

45 Correct answer—**B**

If the patient's blood pressure drops or tachycardia secondary to hemorrhage develops, rapid fluid and blood replacement will be needed.

46 Correct answer—**A**

The earliest response to shock is tachycardia, a compensatory mechanism initiated by the sympathetic nervous system in an attempt to maintain cardiac output and organ perfusion. Later signs include a narrowing pulse pressure, which indicates a falling cardiac output, followed by hypotension and cool, clammy skin.

47 Correct answer—**B**

Further diagnostic testing is needed to determine whether there is internal bleeding. This may be accomplished by either CT scan or peritoneal lavage, depending on physician preference. Neither an immediate operation nor blood replacement is warranted at this time.

48 Correct answer—**D**

Hemorrhage from retroperitoneal structures does not cause bleeding into the abdominal compartment; hence, a false-negative lavage result may occur. A negative lavage yields less than 100,000 red blood cells (RBCs)/mm^3 in the drainage. After injury to the spleen, diaphragm, or bladder (all located in the abdominal cavity), bloody drainage is obtained.

49 Correct answer—**B**

Peritoneal lavage may injure structures and organs of a child. Children are usually observed for clinical change and a drop in hematocrit.

50 Correct answer—**D**

Blood at the meatus, a high-riding prostate on rectal examination, and hematuria all indicate trauma to the genitourinary system. An IVP or abdominal CT scan may be necessary to diagnose the specific site of damage.

51 Correct answer—**C**

The spleen is located in the left upper abdominal quadrant and is the organ injured most commonly in abdominal trauma. It is a highly vascular organ, and trauma may result in intrasplenic bleeding; thus, a large mass may be palpated in the left upper abdominal quadrant. A normal spleen cannot be palpated. The liver is located in the right upper abdominal quadrant. Damage to the small intestine or colon usually is associated with lower quadrant injuries.

Selected References

Brunner, L.S., and Suddarth, D.S. *Textbook of Medical-Surgical Nursing,* 5th ed. Philadelphia: J.B. Lippincott Co., 1984.

Burns, K.R., and Johnson, P.J. *Health Assessment in Clinical Practice.* Englewood Cliffs, N.J.: Prentice-Hall, 1980.

Chalfin, L.M. "Tricks of the Trade," *Emergency Medicine.* April 30, 1986.

Crowley, R., and Dunham, C.M. *Shock-Trauma Critical Care Manual.* Baltimore: University Park Press, 1982.

Lanros, N.E. *Assessment and Intervention in Emergency Nursing.* Bowie, Md.: Robert J. Brady Co., 1979.

Luckmann, J., and Sorensen, K. *Medical-Surgical Nursing—A Psychophysiological Approach,* 2nd ed. Philadephia: W.B. Saunders Co., 1980.

Orr, M.E. *Acute Pancreatic and Hepatic Dysfunction.* New York: John Wiley & Sons, 1984.

Shires, G.T. *Care of the Trauma Patient,* 2nd ed. New York: McGraw-Hill Book Co., 1979.

Strange, J.M. "The Riddle of Abdominal Trauma," *RN* 46:42-49,98,100, March 1983.

Trunkey, D.D., and Lewis, F.R. *Current Therapy of Trauma—2.* Philadelphia: B.C. Decker, 1986.

Chapter 13

Hematologic Emergencies Questions and Answers

You must begin with Question 1 of this chapter and progress in sequence. **Do not skip around.** Subsequent answers build on previous ones.

Patricia Robertazza, RN, MSN, CCRN
Susan Weaver, RN, MSN, CCRN, CEN

SITUATION

A 70-year-old man was admitted to the hospital with a diagnosis of pulmonary embolism. The patient was treated with heparin; he was discharged on warfarin (Coumadin) therapy after the pulmonary embolism was resolved. After the patient had been home for 2 months, he became confused and ingested 100 mg of warfarin. He now is readmitted with hematemesis and bright-red rectal bleeding.

Questions 1 to 5 refer to the above situation.

1 During the initial assessment of this patient, signs and symptoms the emergency department (ED) nurse should be particularly alert for include:

A. Facial flushing
B. Petechiae
C. Pruritus
D. Hypertension

2 During long-term anticoagulant therapy, serious hemorrhagic complications occur most commonly in the:

A. Gastrointestinal (GI) tract
B. Genitourinary tract
C. Respiratory system
D. Capillary vasculature

3 Which therapy should *not* be implemented for the patient with hemorrhagic complications from oral anticoagulants?

A. Volume replacement
B. Whole blood
C. Fresh frozen plasma
D. Protamine sulfate

4 The nurse should teach the patient receiving anticoagulant therapy to:

A. Avoid excessive alcohol intake
B. Avoid electric shaver use
C. Avoid using soft-bristled toothbrushes
D. Trim corns and calluses weekly

5 What should nursing care of the patient receiving heparin therapy include?

A. Observe for hypertensive crisis and hematemesis
B. Monitor prothrombin time (PT) to maintain therapeutic level of anticoagulant
C. Test urine and stool for blood
D. Administer aspirin for leg pain as needed

6 When administering subcutaneous heparin, which action is considered *unsafe*?

A. Change injection site with each dose
B. Use the iliac crest or abdominal fat layer for injection sites
C. Massage the area after injection to facilitate absorption
D. Observe for bleeding at injection sites

7 Which statement regarding heparin administration is *true*?

A. Partial thromboplastin time (PTT) must be checked after each dose
B. Larger heparin doses are required during continuous infusion
C. Major bleeding episodes are more frequent with continuous intravenous (I.V.) infusion than with intermittent I.V. infusion
D. The drip rate must be accurately calculated and controlled

SITUATION

A 4-year-old boy is admitted because of a sudden high fever. His mother notes that he has been generally weak and dyspneic and has had generalized pain and recurrent infections. He is found to have an elevated white blood cell (WBC) count and to be anemic, as well as being thrombocytopenic and tachycardic. A diagnosis of acute lymphocytic leukemia is made.

Questions 8 to 11 refer to the above situation.

8 Acute lymphocytic leukemia is *uncommon* after how many years of age?

A. 20
B. 30
C. 40
D. 50

9 A common complication in the acute phase of leukemia is:

A. Thrombocytosis
B. Polycythemia vera
C. Gram-negative septicemia
D. Seizures

10 Temperature elevations in the leukemic patient should be treated with:

A. Aspirin
B. Acetaminophen (Tylenol)
C. Azathioprine (Imuran)
D. Antibiotics

11 Chemotherapy is used to treat leukemia because it:

A. Destroys abnormal leukemic cells
B. Causes bone marrow recovery
C. Increases the patient's immunologic defense mechanisms
D. Produces granulocytosis

SITUATION

A 17-year-old girl is admitted to the ED 10 days after an abortion. She continues to have heavy bleeding and lower abdominal pain. The physician suspects retained products of conception. While she is in the ED, her laboratory studies reveal a prolonged PTT and PT. A diagnosis of disseminated intravascular coagulation (DIC) is made.

Questions 12 to 16 refer to the above situation.

12 The most significant clinical feature of DIC is:

A. Hemoptysis
B. Petechiae
C. Abnormal bleeding
D. Hematuria

13 Bleeding may be observed from:

A. Mucous membranes
B. Venipuncture sites
C. GI tract
D. All of the above

14 Which obstetric incident leads to the development of DIC?

A. Thromboembolism, resulting from bed rest and microemboli formation
B. Placental and fetal tissue activating the clotting mechanism
C. Fetal enzyme release, resulting in hemolysis of red blood cells (RBCs)
D. Normal thrombocytopenic state accompanying pregnancy

15 Which statement does *not* support the rationale for heparin administration in the treatment of DIC?

A. The antithrombin activity of heparin neutralizes free-circulating thrombin
B. Heparin permits normalization of clotting test results
C. Heparin prevents fibrinogenesis
D. Heparin increases hemorrhage manifestations

16 An *inappropriate* nursing action in the care of the patient with DIC is:

A. Early recognition of abnormal bleeding
B. Prevention of further bleeding
C. Complete bed rest during bleeding episodes
D. Gentle scrubbing of bleeding areas

SITUATION

A 10-year-old boy is brought into the ED after injuring his right knee when he fell from his bicycle. He is known to have hemophilia A and presents symptoms indicating hemarthrosis of the right knee.

Questions 17 to 21 refer to the above situation.

17 Hemophilia A and hemophilia B are bleeding disorders that are indistinguishable clinically but may be separated by laboratory studies. Which is a true statement about these disorders?

A. Hemophilia B is caused by a deficiency of Factor VIII
B. Hemophilia A is caused by a deficiency of Factor IX
C. Hemophilia A is more common than hemophilia B
D. Almost all of the individuals with hemophilia A are female

18 Hemarthrosis, especially of the knees, elbows, and ankles, is a common finding in hemophilia. Other signs and symptoms include:

A. Bruising and bleeding gums
B. Neuropathy and paresthesia
C. Pain and hematuria
D. All of the above

19 The most common cause of death in the hemophiliac patient occurs from bleeding in which site?

A. GI tract
B. Heart
C. Cranium
D. Larynx

20 Diagnosis is based upon the bleeding pattern of the patient, family history, and the physical examination. Laboratory studies will indicate:

A. Factor VIII or Factor IX deficiency
B. Prolonged PT and PTT
C. Increased fibrinogen level
D. Decreased platelet count

21 Priority nursing care of this patient should include all of the following *except*:

A. Immobilizing the right leg
B. Stopping local bleeding
C. Preventing deformity
D. Assisting with immediate aspiration of hemarthrosis

SITUATION

A 40-year-old man with a history of alcohol abuse is admitted to the ED with hematemesis. His blood pressure is 88/56 mm Hg; temperature, 99° F. (37.2° C.); hemoglobin, 8.4 g/dl; and hematocrit, 24%.

Questions 22 to 25 refer to the above situation.

22 This patient's blood is typed and cross-matched for transfusion; his type is designated as group AB. Which statement is *true* of this blood group?

A. The antibodies located in the plasma are A and B
B. The antigens located in the plasma are A and B
C. The antigens located on the red cell membrane are A and B
D. This blood group possesses neither A nor B antigens

23 Packed RBCs are recommended for transfusion. Which statement is *true* regarding packed RBCs and whole blood?

A. Both packed cells and whole blood cause the hemoglobin and hematocrit to increase at the same rate
B. Fresh packed cells provide all the necessary blood components, including platelets and coagulation factors
C. Packed cells decrease the risk of hepatitis transmission
D. Packed cells are indicated for massive hemorrhage and hypovolemia

24 The nurse who administers the transfusion of packed RBCs to this patient must be cognizant of standard transfusion practices. Which statement is *true*?

A. Lactated Ringer's and normal saline are the solutions that may be used when administering blood products
B. During a blood transfusion, it is necessary to assess the patient's vital signs only before and after the transfusion
C. When using a blood warmer, the temperature should not exceed 103.1° F. (38.5° C.)
D. 18- or 20-gauge catheters may be used when administering a blood transfusion

25 One hour after the transfusion has been initiated, the patient complains of chills and headache. His vital signs are checked, and his temperature has increased to 103.1° F. (38.5° C.). This patient most likely is experiencing a:

A. Febrile, nonhemolytic transfusion reaction
B. Hemolytic transfusion reaction
C. Delayed hemolytic transfusion reaction
D. Bacterial transfusion reaction

SITUATION

A 60-year-old man with thrombocytopenia is admitted to the ED because of rectal bleeding.

Questions 26 and 27 refer to the above situation.

26 Which would not cause thrombocytopenia?

A. Chlorothiazide therapy
B. Quinidine (Quinaglute) therapy
C. Splenectomy
D. Viral infection

27 When will the platelet count return to normal following the discontinuation of quinidine therapy in a thrombocytopenic patient?

A. 24 hours
B. 72 hours
C. 1 week
D. 2 weeks

SITUATION

A 28-year-old black man with a history of sickle-cell disease is admitted to the ED. During assessment, the following symptoms are noted: severe pain in abdomen and back, aching joint pain, fever, and dyspnea.

Questions 28 to 31 refer to the above situation.

28 All of the following are forms of sickle-cell crisis *except*:

A. Aplastic crisis
B. Sequestration crisis
C. Painful crisis
D. Anemic crisis

29 This crisis may have been precipitated by any of the following factors *except*:

A. Cigarette smoking
B. Infection
C. Increased fluid intake
D. A strenuous game of tennis

30 One aspect of treatment for this patient in sickle-cell crisis involves hydration, which may be achieved by:

A. Inserting the smallest-possible-gauge I.V. catheter and infusing dextrose 5% in 1/2 normal saline solution ($D_5$1/2NS) at 100 ml/hour
B. Inserting a large-gauge I.V. catheter and infusing normal saline solution at 150 ml/hour
C. Inserting a large-gauge I.V. catheter and infusing lactated Ringer's solution at 300 ml/hour
D. Having the patient drink 4 to 6 quarts (3.8 to 5.7 liters) of liquid in the next 24 hours

31 Providing analgesia for this patient in a painful crisis is another critical aspect of treatment in the ED. All of the following medications are recommended for analgesia, *except*:

A. Meperidine (Demerol)
B. Morphine sulfate
C. Aspirin
D. Codeine

Answer Sheet

	A	B	C	D		A	B	C	D
1	○	○	○	○	31	○	○	○	○
2	○	○	○	○					
3	○	○	○	○					
4	○	○	○	○					
5	○	○	○	○					
6	○	○	○	○					
7	○	○	○	○					
8	○	○	○	○					
9	○	○	○	○					
10	○	○	○	○					
11	○	○	○	○					
12	○	○	○	○					
13	○	○	○	○					
14	○	○	○	○					
15	○	○	○	○					
16	○	○	○	○					
17	○	○	○	○					
18	○	○	○	○					
19	○	○	○	○					
20	○	○	○	○					
21	○	○	○	○					
22	○	○	○	○					
23	○	○	○	○					
24	○	○	○	○					
25	○	○	○	○					
26	○	○	○	○					
27	○	○	○	○					
28	○	○	○	○					
29	○	○	○	○					
30	○	○	○	○					

Answer Sheet

	A	B	C	D		A	B	C	D
1	○	○	○	○	31	○	○	○	○
2	○	○	○	○					
3	○	○	○	○					
4	○	○	○	○					
5	○	○	○	○					
6	○	○	○	○					
7	○	○	○	○					
8	○	○	○	○					
9	○	○	○	○					
10	○	○	○	○					
11	○	○	○	○					
12	○	○	○	○					
13	○	○	○	○					
14	○	○	○	○					
15	○	○	○	○					
16	○	○	○	○					
17	○	○	○	○					
18	○	○	○	○					
19	○	○	○	○					
20	○	○	○	○					
21	○	○	○	○					
22	○	○	○	○					
23	○	○	○	○					
24	○	○	○	○					
25	○	○	○	○					
26	○	○	○	○					
27	○	○	○	○					
28	○	○	○	○					
29	○	○	○	○					
30	○	○	○	○					

1 Correct answer—**B**

Signs and symptoms of anticoagulant overdose include petechiae, tachycardia, hypotension, hematuria, epistaxis, bleeding gums, ecchymoses, tarry stools, and coffee-grounds vomitus.

2 Correct answer—**A**

During long-term therapy, serious hemorrhagic complications occur intracranially and in the GI tract. Bleeding in these sites accounts for 90% of serious hemorrhagic episodes. GI hemorrhage is most commonly associated with underlying lesions (e.g., ulcers). Minor bleeding is caused by capillary rupture and may include epistaxis and hematuria. Genitourinary and pulmonary bleeding are rare and may occur after instrumentation.

3 Correct answer—**D**

Protamine sulfate neutralizes the effects of parenteral anticoagulant heparin and is used to treat heparin overdose. Therapy for hemorrhagic complications from oral anticoagulants includes volume replacement, clotting factor replacement, vitamin K administration, and infusions of fresh frozen plasma and whole blood. Vitamin K acts as a pharmacologic antagonist to oral anticoagulants and may be given orally or parenterally.

4 Correct answer—**A**

Excessive alcohol intake should be avoided. Patients on anticoagulant therapy should also be cautioned to wear gloves while gardening, to use an electric shaver rather than straight-edged blades, and to use soft-bristled toothbrushes. Medical identification bracelets should be worn, and corns or calluses should not be trimmed.

5 Correct answer—**C**

Urine and stool should be checked for blood. The patient should also be observed for other signs and symptoms of GI hemorrhage, including tachycardia, hypotension, and hematemesis. The partial thromboplastin time (PTT) should be monitored to maintain therapeutic anticoagulation. The therapeutic range should be 1.5 to 2.5 times the patient's control. Warfarin anticoagulation is monitored by PT. Aspirin should be avoided because it aggravates bleeding tendencies.

6 Correct answer—**C**

Injection sites should not be massaged before or after injection. Optimal sites for subcutaneous administration of heparin include the iliac crest and abdominal fat layer; use of these sites will minimize trauma. Sites should be changed to prevent massive hematoma and should be observed for prolonged bleeding.

7 Correct answer—**D**

The disadvantage of continuous administration is that the drip rate must be accurately calculated and controlled. Intermittent infusion requires larger doses and frequent injections. The PTT must be checked just before the next scheduled dose. Major bleeding episodes occur more commonly with intermittent I.V. infusion than with continuous I.V. infusion.

8 Correct answer—**A**

Acute lymphocytic leukemia is a disease of young children and is uncommon after age 20. Children between ages 2 and 5 years account for approximately 80% of all cases.

9 Correct answer—**C**

The major causes of death in acute leukemia are infection and bleeding from anemia, and thrombocytopenia. Infection is commonly caused by gram-negative sepsis. Frequent cultures are necessary, and treatment with appropriate antibiotics is required. The patient may require placement in a protected environment. Seizures are rare.

10 Correct answer—**B**

Fever may be the most important sign of infection; judicious use of analgesic and antipyretic medications is appropriate. Granulocytosis and inflammation are commonly absent. Bleeding is another major complication; therefore, aspirin must be used cautiously because of its antiplatelet activity and the risk of Reye's syndrome.

11 Correct answer—**A**

Chemotherapy destroys abnormal leukemic cells, causes bone marrow depression, and depresses the patient's immunologic defense mechanisms. Chemotherapy produces granulocytopenia, so the patient must be observed for the first signs of infection.

12 Correct answer—**C**

The most significant clinical feature of DIC is abnormal bleeding such as hemoptysis, petechiae, or hematuria, without history of a serious bleeding disorder. Other signs and symptoms include a prolonged PT, a prolonged PTT, decreased fibrinogen levels, decreased platelet count, increased fibrin degradation products, and an elevated blood urea nitrogen (BUN) level.

13 Correct answer—**D**

Bleeding may occur from mucous membranes, venipuncture sites, and the GI and genitourinary tracts. Widespread clotting occurs in small blood vessels, leading to the consumption of clotting factors as well as platelets, which then leads to a bleeding disorder.

14 Correct answer—**B**

Obstetric incidents leading to the development of DIC are caused by activation of the clotting mechanism via fetal and placental tissue. In pregnancy, a normally hypercoagulable state, amniotic fluid causes clot-promoting activities. However, dead fetal and placental tissues also cause clot-promoting activities, and clots may be released into the maternal circulation in such conditions as retained dead fetus and abruptio placentae. In these conditions, the incidence of DIC approaches 50%. Treatment involves blood factor replacements and removal of fetal material.

15 Correct answer—**D**

Because heparin therapy retards the coagulation process, it will decrease hemorrhagic manifestations and also will permit normalization of clotting test results. Its antithrombin activity neutralizes free-circulating thrombin, thus preventing proliferation of thrombin and further blood clotting.

16 Correct answer—**D**

Bleeding areas should not be scrubbed, which could dislodge clots and cause fresh bleeding. Care of the patient with DIC includes early recognition of abnormal bleeding, treatment of underlying disorders, and prevention of further bleeding. Pressure, cold compresses, and topical hemostatic agents may be used to control bleeding. Protecting the patient from injury includes placing her on complete bed rest during bleeding episodes. All I.V. and venipuncture sites should be checked for at least 10 minutes. Also observe for bleeding from the GI and genitourinary tracts.

17 Correct answer—**C**

Hemophilia A (a deficiency of Factor VIII) is five times more common than hemophilia B (a deficiency of Factor IX). Both types are inherited as X-linked traits; therefore, almost all affected individuals are male. Their mothers and some of their sisters may be carriers, but remain asymptomatic.

18 Correct answer—**D**

Bleeding near peripheral nerves causes neuropathy, pain, paresthesia, and muscle atrophy. Bleeding gums and hematuria, unrelated to trauma, are very common. Abnormal bleeding occurs through the absence or deficiency of a specific clotting factor. About one-half of all hemophiliacs have severe, spontaneous bleeding into joints. This can lead to crippling and deformity.

19 Correct answer—**C**

The most common cause of death is intracranial hemorrhage. Shock and death occur as a result of intracranial and intracerebral bleeding. Other areas of bleeding include the GI and genitourinary tracts, as well as pharyngeal and intracardiac hemorrhage.

20 Correct answer—**A**

Laboratory studies will indicate a Factor VIII or IX deficiency, a prolonged PTT, normal PT, normal fibrinogen level, and normal platelet count. Von Willebrand's disease has a deficiency in Factor VIII and platelet dysfunction. This is an autosomal disease that occurs in both sexes.

21 Correct answer—**D**

Hemarthroses are not aspirated unless acute pain and pressure are present, because aspiration may cause additional bleeding and carries the risk of introducing infection. Treatment is aimed at preventing crippling deformities while also prolonging life expectancy. Joint bleeding is initially managed by immobilization of the affected limb and application of ice packs to diminish swelling and reduce pain. The plasma level of the deficient factor must be raised. An immediate infusion of cryoprecipitate (factors VIII, XIII, and fibrinogen) may be necessary. Hemarthroses are not seen in von Willebrand's disease.

22 Correct answer—**C**

The antigens located on the red cell membrane are A and B. The four main blood groups of the ABO system are A, B, AB, and O. The antigens for this system are located on the red cell membrane and are the same as the blood group. The antibodies of the ABO system are located in the serum. These antibodies do not correspond to the antigens on the red cell membrane, since antibodies cannot be produced against the present antigens. The table below lists the antigens and antibodies of the ABO system.

BLOOD GROUP	RED CELL ANTIGEN	SERUM ANTIBODY
A	B	B
B	AB	A
AB (Universal Recipient)	—	—
O (Universal Donor)	A	AB

23 Correct answer—**C**

Packed RBCs decrease the risk of hepatitis transmission. A unit of whole blood, which contains all the necessary blood components, including platelets and coagulation factors, is centrifuged to separate the RBCs from the plasma. The packed cells consist of the same RBC mass as whole blood with only small amounts of plasma, leukocytes, and platelets. Because only a small amount of plasma is present, the risk of hepatitis and plasma protein reaction decreases. A transfusion of packed RBCs causes the hemoglobin and hematocrit levels to rise faster than a whole blood transfusion does. In the average patient, the hemoglobin rises 1 g/dl, and the hematocrit rises 2% to 3%. With a whole blood transfusion, a similar increase will be seen; however, it will occur 24 hours after administration. Packed RBCs restore or maintain oxygen-carrying capacity and are indicated in anemia or surgical blood loss or to increase RBC mass. Whole blood is indicated when massive hemorrhage is present.

24 Correct answer—**D**

When administering blood transfusions, 18- or 20-gauge catheters may be used. To prevent hemolysis, 18-gauge catheters are recommended for most blood transfusions. However, 20-gauge catheters are acceptable for average transfusion rates. Only normal saline solution may be used when administering blood products. Lactated Ringer's solution causes agglutination, and dextrose 5% in water (D_5W) causes hemolysis. During a blood transfusion, the patient's vital signs should be assessed before initiation of the transfusion, 15 minutes after initiation, and after completion of the transfusion. Assessing the vital signs at these times enables the nurse to detect any adverse effects. It is particularly important to assess the vital signs 15 minutes after the initiation of the transfusion, because this is when most severe reactions occur. When using a blood warmer, the temperature should not exceed 98.6° F. (37° C.). Red blood cells heated above 37° C. may hemolyze.

25 Correct answer—**A**

Febrile, nonhemolytic transfusion reactions are the most common of the immediate reactions. Signs and symptoms include fever, chills, headache, hypotension, lumbar pain, palpitations, and malaise. The fever usually occurs 1 to 6 hours after the transfusion has been initiated. This reaction typically occurs in patients who have received multiple transfusions. The hemolytic transfusion reaction is the most acute and the most dreaded adverse effect of a transfusion. This reaction occurs because of ABO blood group incompatibility. The signs and symptoms develop immediately and include fever that may exceed 104.9° F. (40.5° C.), facial flushing, chills, lumbar pain, hypotension, headache, chest pain, dyspnea, oliguria, and shock. A bacterial transfusion reaction is rare and is caused by bacterial contamination of the blood product. The signs and symptoms are high fever, severe hypotension, dry flushed skin, pain in the abdomen and extremities, vomiting, and bloody diarrhea. The delayed hemolytic transfusion reaction will occur 2 or more days after a transfusion. This reaction typically occurs in patients who have received previous transfusions. The signs and symptoms include continued anemia, decreased hemoglobin level, hemoglobinuria, and bilirubinuria.

26 Correct answer—**C**

A splenectomy would cause the platelet count to increase. This thrombocytosis is attributed to the fact that the spleen collects one-third of all the platelets, and its removal eliminates the site of platelet antibody production, thus decreasing platelet destruction. Chlorothiazide and quinidine therapy may cause thrombocytopenia because of platelet antibody formation. Additionally, chlorothiazide suppresses thrombocyte production. Viral infections may cause thrombocytopenia, because the virus can actually destroy circulating platelets. Viral infections may also impair platelet production.

27 Correct answer—**C**

As soon as quinidine therapy is stopped, a normal platelet count will be restored within 1 week. One in 100,000 persons taking quinidine develops this idiosyncratic reaction of platelet antibody formation, with the resultant thrombocytopenia. Within 12 hours after quinidine therapy is started, thrombocytopenia may develop. When the therapy is halted, thrombocytopenia recedes within 24 hours. A normal platelet count and even mild thrombocytosis will occur within 1 week.

28 Correct answer—**D**

Anemic crisis is not a type of sickle-cell crisis. Three forms of sickle-cell crisis exist: aplastic, sequestration, and painful crisis. In aplastic crisis, the bone marrow stops producing RBCs and the hemoglobin level drops. A sequestration crisis, which is caused by splenic blockage, involves a sudden, large pooling of blood in the spleen. The painful crisis or the painful episode is the most common form of crisis. In the painful crisis, sickle cells occlude the blood vessels, decreasing blood flow and producing ischemia and infarction.

29 Correct answer—**C**

Increased fluid intake will actually prevent sickle-cell crisis by preventing dehydration. Cigarette smoking, infection, and physically demanding activities, such as tennis, do have the potential for precipitating a painful episode of sickle-cell crisis. Cigarette smoking contributes to sickle-cell crisis by interfering with oxygen exchange. The precise relationship between infections and sickle-cell crisis has not been identified. It is uncertain whether the decreased oxygen state is caused by infection, or if the crisis encourages infection.

Physically demanding activities, such as tennis, lead to overexertion and dehydration. The dehydration potentiates the sickling process, thus causing a crisis.

30 Correct answer—**A**

Inserting the smallest-possible-gauge I.V. catheter and infusing D_5½NS at 100 ml/hour would be the best way to maintain hydration in this patient. Inserting a small-gauge I.V. catheter, such as a 21- or 23-gauge catheter, will minimize trauma and reduce tissue scarring. Patients with sickle-cell anemia have a lifelong illness in which venous access must be preserved. The recommended I.V. solutions for hydration of patients in sickle-cell crisis include D_5W, D_5 ½NS, and lactated Ringer's solution. To avoid fluid overload and congestive heart failure, the recommended rate of infusion is 100 to 150 ml/hour. Patients with sickle-cell anemia should normally consume 4 to 6 quarts (3.8 to 5.7 liters) of liquid in 24 hours. In sickle-cell crisis, adequate hydration is critical because it assists in halting the sickle cycle by decreasing blood viscosity.

31 Correct answer—**B**

Morphine sulfate is not the ideal medication for providing analgesia to patients in a painful crisis because it produces respiratory depression. Meperidine (Demerol), aspirin, and codeine are used to provide analgesia for these patients. The analgesic used varies with the severity of the crisis; typically, oral analgesics will be ordered before intramuscular (I.M) or I.V. agents.

Selected References

Alspach, T.G., and Williams, S.M. *Core Curriculum for Critical Care Nursing,* 3rd ed. Philadelphia: W.B. Saunders Co., 1985.

The Committee on Transfusion Practices. "The Latest Protocols for Blood Transfusions," *Nursing 86* 16:34-41, October 1986.

Cosgriff, T.H., and Anderson, D.L. *The Practice of Emergency Care,* 2nd ed. Philadelphia: J.B. Lippincott Co., 1984.

Lamb, C. "Managing Sickle Cell Emergencies," *Patient Care* 19:92-95, 98, 103-105, January 15, 1985.

Pauley, S.Y. "Transfusion Therapy for Nurses: Part 1," *NITA 7:* 501-511, November/December, 1984.

Pauley, S.Y. "Transfusion Therapy for Nurses: Part 2," *NITA 8:* 51-60, January/February 1985.

Rozzell, M.S., et al. "The Painful Episode," *Nursing Clinics of North America 18*:185-199, 1983.

Sheehy, S.B., and Barber, T. *Emergency Nursing: Principles and Practice,* 2nd ed. St. Louis: C.V. Mosby Co., 1985.

Warner, C.G. *Emergency Care: Assessment and Interventions,* 3rd ed. St. Louis: C.V. Mosby Co., 1983.

Chapter 14

Behavioral Emergencies Questions and Answers

You must begin with Question 1 of this chapter and progress in sequence. **Do not skip around.** Subsequent answers build on previous ones.

Linda Reese, RN, MA
Nancy C. Seddio, RN, CS, PhD

SITUATION

A 32-year-old man, accompanied by two police officers, is brought to the emergency department (ED) in handcuffs. He had been standing on the rooftop of a six-story office building shouting obscenities and yelling, "You are all doomed to die for what you've done to me."

Questions 1 to 5 refer to the above situation.

1 The priority assessment at this time is to evaluate the patient's:

A. Orientation to time, place, and person
B. Vital signs
C. Threat to the safety of self and others
D. History of psychiatric illness

2 The patient is agitated and complains about the handcuffs and the presence of the police officers. The most helpful approach is to be:

A. Calm and firm, but nonthreatening
B. Relaxed, casual, and friendly
C. Authoritarian and directive
D. Permissive and comforting

3 After evaluation by the nurse and the psychiatric resident, a decision is made to remove the handcuffs. The patient should be told:

A. "If you promise to be good, we won't have to restrain you anymore."
B. "We will remove the handcuffs now. You will not be restrained as long as you are able to control yourself."
C. "I know the handcuffs are uncomfortable, so we will take them off now."
D. "Since you have calmed down, we will remove the handcuffs."

4 The patient appears anxious and guarded during the interview. His anxiety may be reduced by:

A. A detailed explanation of the entire admission procedure
B. A confident manner and simple, direct explanations
C. Limited interaction and focus on physical assessment rather than conversation
D. An attitude of warmth and the use of touch to demonstrate caring

5 A decision to admit the patient for psychiatric observation is most likely made on the basis of:

A. History of previous psychiatric hospitalizations
B. Anxiety level
C. The need to evaluate his homicidal and suicidal ideation more thoroughly
D. The fact that he was brought in by the police

SITUATION

A 30-year-old woman is brought to the ED by her husband. He reports that she has not eaten or slept in 7 days, and that she has become more and more elated over the past 3 weeks.

Questions 6 to 10 refer to the above situation.

6 The patient is wearing shorts and a halter top even though it is 20° F. (-6.7° C.) outside. When confronted about this, she says, "Well, it must be summer somewhere, and that's where I want to be." Which of the following is the best response?

A. "It is obvious that your judgment is impaired. You are dressed inappropriately."
B. "Where would you like to be, instead of here?"
C. "Please put this robe on. You don't want to catch pneumonia, do you?"
D. "You appear chilled, and you are shivering. Put this robe on."

7 While waiting to be examined, the patient begins singing loudly and starts walking around "entertaining" other patients. The best approach at this time is to:

A. Assign three available nursing assistants to keep the patient from annoying others
B. Recognize that this behavior is characteristic of bipolar disorder
C. Lead the patient to a quiet area in order to decrease her stimulation, and stay with her
D. Obtain an order for p.r.n. medication to control her behavior

8 During the admission interview, the patient is asked about her sleeping and eating patterns. She replies, "I live on love. I thank the stars above. Sleep is cheap. Food ruins the mood." This response shows evidence of:

A. Grandiose delusions
B. Auditory hallucinations
C. Word salad
D. Clang association

9 An admitting diagnosis of bipolar disorder, manic, is made. Signs and symptoms supporting this diagnosis include:

A. Looseness of association, agitation, suspiciousness, and irregular menses
B. Flight of ideas, hyperactivity, social isolation, and increased appetite
C. Rhyming, grandiosity, insomnia, and decreased appetite
D. Pressured speech, anxiety, delusions and persecution, and refusal to eat or drink

10 While awaiting admission, an appropriate medication order is:

A. Chlorpromazine (Thorazine) 100 mg P.O.
B. Lithium (Eskalith) 300 mg P.O.
C. Imipramine (Tofranil) 50 mg I.M.
D. Chlordiazepoxide (Librium) 25 mg P.O.

SITUATION

A 30-year-old man is brought to the ED by the police. He had been in a local bar when he suddenly began screaming at several male patrons, accusing them of wanting to have sex with him. The owner called the police, who found the patient huddled in a corner mumbling, "I'm not gay, I'm not gay. Don't call me a fag."

Questions 11 to 15 refer to the above situation.

11 In the waiting area, the patient is lying on a couch in a fetal position. The best initial approach to get him into the examining room is to:

A. Gently say, "Would you like to talk to the doctor now?"
B. Say, "Mr. ___________, I am a nurse here at City Hospital. Please come with me so we can understand how to help you."
C. Matter-of-factly state, "It is time to see the doctor. You must come with me now."
D. Ask the police officers to take the patient by the arms and escort him to the examining room

12 In the examining room, the patient stares blankly ahead; his affect is flat, and he barely responds to questions. His arm remains outstretched after his pulse is taken. This is called:

A. Resistance
B. Waxy flexibility
C. Stupor
D. Tenacity

13 The patient's behavior is consistent with:

A. A refusal to cooperate with the admission interview
B. An inability to accept his own homosexuality
C. An extreme withdrawal from an anxiety-provoking situation
D. A drug-induced lethargy

14 What statement is true regarding the remainder of the admission interview with this patient?

A. Although the patient does not respond verbally, the nurse should continue to explain in simple terms what is being done
B. Talking to the patient should be avoided at this time
C. The patient must be told what to do in a firm, directive manner
D. The patient's withdrawal is a defense mechanism and therefore should be supported until he is comfortable

The patient's parents arrive at the ED. They report that he has been increasingly withdrawn over the last several weeks. His mother adds that he "had a similar nervous breakdown 2 years ago and had to stay in the hospital for 6 months. He never seemed the same after that."

15 Based on the presenting symptoms and history, which is the most likely diagnosis?

A. Schizophrenia, disorganized type
B. Schizophrenia, residual type
C. Schizophrenia, catatonic type
D. Panic disorder

SITUATION

A 40-year-old woman walks into the ED and says to the clerk, "Are there any doctors here who can take the radio out of my brain?" The clerk tells her to have a seat and calls the nurse.

Questions 16 to 20 refer to the above situation.

16 While sitting in the waiting area, the patient strikes herself in the head, saying, "Somebody has to help me. I can't take this any longer." Which action is most appropriate at this point?

A. Alert the security guards that the patient may become agitated and to keep an eye on her
B. Approach the patient with two other staff as back-up and ask, "What seems to be the problem?"
C. Walk over to the patient and say, "I understand you think there is a radio in your brain. How did that happen?"
D. Sit next to the patient and say, "I'm a nurse here. I saw you hitting your head. Can you tell me what you are experiencing right now?"

17 In a more agitated manner, she begins pacing the floor and hitting her head harder as she yells, "Stop it. I'm a good girl. Stop saying those things about me." The patient is experiencing:

A. Auditory hallucinations
B. Delusions of persecution
C. Obsessive ideation
D. Looseness of associations

18 At this time, further assessment will focus on the patient's:

A. Vital signs
B. Orientation to time, place, and person
C. Receptivity to treatment
D. Content of thought

19 Should the patient's agitation increase to a point where she becomes out of control and requires restraint, the best approach is to:

A. Address her in a warm, reassuring manner
B. Use two hospital security guards to restrain her until medication is administered
C. Use at least four trained personnel to handle the patient
D. Administer medication to avoid restraint

20 The nursing care for a patient who is restrained includes:

A. Allowing the patient to rest undisturbed until calm
B. Talking to the patient about what precipitated the restraint
C. Constant observation and monitoring of vital signs
D. Doing range-of-motion exercises every ½ hour until the patient is released from restraints

SITUATION

A 30-year-old man is brought to the ED by his mother. She states that she can no longer manage him at home. He has been in and out of psychiatric hospitals since he was age 19. She says that he "acts like a baby." He will not dress or wash without her help and is frequently incontinent of urine and feces.

Questions 21 to 25 refer to the above situation.

21 In the examining room, the patient grimaces and poses in front of a glass cabinet. He does not respond when his name is called. Which is the best way to approach this patient?

A. Walk over to him, place a hand on his shoulder, and repeat his name
B. Say, "What are you doing?"
C. Tell him to stop making faces and talk to you
D. Repeat his name more loudly, move closer to him, and then wait for a sign that he is aware of your presence

22 When questioned about the reasons his mother brought him to the hospital, the patient replies, "I had to go on a trip. The sky is empty now. The man's name is Big Bob." This response shows evidence of:

A. Looseness of association
B. Flight of ideas
C. Neologisms
D. Echolalia

23 During the admission interview, the patient is incontinent of urine. The best way to handle this situation is to:

A. Ignore the incontinence to avoid embarrassing him
B. Firmly remind him that "grown men do not urinate in their pants."
C. Have him take off his wet pants and put on a gown and a diaper to "prevent further accidents"
D. Say, "You are wet. Let me help you change into this dry gown."

24 The patient says to the nurse, "Is it better to eat or to drink? To sleep or to wake? To sing or to dance? Which is better?" These questions demonstrate:

A. Ambivalence
B. Confusion
C. Autism
D. Regression

25 The patient's mother tells the nurse she feels guilty about bringing her son back to the hospital. She says, "He doesn't like to be here; he always begs me to take him out. Why can't I take care of him at home?" Which statement best expresses support for the mother?

A. "Don't feel guilty. You've certainly done your best for him. Let us help him now."
B. "I understand how much you care about him. You are able to recognize when you need help in dealing with him."
C. "Patients like your son never really recover; they frequently need repeated hospitalizations."
D. "It must be an awful strain taking care of him all these years. You should consider a group home."

SITUATION

A 45-year-old man is brought to the ED by his wife. He had been well until 2 months ago when his wife began to notice changes in his personality and thinking. He also had mood changes. On admission, the patient appears disheveled and assumes bizarre postures. He does not respond to questions and cannot describe his feelings; his speech is only partly understandable. Thoughts are dominated by delusions of being controlled by Jesus Christ. He states that he has heard the voice of Jesus and President Reagan speaking to him. He believes the FBI is following him and that the nurses are secret agents who plan to destroy him. A diagnosis of schizophrenia, paranoid type, is made.

Questions 26 to 32 refer to the above situation.

26 Schizophrenia is one of a group of psychotic reactions characterized by:

A. Marked psychomotor disturbance, which may involve stupor, negativism, excitement, rigidity, or posturing
B. Incoherence, grossly disorganized actions, prominent delusions, and hallucinations
C. Prominent psychotic symptoms followed by an episode without symptoms
D. Basic disturbances in the individual's relationships with others, and an inability to communicate and think clearly

27 Nursing assessment of this patient requires careful inquiry and observation of the patient's:

A. Reality points and situations, and his ability to communicate on multiple levels
B. Communication changes in his relationships when he becomes totally absorbed in his thoughts and experiences
C. Thinking, perceiving, symbolizing, communicating, and decision-making skills and abilities
D. Blunted or inappropriate affect, social withdrawal, loosening of associations, and eccentric behavior with illogical thinking

28 The major assessment area regarding content of thought is the:

A. Presence of delusions
B. Presence of complex fantasies and preoccupation with self
C. Degree of negative verbalization toward significant others
D. Objective data elicited from the patient's psychiatric history

29 During the interview, the patient is asked questions such as, "Do you dream vividly? Do you see flashes of light, or figures that others cannot see? Do you hear voices when no one is present? If so, whose voice? Is it clear? Abusive? Accusatory? Can you stop the voices?" These questions are important because:

A. The major mechanisms of defense used by the patient are an indication of the level of his psychosis
B. The assessment for perceptual changes includes evaluating for the presence of hallucinations
C. The emotional responses elicited provide an assessment of the appropriateness of the patient's affect (mood)
D. The psychotic patient can never distinguish between what is real and what is not real

30 When caring for a psychotic patient, the ED nurse must be:

A. Nonthreatening, so that the patient will demonstrate an increased ability to express emotions appropriately
B. Goal-directed, so that data essential for the treatment plan is elicited
C. Nonjudgmental, to provide an atmosphere conducive to trust and communication
D. Flexible, to adjust nursing care as the situation demands

31 Two major theories about the etiology of schizophrenia are currently under study. These are the biological, including genetic, biochemical, and physiologic theories; and the psychosocial, including behavioral, psychoanalytic, and socioepidemiologic theories. Two current theories about the biological factors of schizophrenia are:

A. The cortisol suppression hypothesis, and the dexamethasone suppresson hypothesis
B. The endocrine hypothesis and the serotonin hypothesis
C. The chemical imbalance hypothesis, involving four specific agents, and the genetic transmission hypothesis
D. The transmethylation hypothesis and the dopamine hypothesis

32 Since schizophrenia is considered primarily a thought disorder, emotional changes may sometimes be overlooked by the examining practitioner. The more withdrawn the patient, the more the dynamics of the psychotic process apply to the patient. The affect disorders typical of schizophrenia are:

A. Limited movement of affect; slow to express feeling state in a situation; apathy, distance, seriousness, lack of spontaneous warmth
B. Limited capacity for expressing wide range of emotions; reserved and distant in interpersonal relationships
C. Abrupt mood fluctuations; lack of smooth transition when expressing several feeling states; may move suddenly into extremes of behavior
D. Consistency between ideas and emotional responses present at times

SITUATION

A 30-year-old woman is brought to the ED anxious, trembling, and crying. She states her depression and lack of interest in life began 1 year ago after being told by her husband that he wanted a divorce, because of his relationship with another woman. The couple had been married for 10 years. She was not angry with her husband, but blamed herself for his infidelity. During the marriage, she developed few personal interests, having little time between working and domestic responsibilities. After her husband began divorce proceedings, she became aware of intense feelings of sadness, fatigue, grief, hopelessness, worthlessness, and recurrent thoughts of death. The patient's mother was chronically ill with depression. A diagnosis of distorted grief reaction, major depression, is made.

Questions 33 to 39 refer to the above situation.

33 Grief is a process that accompanies all loss. A maladaptive or pathologic response to loss occurs when the person:

A. Does not successfully complete the process of physical and psychological distress over the loss
B. Does not resolve the social situations that caused the feelings of powerlessness and low self-esteem
C. Cannot successfully utilize coping mechanisms and ego strengths
D. Does not successfully balance intrapersonal and interpersonal needs

34 Two current biological theories have been proposed to explain the high incidence of depression in women, as compared to men. These two theories are based on:

A. Opiate-receptor and endorphin studies
B. Nutritional deficiency and neurologic studies
C. Postpartum and metabolic studies
D. Genetic and endocrine studies

35 In the last decade, major advances in the diagnosis of depression through biochemical means have occurred. Which test is used?

A. Serotonin level test
B. Serotonin suppression test
C. Dexamethasone suppression test
D. Monoamine oxidase (MAO) inhibitor suppression test

36 For a delayed or distorted grief reaction to be dealt with successfully, the patient must experience the feelings and thoughts that were initially avoided. The best way to assist with this regrief process is to:

A. Encourage the patient to engage in therapy with her former husband to work through her loss
B. Gently encourage the patient to discuss the loss and then be with her during the grief process
C. Encourage the patient to increase her social contacts and realistically accept her ego strengths
D. Communicate to the patient that grieving is time limited and that the emotional pain will resolve as time passes

37 The patient tells the ED nurse that she is afraid to face her feelings and express any emotions; she fears that her condition will worsen if she remembers the past and the accompanying pain. When educating the patient about the grieving process:

A. Reassure her that she will not cry forever, permanently lose control, or go crazy if she grieves
B. Reassure her that the expression of active feelings is a natural part of the process
C. Encourage the patient not to blame herself for the divorce
D. Encourage the patient to express repressed feelings toward herself and her former husband by using role-playing

38 In grief and depression, sadness is the major affect. Other affects that may be noted include:

A. Euphoria, with varying degrees of dysphoria
B. Panic, preoccupation with self, withdrawal, crying, psychomotor agitation or psychomotor retardation, apathy
C. Irritability, agitation, hostility, anger, apathy, lethargy, shame, self-doubts, and lack of humor (anhedonia)
D. Agitation, low energy, withdrawal; demanding, regressive, and infantile behavior with occasional periods of crying

39 The physician orders phenelzine (Nardil) 10 mg P.O. stat. The patient is given a prescription for Nardil 10 mg P.O. q.i.d. and an appointment with the outpatient mental health department in 2 weeks. Patient teaching by the ED nurse must include:

A. Instruction and follow-up, which may include a physical examination and psychotherapy
B. Possible adverse effects, such as blurred vision, constipation, tachycardia, delayed micturition
C. Possible adverse effects, especially toxic effects, such as hypothalamic crises and hyperglycemia
D. Dietary information

SITUATION

A 45-year-old man is brought to the ED by police. He had been standing at the corner of a busy intersection throwing rocks at pedestrians and passing cars. He says he did this because he was just fired from his job. He also says that his wife left him because he hit her on several occasions. He is angry about being brought to the hospital and is verbally abusive to nursing and medical staff. He belligerently demands to be discharged. When asked to remove his jacket so that vital signs could be obtained, he throws a chair against the wall. He threatens anyone who gets close to him, saying, "I'll break every bone in your body." A team of five staff members calmly enters the room and removes him to a seclusion room where he is given haloperidol (Haldol) 5 mg I.M. and is isolated until he regains control of his behavior. Approximately 2 hours later, he is still upset and angry but no longer verbally or physically violent. During the course of the interview, he says, "I hope I didn't hurt anyone before, but at times my mind loses control and I can't help myself. I don't mean to be violent, it just happens from time to time."

Questions 40 to 47 refer to the above situation.

40 Assaultive or violent behavior is primarily the result of:

A. A psychotic state, an organic condition, a depressive state, or a disorder of impulse control
B. Repressed frustration, psychoses (e.g., hallucinations and voices), substance abuse
C. Psychoses, impulse control, history of abuse as a child
D. Alcohol intoxication, depression, loss of ego and superego control

41 Violent or assaultive and homicidal behaviors occur because:

A. Patients who have been incarcerated in hospitals possess explosive personalities
B. The patient imagines being threatened by outside forces
C. The patient acts out of rage, frustration, and anger because he cannot think before acting
D. The patient gives in to impulses to get what he wants (often repeating old conflict patterns)

42 Patients who present the greatest danger of exhibiting violent behavior are:

A. Those with a diagnosis of organic brain syndrome
B. Criminals
C. Substance abusers
D. Psychotics

43 The best means by which to predict the threat of violent behavior is via:

A. Patient's psychomotor activity
B. Patient's affect and accompanying changes in speech and motor activity
C. Amount of violence to which the patient has been subjected (e.g., child abuse, spouse abuse, or the patient's history of violent behavior)
D. One's own senses: sight, hearing, touch, and gut reactions

44 The major criteria used to determine that a patient is potentially assaultive are:

A. Disorientation, visual hallucinations, memory impairment, and auditory hallucinations
B. Diagnosis of psychoses and history of violent behavior; in particular, history of recent criminal incarceration
C. Diagnosis of manic depression with psychotic features, and possession of a weapon, such as a gun or knife
D. Increase in motor agitation, threatening verbalization or gestures, intensification of affect, history of assaultive behavior, use of alcohol or addictive drugs, and acute organic brain syndrome

45 The immediate goals of nursing intervention for assaultive or homicidal patients are to:

A. Administer fast-acting sedation, as ordered by physician
B. Restore control or prevent further loss of control
C. Restrain according to hospital policy and help patient regain control
D. Provide patient with opportunities for appropriate release of frustrations

46 The best approach for dealing with an overtly violent patient is:

A. Calm and firm manner
B. A team of trained staff
C. The patient's psychiatrist and a family member who represents a support system to the patient
D. Psychotropic medication

47 The mental hygiene law in most states is quite specific about how long a patient may legally be restrained. Most laws stipulate that restraints:

A. Cannot be used for longer than 24 hours
B. Cannot be used if the patient has cardiac or respiratory disease or insufficiency
C. Can be used only after the patient is evaluated by a psychiatrist
D. May be applied if the patient is a danger to self or others, but this danger must be reevaluated every few hours

SITUATION

A 50-year-old female secretary is brought to the ED after a suicide attempt. She lives in an apartment which she shared with her sister until her sister's death 1 year ago. The patient divorced her husband 5 years ago. The patient has seen several internists during the past several months for various somatic complaints, which gradually caused her to lose much time from work. She also began to lose interest in her appearance and her job. After a meeting with her supervisor last week when she was placed on probation, she went home and has not left her apartment. Her supervisor tried numerous times to call her, but the patient did not answer the phone. When found by the police, she was lying on the floor of her apartment and slashing at both wrists with a razor blade. On arrival, her cuts are found to be superficial and vital signs stable. While the ED nurse applies sterile dressings to the wounds, the patient says, "It makes sense. I don't have anybody. I want to put myself out of this misery. Next time, I will succeed."

Questions 48 to 55 refer to the above situation.

48 Which is essential during the initial interview of this patient?

A. Assist the patient in reevaluating her life situation and in making immediate realistic changes
B. Inform the patient that a professional mental health practitioner will take responsibility to care for and watch over her
C. Assess the need for psychotropic medications
D. Listen very carefully to what she says about the nature of the suicidal intent

49 When assessing this patient's behavior, emphasis should be placed on the suicide method because:

A. Certain attempts are referred to as suicide gestures, a means for the patient to engage in attention-seeking behavior, and are not meant to be taken seriously
B. Some nonlethal behaviors represent a patient's intrapsychic hope that someone will recognize the danger and rescue the person from self-destruction
C. Although all suicide threats and attempts are to be taken seriously, more vigorous and vigilant nursing attention is indicated when the person is planning or tries a highly lethal means, such as shooting, hanging, or jumping from a high place
D. Some behaviors represent a dysfunctional approach by which the patient tries to discover whether anyone cares enough to prevent his self-destruction

50 The person most likely to attempt suicide is one who:

A. Plans a violent death, has a specific plan, and has the means readily available
B. Thinks about taking a bottle of aspirin if the situation at work does not improve soon
C. Gives away all possessions, appears despondent, and has frequent thoughts of dying
D. Gives away all possessions, is preoccupied with morbid thoughts, and verbalizes the wish to die

51 All of the following are true statements about suicide *except:*

A. People who talk about suicide don't commit suicide; suicidal people are fully intent on dying
B. Suicide is an individual pattern that does not run in families; it occurs equally among all levels of society
C. Most suicides occur within 3 months after the beginning of improvement, when the individual has the energy to put morbid thoughts and feelings into action
D. Although the suicidal person is extremely unhappy, he is not necessarily mentally ill

52 Individuals who are severely depressed are always suicide risks. When investigating the source of depression, do not overlook the possibility that the patient's medication may be responsible. Some of the commonly used prescription drugs whose adverse effects include depression are:

A. Diazepam (Valium), chlordiazepoxide (Librium), tetracycline (Achromycin), imipramine (Tofranil), amitriptyline (Elavil), doxepin (Sinequan), isocarboxazid (Marplan)
B. Chloramphenicol (Chloromycetin), clonidine (Catapres), indomethacin (Indocin), methyldopa (Aldomet), propranolol (Inderal), reserpine (Serpasil), trimethobenzamide (Tigan)
C. Methylphenidate (Ritalin), Catapres, Valium, protriptyline (Vivactil)
D. Loxapine (Loxitane), chlorpromazine (Thorazine), phenelzine (Nardil), tranylcypromine (Parnate), Tofranil, Elavil

53 The ED nurse and the physician have assessed the patient and determined that hospitalization is required, because she cannot control her destructive impulses without assistance. Which measure designed to assess physical safety should be instituted?

A. Provide the patient with a quiet room to decrease stimuli
B. Place the patient on suicide precautions
C. Place the patient on one-to-one observation
D. Administer psychotropic medications as ordered by the physician to help the patient gain more control and reduce her self-destructive impulses

54 One of the most commonly encountered features of suicidal persons is that they are:

A. Psychotic
B. Guilty
C. Ambivalent
D. Angry

55 Individuals in certain population groups are more likely to become self-destructive than others. Some of the groups at highest risk include:

A. Alcoholics, police, physicians, previous attempters, adolescents, terminally ill patients, elderly people, members of minority groups, and psychotic patients
B. Adolescents, psychotic patients, and substance abusers
C. Psychotic patients, previous attempters, clergy members, adolescents, and terminally ill patients
D. Psychotic patients, depressed individuals, and adolescents

Answer Sheet

	A	B	C	D		A	B	C	D
1	○	○	○	○	31	○	○	○	○
2	○	○	○	○	32	○	○	○	○
3	○	○	○	○	33	○	○	○	○
4	○	○	○	○	34	○	○	○	○
5	○	○	○	○	35	○	○	○	○
6	○	○	○	○	36	○	○	○	○
7	○	○	○	○	37	○	○	○	○
8	○	○	○	○	38	○	○	○	○
9	○	○	○	○	39	○	○	○	○
10	○	○	○	○	40	○	○	○	○
11	○	○	○	○	41	○	○	○	○
12	○	○	○	○	42	○	○	○	○
13	○	○	○	○	43	○	○	○	○
14	○	○	○	○	44	○	○	○	○
15	○	○	○	○	45	○	○	○	○
16	○	○	○	○	46	○	○	○	○
17	○	○	○	○	47	○	○	○	○
18	○	○	○	○	48	○	○	○	○
19	○	○	○	○	49	○	○	○	○
20	○	○	○	○	50	○	○	○	○
21	○	○	○	○	51	○	○	○	○
22	○	○	○	○	52	○	○	○	○
23	○	○	○	○	53	○	○	○	○
24	○	○	○	○	54	○	○	○	○
25	○	○	○	○	55	○	○	○	○
26	○	○	○	○					
27	○	○	○	○					
28	○	○	○	○					
29	○	○	○	○					
30	○	○	○	○					

Answer Sheet

	A	B	C	D
1	○	○	○	○
2	○	○	○	○
3	○	○	○	○
4	○	○	○	○
5	○	○	○	○
6	○	○	○	○
7	○	○	○	○
8	○	○	○	○
9	○	○	○	○
10	○	○	○	○
11	○	○	○	○
12	○	○	○	○
13	○	○	○	○
14	○	○	○	○
15	○	○	○	○
16	○	○	○	○
17	○	○	○	○
18	○	○	○	○
19	○	○	○	○
20	○	○	○	○
21	○	○	○	○
22	○	○	○	○
23	○	○	○	○
24	○	○	○	○
25	○	○	○	○
26	○	○	○	○
27	○	○	○	○
28	○	○	○	○
29	○	○	○	○
30	○	○	○	○

	A	B	C	D
31	○	○	○	○
32	○	○	○	○
33	○	○	○	○
34	○	○	○	○
35	○	○	○	○
36	○	○	○	○
37	○	○	○	○
38	○	○	○	○
39	○	○	○	○
40	○	○	○	○
41	○	○	○	○
42	○	○	○	○
43	○	○	○	○
44	○	○	○	○
45	○	○	○	○
46	○	○	○	○
47	○	○	○	○
48	○	○	○	○
49	○	○	○	○
50	○	○	○	○
51	○	○	○	○
52	○	○	○	○
53	○	○	○	○
54	○	○	○	○
55	○	○	○	○

1 Correct answer—**C**

The safety of the patient and others is always a priority, although the patient's orientation, vital signs, and history are part of the total assessment.

2 Correct answer—**A**

A calm, firm, nonthreatening approach helps to lessen fears and anxiety. Other approaches may be viewed with suspicion or as threatening.

3 Correct answer—**B**

The nurse should say, "We will remove the handcuffs now. You will not be restrained as long as you are able to control yourself." A clear statement of what is to be done, as well as of the limits for its continuance, is best. Do not ask for promises the patient may be unable to keep, and avoid explanation of what is expected.

4 Correct answer—**B**

The patient will feel more secure with simple, direct explanations, confidently given. Anxiety interferes with the ability to concentrate and comprehend complex information. Touch should be avoided, because it is often interpreted as intrusive and threatening, as would a physical examination at this time.

5 Correct answer—**C**

Because the patient was threatening others, it is necessary to evaluate his homicidal and suicidal ideations thoroughly. When taken alone, the patient's history of previous psychiatric hospitalizations and the fact that he was brought in by police are not usually sufficient to warrant admission.

6 Correct answer—**D**

The nurse should say, "You appear chilled, and you are shivering. Put this robe on." The nurse makes an observation and suggests an appropriate behavior in a matter-of-fact, nonjudgmental way. To say that her judgment is impaired degrades the patient; asking where she would like to be will provide no meaningful information.

7 Correct answer—**C**

To reduce hyperactivity, decrease stimulation from the environment and provide constant supervision. Three people will provide too much stimulation. Medication should be avoided until the patient has been thoroughly evaluated.

8 Correct answer—**D**

This response shows evidence of clang association. Clanging rhyme is common in mania. Auditory hallucinations and word salad (meaningless combination of words) are seen in schizophrenia. Grandiose delusions are not evident here.

9 Correct answer—**C**

Rhyming, grandiosity, insomnia, and decreased appetite are all signs and symptoms of a manic disorder. Those signs and symptoms that are *not* characteristic of mania are social isolation, increased appetite, looseness of associations, suspiciousness, delusions of persecution, or refusal to eat or drink (although usually too busy, manic patients will eat on the run).

10 Correct answer—**A**

Thorazine is used to control hyperactivity. Lithium, used to prevent or control mania, takes 7 to 10 days to reach a therapeutic blood level. Tofranil is an antidepressant.

11 Correct answer—**B**

The nurse addresses the patient by name, states who she is, and offers to help. The patient cannot make decisions and therefore should not be asked to do so. Responses that would probably be threatening to the patient in his frightened state should be avoided.

12 Correct answer—**B**

Waxy flexibility is a condition in which the limbs have a waxlike rigidity and remain as placed for a long time.

13 Correct answer—**C**

It is consistent with withdrawal from an anxiety-provoking situation. Understanding the patient's behavior as a protection from a threatening reality is important. No evidence exists at this time to support the inability of the patient to accept his own homosexuality, or that he has a drug-induced lethargy.

14 Correct answer—**A**

Although the patient does not respond, the nurse should continue to explain in simple terms what is being done. The patient is usually aware of what is going on despite his nonresponsiveness and should be treated respectfully. Although recognizing the dynamics of the withdrawal is important, supporting the withdrawal is not helpful. The nurse must not increase the patient's suspicion.

15 Correct answer—**C**

The diagnostic criteria for schizophrenia, catatonic type, are present. Disorganized type shows more autistic, bizarre delusions; agitation; and silliness. The diagnosis schizophrenia, residual type, is used to describe symptoms remaining in compensated patients.

16 Correct answer—**D**

The nurse should sit next to the patient and say, "I'm a nurse here. I saw you hitting your head. Can you tell me what you are experiencing right now?" Direct intervention is needed. The nurse should introduce herself, identify the patient's distress, and want to understand it. Measures that place the patient on the defensive must be avoided.

17 Correct answer—**A**

The patient is experiencing auditory hallucinations. She is obviously responding to what she is hearing.

18 Correct answer—**D**

Assess the content of hallucinations to protect the patient and others from possible command hallucinations or violent outbursts.

19 Correct answer—**C**

Restraints are used to protect the safety of the patient and staff. At least four persons trained in restraining patients can do this safely and efficiently. Medication should have been given earlier in an attempt to prevent escalation of patient's agitated behavior to the point where she required restraints.

20 Correct answer—**C**

Restrained patients should not be left alone and must be monitored closely for changes in vital signs. Talking about the event at this point will further agitate the patient rather than calm her. Range-of-motion exercises are not as important as checking for circulation, respirations, and hydration.

21 Correct answer—**D**

The nurse should repeat the patient's name more loudly, move closer to him, and wait for a sign that the patient is aware of the nurse's presence. The nurse can avoid startling the patient by not touching him, or asking questions, before identifying herself and establishing the relationship.

22 Correct answer—**A**

The links between this patient's thoughts are obscure; this is called looseness of association. In flight of ideas, the links, although weak, are more evident. No new words (neologisms) or repetitious speech (echolalia) is present.

23 Correct answer—**D**

The nurse should say, "You are wet. Let me help you change into this dry gown." Be aware of the patient's fragile self-esteem during regressive episodes. Sensitively helping the patient change his clothes is the best approach. Avoiding the issue may be interpreted as not caring.

24 Correct answer—**A**

Ambivalence is evident in the statements of opposing or dual behaviors.

25 Correct answer—**B**

Acknowledge the mother's concern and decision to bring her son to the hospital. The nurse must not deny the mother's feelings, imply that there is no hope, or increase her guilt rather than ease it.

26 Correct answer—**D**

Schizophrenia is one of a group of psychotic reactions characterized by basic disturbances in the individual's relationships with others and an inability to communicate and think clearly. The person's thoughts, feelings, and behavior are often evidenced by withdrawal, fluctuating moods, disordered thinking, and regressive tendencies.

27 Correct answer—**C**

Nursing assessment of a patient who is psychotic requires careful inquiry and observation of the patient's thinking, perceiving, symbolizing, communicating, and decision-making skills and abilities. Assessment is made in each of the following areas: alterations in thought content, thought process, perception, affect (mood), and psychomotor behavior; changes in personality, coping styles, and sense of self; lack of self-motivation; psychosocial stressors; and degeneration of adaptive functioning.

28 Correct answer—**A**

Delusions constitute the major disturbance in the content of thought. Patients may report delusions spontaneously, but usually specific questioning is required. Clues suggesting delusions include evasiveness, suspicion, and other indications of sensitivity regarding aspects of the interview.

29 Correct answer—**B**

The assessment for perceptual changes includes evaluating for hallucinations, the major disturbance in perception. The most common forms are auditory and visual. The voices may be those of either family members or strangers, and they often make derogatory or insulting remarks. Command hallucinations may be obeyed, having the capacity to create danger for the patient or others.

30 Correct answer—**D**

The ED nurse must be flexible when caring for a patient who behaves in a suspicious, withdrawn, regressed way or who has a thought disorder. Because the patient communicates at various levels and is in control of himself at various times, the nurse must adjust the care as the situation demands.

31 Correct answer—**D**

Currently, two theories relating to the biological factors of schizophrenia exist: the transmethylation hypothesis and the dopamine hypothesis. The transmethylation hypothesis results from recent findings of a significantly diminished level of monoamine oxidase in the platelets of schizophrenic patients. The dopamine hypothesis relates to pharmacology studies that investigated the mechanism of action of drugs that reduced the disorder, and drugs that produced or mimicked the disorder.

32 Correct answer—**C**

The psychotic patient displays a constricted range of affect that expresses few emotional extremes. Fixation at one end of the emotional continuum occurs; the patient is usually withdrawn and introverted rather than extroverted; mood fluctuations are abrupt; the person lacks smooth transitions when expressing several feeling states and may move suddenly into extremes of behavior range, i.e., sudden sadness, joy, rage, submission.

33 Correct answer—**A**

A maladaptive or pathologic response to loss implies that something has prevented it from running its course. Two types of pathologic grief reactions exist: the delayed reaction and the distorted reaction. Depression is a type of distorted grief reaction in which the individual does not successfully engage in the physical and psychological distress over the loss. Depression is an abnormal extension or overelaboration of sadness and grief.

34 Correct answer—**D**

Genetic and endocrine studies are currently being researched to explain the high incidence of depression in women as compared to men. Most genetic studies are concerned with evidence suggesting that the risk of depression increases in first-generation relatives of diagnosed depressives as compared to the general population; and that a higher concordance rate occurs in monozygotic (identical) twins than in dizygotic (fraternal) twins. Endocrine theories of depression reveal a relationship with sex hormones. Clinical depression tends to occur with events in the reproductive cycle, such as menstruation, use of contraceptive drugs, postpartum, and menopause.

35 Correct answer—**C**

The dexamethasone suppression test has gained considerable attention as a diagnostic marker for endogenous depression, as well as for its implications for treatment and prognostic factors. Most studies have found that 40% to 50% of patients suffering from endogenous depression, or from major depressive disorders with melancholia, show early recovery from cortisol suppression after the administration of dexamethasone.

36 Correct answer—**B**

Gently encourage the patient to discuss the loss and then be with her during the grief process. Help can be provided for the large number of people who fail to grieve because they have no available and supportive social matrix. The grieving person will carefully but subtly scrutinize to see whether strength, respect, and kindness are available.

37 Correct answer—**A**

Educate and reassure the patient as to what is expected. Reassure her that she will not cry forever, or permanently lose control, or go crazy if she grieves. These untoward consequences may occur only when there is a failure to grieve. If the patient complains that the past is the past and should remain buried, reply that the past is very much in the present because it has not really been buried. Grieving is necessary to put the past in its proper perspective.

38 Correct answer—**C**

Other characteristics to look for include irritability, agitation, hostility, anger, apathy, lethargy, shame, self-doubt, and lack of humor (anhedonia). The mental status examination of a depressed patient includes a careful assessment of mood. Ambivalence and hopelessness need to be identified as dire feelings of emptiness, worthlessness, and a lack of self-respect and confidence. Self-blame and low self-esteem are also present. The patient may be emotionally labile, crying easily one moment and laughing the next.

39 Correct answer—**D**

The nurse must instruct the patient about dietary precautions. Because of the dangers of hypertensive reactions resulting from the tyramine content, the following foods must be avoided by patients taking MAO inhibitors: aged cheese, sour cream, beer, wine (especially Chianti), yogurt, yeast, pickled herring, aged meat, meat tenderizer, and chicken liver. Chocolate and caffeine have also been implicated in blood pressure elevations. The patient should be advised to note and report early signs of an impending hypertensive reaction (headache, palpitations, neck stiffness, sweating, nausea, and photophobia).

40 Correct answer—**A**

Assaultive behavior is primarily from a psychotic state, an organic condition, a depressive state, or a disorder of impulse control or way of acting out.

41 Correct answer—**B**

In acute psychotic or organic states, violent or assaultive and homicidal behaviors occur because the patient imagines being threatened by outside forces. The patient cannot perceive the reality of the environment correctly. The violent behavior stems from the patient's perception of real or imagined threats.

42 Correct answer—**D**

Acute attacks of paranoia are psychotic episodes that can result from a functional mental disorder or from an organic brain syndrome. These patients represent the greatest danger to others. The pattern of thought is projective and leads to the development of delusions, which are usually persecutory in nature. In this disorder, reality testing is impaired. If it remains uncorrected, the delusions persist, causing the patient to perceive the environment as hostile and destructive. The patient then becomes violent in an effort to protect the self.

43 Correct answer—**D**

The nurse's actions should be based on the nurse's perceptions, thoughts, and feelings in response to given stimuli; in this case, the patient's behavior. The patient who is violent or threatening violence is a given stimulus. The nurse perceives the threat via the senses: sight, sound, touch, and gut reaction. When a patient suddenly begins to pace and mumble angrily, the nurse senses that the patient is behaving strangely, that people nearby may be in danger, or that the patient may be self-destructive. The potential for danger is assessed not only on the basis of the perceived external reality, but also in terms of the nurse's prior experience, and how the nurse's "insides feel." Thus, nurses who have seen those warning signs before will sense danger more readily than inexperienced nurses will.

44 Correct answer—**D**

Six criteria by which to identify a potentially assaultive patient are increase in motor agitation, threatening verbalization or gestures toward real or imagined objects, intensification of affect, history of assaultive behavior, use of alcohol or addictive drugs, and presence of acute organic brain syndrome.

45 Correct answer—**B**

The immediate goals of nursing intervention for assaultive or homicidal patients are to prevent further loss of control, or to restore control in patients already behaving in a violent or assaultive manner.

46 Correct answer—**B**

The team approach is recommended because it is a constant sign of external control for the patient. The goal of the team is to bring into disciplined play the understanding of feelings. In general, this is done by assisting the patient to control or set limits on impulsive aggressive behavior, examine the immediate situation that prompted the impulse reaction, and learn alternative methods of reacting in similar situations or other ways to discharge aggressive energies on an ongoing basis.

47 Correct answer—**D**

Most laws stipulate that restraints may be applied if the patient is a danger to self or others, but this danger must be reevaluated every few hours and restraints continued only until more humane methods (e.g., medication) become effective. This becomes a problem treating violent patients who are intoxicated or overdosed on drugs, because it is usually not possible to give any sedation until the alcohol or drug is metabolized; in such instances, restraints with continued observation are necessary. In many states, the only legal form of restraint is the camisole (straitjacket) or restraining sheet. Four-point restraint (both wrists and ankles tied separately) is illegal in many states. However, when no other method works, four-point restraint may be used with the condition that one limb be untied at a specified interval and the restraints rotated, much in the matter of rotating tourniquets. Handcuffs, which are commonly used by the police to restrain such patients, may *never* be used by health professionals.

48 Correct answer—**D**

During the initial interview, listen carefully to what the person says about the nature of the suicidal intent. After the information is evaluated, it is important to assess the patient's feelings of inadequacy in coping with the immediate and chronic stresses in her life, her level of hope, and her view of the situation as intolerable. The nurse listens and tries to understand the patient's view of her existence at that moment.

49 Correct answer—**C**

In the assessment of suicidal behavior, much emphasis is placed on how lethal the suicidal method that is threatened or used is. Although all suicide threats and attempts should be taken seriously, more vigorous and vigilant nursing attention is indicated when the patient is planning or tries a highly lethal means, such as shooting, hanging, or jumping. Less lethal means include carbon monoxide poisoning and drug overdose, which allow time for discovery once the suicidal action has been taken. Assessment should also include whether the person has made a specific plan and whether the means to carry out the plan are available.

50 Correct answer—**A**

The most suicidal person is one who plans a violent death (e.g., gunshot to the head), has a specific plan (e.g., as soon as his wife goes shopping), and has the means readily available (e.g., a loaded gun in the desk drawer). Such a person appears serious about the plan. On the other hand, the person who thinks about taking a bottle of aspirin if the work situation does not improve is communicating an element of hope and is really asking for help in coping with his work situation.

51 Correct answer—**A**

Myth: People who talk about suicide don't commit suicide. The fact is that of any 10 persons who kill themselves, 8 have given definite warnings of their suicidal intentions. Myth: Suicidal people are fully intent on dying. The fact is that most suicidal people are undecided about living and dying and they "gamble with death," leaving it to others to save them. Almost no one commits suicide without letting others know how he is feeling.

52 Correct answer—**B**

When investigating the source of a patient's depression, do not overlook the possibility that the medications may be responsible. The adverse effects of the following agents include depression: Aldomet, asparaginase (Elspar), baclofen (Lioresal), carisoprodol (Soma), Chloromycetin, Catapres, dantrolene (Dantrium), diethylstilbestrol (DES), gentamicin (Garamycin), guanethidine (Ismelin), hydralazine (Apresoline), Indocin, Inderal, pentazocine (Talwin), phenytoin (Dilantin), Serpasil, tamoxifen (Nolvadex), Tigan, and Valium, as well as anorexiants, barbiturates, estrogen-containing products, and sulfonamides.

53 Correct answer—**B**

The patient is placed on suicide precautions, treatment orders designed to ensure physical safety, such as (1) search personal effects for toxic agents (such as drugs or alcohol); (2) remove sharp instruments (e.g., razor blades, knives, letter openers, glass bottles); (3) remove straps from clothing (e.g., belts, neckties, stockings or pantyhose); (4) place on one-to-one observation.

54 Correct answer—**C**

One of the most common features of suicidal persons is that they are ambivalent. Within each patient is a struggle between self-preserving and self-destructing forces. Ambivalence is apparent when people threaten or attempt suicide and then try to get help. When patients discuss possible outcomes of suicide, it is remarkable how often they talk of life-related outcomes, such as relief from an unhappy situation. Although many people ponder suicide as an alternative to the way they are living, they may not consider death as the outcome.

55 Correct answer—**A**

Rates are highest among certain sections of the population: alcoholics, police, physicians, previous attempters, adolescents, terminally ill patients, elderly people, members of minority groups, and psychotic patients. As the suicide rates indicate, certain groups of the population are more likely to become self-destructive than others. Among those who commit suicide, about three times as many men die as women; although more women attempt to kill themselves, they typically choose less effective means than men do.

Selected References

Adams, C.G., and Macione, A. *Handbook of Psychiatric and Mental Health Nursing.* New York: John Wiley & Sons, 1983.

Altschul, A.T., ed. *Psychiatric Nursing.* New York: Churchill Livingstone, 1985.

Backer, B.A., et al. *Psychiatric Mental Health Nursing: Contemporary Readings.* Boston: Jones & Bartlett, 1985.

Barker, P.J. *Patient Assessment in Psychiatric Nursing.* Wolfeboro, N.H.: Longwood Publishing Group, 1985.

Beck, C.M., and Rawlins, R.P. *Mental Health-Psychiatric Nursing: A Holistic Life-Cycle Approach.* St. Louis: C.V. Mosby Co., 1984.

Brooking, J., ed. *Psychiatric Nursing Research.* New York: John Wiley & Sons, 1986.

Burgess, A.W. *Psychiatric Nursing in the Hospital and the Community.* Englewood Cliffs, N.J.: Prentice-Hall, 1985.

Cain, H. *Flint's Emergency Treatment and Management,* 7th ed. Philadelphia: W.B. Saunders Co., 1985.

Carr, P.J., et al. *Community Psychiatric Nursing.* New York: Churchill Livingstone, 1980.

Comstock, B., et al., eds. *Phenomenology and Treatment of Psychiatric Emergencies.* Jamaica, N.Y.: SP Medical & Science Books, 1984.

Crawford, A.L., and Kilander, V.C. *Psychiatric Nursing & Mental Health Nursing: A Basic Manual.* Philadelphia: F.A. Davis Co., 1984.

DeCastro, N.S. *Mental Health Nursing.* Dubuque, Iowa: Kendall-Hunt, 1984.

Emergencies. Nurse's Reference Library Series. Springhouse, Pa.: Springhouse Corporation, 1985.

Fitzpatrick, J., et al., *Nursing Models & Their Psychiatric Mental Health Applications.* Bowie, Md.: Robert J. Brady Co., 1981.

Haber, J., et al. *Comprehensive Psychiatric Nursing,* 3rd ed. New York: McGraw-Hill Book Co., 1987.

Harris, A.C., and McCarthy, K. *Mental Health Practice for Community Nurses.* New York: Springer Publishing Co., 1981.

Janosik, E.H., and Davies, J.L. *Psychiatric Mental Health Nursing.* Philadelphia: Wadsworth Health, 1986.

Joel, L.A., and Collins, D.L. *Psychiatric Nursing: Theory & Application.* New York: McGraw-Hill Book Co., 1978.

Johnson, B.S. *Psychiatric-Mental Health Nursing: Adaption & Growth.* Philadelphia: J.B. Lippincott Co., 1986.

Kalkman, M.E., and Davis, A.B. *New Dimensions in Mental Health-Psychiatric Nursing.* New York: McGraw-Hill Book Co., 1979.

Kaplan, H.I., and Sadock, B.J., eds. *Comprehensive Textbook of Psychiatry IV* (Vol. 2), 4th ed. Baltimore: Williams & Wilkins, 1985.

Kyes, J.J., and Hofling, C.K. *Basic Psychiatric Concepts in Nursing.* Philadelphia: J.B. Lippincott Co., 1980.

Lanros, N. *Assessment and Intervention in Emergency Nursing,* 2nd ed. Bowie, Md.: Robert J. Brady Co., 1983.

Lego, S. *The American Handbook of Psychiatric Nursing.* Philadelphia: J.B. Lippincott Co., 1984.

McFarland, G.K., and Wasli, E.L. *Nursing Diagnosis & Process in Psychiatric-Mental Health Nursing.* Philadelphia: J.B. Lippincott Co., 1986.

Maddison, D., et al. *Psychiatric Nursing.* New York: Churchill Livingstone, 1982.

Pasquali, E.A., et al. *Mental Health Nursing: A Holistic Approach.* St. Louis: C.V. Mosby Co., 1985.

Redmond, G.T., and Ouellette, F. *Concept & Case Studies Nursing: A Life Cycle Approach.* Menlo Park, Calif.: Addison-Wesley Publishing Co., 1982.

Robinson, L. *Psychiatric Nursing As A Human Experience.* Philadelphia: W.B. Saunders Co., 1983.

Shives, L.R. *Basic Concepts of Psychiatric-Mental Health Nursing.* Philadelphia: J.B. Lippincott Co., 1986.

Smoyak, S.A., and Rouline, S., eds. *A Collection of Classics in Psychiatric Nursing Literature.* Thorofare, N.J.: Charles B. Slack, 1982.

(continued)

Selected References (continued)

Stockwell, F. *The Nursing Process in Psychiatric Nursing.* Wolfeboro, N.H.: Longwood Publishing Group, 1985.

Stuart, G.W., and Sundeen, S.J. *Principles & Practice of Psychiatric Nursing.* St. Louis: C.V. Mosby Co., 1983.

Warner, C., ed. *Emergency Care: Assessment and Intervention,* 3rd ed. St. Louis: C.V. Mosby Co., 1983.

Wells, L.A. *Psychiatric Nursing Handbook.* St. Louis: Warren H. Green, 1986.

Wilson, H.S., and Kneisl, C.R. *Psychiatric Nursing.* Menlo Park, Calif.: Addison-Wesley Publishing Co., 1983.

Chapter 15

Abuse/Neglect/Sexual Assault Questions and Answers

You must begin with Question 1 of this chapter and progress in sequence. **Do not skip around.** Subsequent answers build on previous ones.

Mary Blum, RN, MSN
Catherine T. Kelly, RN, MSN, EMT-P, CCRN, CEN

1 The most common cause of death from acute alcohol intoxication is:

A. Respiratory depression or arrest
B. Aspiration of vomitus
C. Gastrointestinal bleeding
D. Accidental injury

2 Alcohol intoxication can often be confused with which of the following:

A. Diabetic reactions
B. Head injury
C. Drug overdose
D. All of the above

3 All of the following are indicated in the management of the acutely intoxicated adult patient *except*:

A. Thiamine 100 mg I.M.
B. Chlordiazepoxide (Librium) 100 mg I.M. every 2 to 4 hours as needed
C. Diazepam (Valium) 5 to 10 mg I.V. bolus for seizure management
D. I.V. of normal saline solution

4 To implement a plan of care for a patient with alcohol intoxication, the nurse understands that delirium tremens:

A. Is not a significant cause of death
B. Starts 6 to 72 hours after the last alcohol ingestion
C. Lasts up to 12 hours after withdrawal
D. Is best managed by restricting fluid intake

5 Many patients undergoing therapy for alcohol abuse use disulfiram (Antabuse). Emergency management of an Antabuse–alcohol reaction includes:

A. Initiation of an I.V. infusion of normal saline solution
B. Administration of diphenhydramine (Benadryl) 50 mg
C. Administration of chlorpheniramine (Chlor-Trimeton) or similar drug
D. All of the above

SITUATION

A 20-year-old woman walks into the emergency department (ED) and states, "I was raped." Her clothes are torn and several bruises on her face are noted. Trembling and withdrawn, she avoids eye contact with immediate personnel and is escorted by a nurse to a private room.

Questions 6 to 10 refer to the above situation.

6 The *most* important message that the receiving nurse can convey to the victim of sexual assault is:

A. All medical tests will be handled confidentially
B. The examination will be done quickly
C. The patient is now in a safe, secure environment
D. There are medications to prevent pregnancy

7 When collecting the victim's clothing, you would:

A. Have the victim place all her clothing together in a plastic bag
B. Have the victim fold each piece of clothing inward and place each article in a separate paper bag
C. Shake each piece of clothing separately, then place all articles together in a paper bag
D. Not collect the clothing of the victim who had been totally undressed before the assault

8 The rape victim should be advised to return to her physician for a repeat serologic test for syphilis (Venereal Disease Research Laboratory [VDRL] test) within how many weeks?

A. 1 to 2
B. 2 to 4
C. 4 to 6
D. 6 to 8

9 What should be provided to the victim upon discharge?

A. Written discharge instructions
B. Suitable clothing, if hers had been retained for evidence
C. A list of referral telephone numbers
D. All of the above

10 When interviewing the victim, you will need to know if she has done which of the following since the assault?

A. Urinated or defecated
B. Changed clothes
C. Rinsed her mouth
D. All of the above

11 The age-group of children most likely to be physically abused is:

A. Infants
B. Toddlers
C. School-age children (ages 5 to 12)
D. Adolescents

12 The abused child in a hospital setting may commonly exhibit all of the following behaviors *except:*

A. Always wants to know what's going to happen next
B. Seems constantly alert to possible danger
C. Looks to adults for reassurance
D. Seems less afraid of other children

13 All of the following increase a child's risk of being abused *except:*

A. Mental retardation
B. Physical handicap
C. Prematurity
D. Being the first-born child

14 Child abuse or neglect should be suspected in which 2-year-old child?

A. With symmetrical bruises on both knees
B. With a finger laceration; the child clings to the mother
C. With bruises in various stages of healing on both arms
D. With a partial-thickness burn to the fingers of one hand

15 The most common cause of death in child abuse is:

A. Abdominal trauma
B. Asphyxiation
C. Head trauma
D. Malnutrition

16 Forms of child neglect include:

A. Educational neglect
B. Lack of supervision
C. Failure to thrive
D. All of the above

17 Which statement is *true* regarding child sexual abuse?

A. Incest that occurs during adolescence is easier for the victim to manage than incest occurring before adolescence
B. Children recover more easily from the experience if the abuser is a family member
C. Boys who are sexually abused have greater adjustment problems than girls
D. Boys receive more support from the family than girls when incest is discovered

SITUATION

A 12-year-old girl is seen in the ED with dysuria, scant vaginal bleeding, and a 2-cm linear laceration on the posterior aspect of the left thigh. She has not had menarche. The mother reports that her daughter has a poor relationship with her peers and that she has recently become more withdrawn. The parents are divorced; the patient and her mother recently moved in with a maternal uncle to help ease financial difficulties. Child abuse is suspected.

Questions 18 to 21 refer to the above situation.

18 Which assessment data indicate possible child abuse?

A. Occasional accidents from lack of adult supervision
B. Venereal disease in a young child
C. Pregnancy in late adolescence
D. Excessive anger by a daughter toward her father

19 Which should be the nurse's primary concern when caring for the abused child?

A. Establishment of peer relationships
B. Continuation of parental contact
C. Demonstrated acceptance and affection of the child
D. Behavior modification for the child

20 The nurse should consider which problem when planning the care of the child admitted to the hospital because of sexual abuse?

A. The nurse's personal feelings toward the parents and parental expectations
B. The child's developmental level and parental desires for contact
C. The child's sibling and peer relationships
D. Community support and foster parent needs

21 Which is the most appropriate nursing action when child abuse is suspected?

A. Assume that the physician caring for the child will suspect abuse and report it to the appropriate agency
B. Confront the parents directly and report findings to the appropriate agency
C. Assume responsibility for reporting suspected abuse to the appropriate agency
D. Assign responsibility for reporting suspected abuse to a social worker

22 A common characteristic of parents who abuse their children is that they:

A. View violence as an acceptable method of behavior modification
B. Are socially involved with their neighbors
C. Have had good relationships with their parents
D. Are self-sufficient

23 Which statement regarding abuse or neglect is true?

A. A neglectful parent is likely to restrict a child's social activities
B. An abusive parent is not likely to restrict a child's social activities
C. Only a small number of children who are neglected are abused
D. All of the above

24 The treatment objectives for the abused child and family include all of the following *except:*

A. Helping the parents understand their own needs
B. Teaching the child to express his needs in a direct manner
C. Encouraging the parents and child to increase their isolation and focus upon themselves
D. Redistributing power within the family so that no one assumes total control

25 A 19-year-old man comes to the ED exhibiting confusion, lethargy, dysarthria, and emotional instability. Which drug is most likely to produce these symptoms?

A. Phencyclidine (PCP)
B. Barbiturate
C. Amphetamine
D. Cocaine

26 Naloxone (Narcan) is the narcotic antagonist of choice for patients who overdose on opiates. After administration, the danger of respiratory depression is still present for how many hours?

A. 1
B. 2
C. 3
D. 4

27 A 22-year-old man comes to the ED for treatment of PCP ingestion. What should be avoided when caring for this patient?

A. Constant verbal reassurance
B. Phenothiazines
C. Tactile stimulation
D. All of the above

28 Symptoms from methadone withdrawal usually appear within how many hours?

A. 8 to 10
B. 12 to 24
C. 24 to 36
D. 36 to 48

29 Gastric lavage in the management of the unconscious overdose patient includes:

A. Instillation of 200 ml of warmed normal saline solution via nasogastric tube, drained by gravity
B. Instillation of iced normal saline solution
C. Lavage before endotracheal intubation
D. Lavage with a 50% normal saline, 50% magnesium sulfate solution

SITUATION

A 24-year-old man is brought to the ED by family members who found him slumped over in a chair at home. An empty prescription bottle for thirty 100-mg amitriptyline (Elavil) tablets, with an issue date of 5 days before, was found near the patient. He is unresponsive except to deep pain, which elicits purposeful movements. Lungs are clear, and his vital signs are blood pressure, 160/96 mm Hg; pulse, 140 beats/minute; and respirations, 14 breaths/minute.

Questions 30 to 34 refer to the above situation.

30 Tricyclic antidepressants are chiefly used in the treatment of:

A. Psychotic disorders
B. Anxiety-related neurosis
C. Chronic paranoia
D. Depression

31 The nursing action having the highest priority for the initial management of tricyclic antidepressant overdose is:

A. Cardiac monitoring
B. Neurologic assessment
C. Protection from aspiration
D. Infusion of normal saline solution

32 In the initial care of this patient, management should include:

A. Evacuation of gastric contents
B. Insertion of an indwelling (Foley) catheter
C. Parenteral infusion of physostigmine (Antilirium)
D. Administration of quinidine (Cardioquin) for dysrhythmia control

33 Which assessment finding is *not* seen in the early manifestations of tricyclic antidepressant overdose?

A. Agitation
B. Diaphoresis
C. Dilated pupils
D. Exaggerated reflexes

34 The most effective and conservative treatment for the patient who has overdosed with a tricyclic antidepressant and develops severe tachycardia is the administration of:

A. Sodium bicarbonate
B. Magnesium sulfate
C. Diazepam (Valium)
D. Phenytoin (Dilantin)

35 When a nurse is referring a child who has been sexually abused to the community health nurse, which observation should be included?

A. Procaine penicillin 50,000 units/kg I.M.
B. VDRL was obtained and no further studies are indicated
C. Urine for human chorionic gonadotropin (HCG) levels was obtained for pregnancy testing
D. The pelvic examination revealed an intact hymen

Answer Sheet

	A	B	C	D
1	○	○	○	○
2	○	○	○	○
3	○	○	○	○
4	○	○	○	○
5	○	○	○	○
6	○	○	○	○
7	○	○	○	○
8	○	○	○	○
9	○	○	○	○
10	○	○	○	○
11	○	○	○	○
12	○	○	○	○
13	○	○	○	○
14	○	○	○	○
15	○	○	○	○
16	○	○	○	○
17	○	○	○	○
18	○	○	○	○
19	○	○	○	○
20	○	○	○	○
21	○	○	○	○
22	○	○	○	○
23	○	○	○	○
24	○	○	○	○
25	○	○	○	○
26	○	○	○	○
27	○	○	○	○
28	○	○	○	○
29	○	○	○	○
30	○	○	○	○
31	○	○	○	○
32	○	○	○	○
33	○	○	○	○
34	○	○	○	○
35	○	○	○	○

Answer Sheet

	A	B	C	D		A	B	C	D
1	○	○	○	○	31	○	○	○	○
2	○	○	○	○	32	○	○	○	○
3	○	○	○	○	33	○	○	○	○
4	○	○	○	○	34	○	○	○	○
5	○	○	○	○	35	○	○	○	○
6	○	○	○	○					
7	○	○	○	○					
8	○	○	○	○					
9	○	○	○	○					
10	○	○	○	○					
11	○	○	○	○					
12	○	○	○	○					
13	○	○	○	○					
14	○	○	○	○					
15	○	○	○	○					
16	○	○	○	○					
17	○	○	○	○					
18	○	○	○	○					
19	○	○	○	○					
20	○	○	○	○					
21	○	○	○	○					
22	○	○	○	○					
23	○	○	○	○					
24	○	○	○	○					
25	○	○	○	○					
26	○	○	○	○					
27	○	○	○	○					
28	○	○	○	○					
29	○	○	○	○					
30	○	○	○	○					

1 Correct answer—**A**

The most common cause of death is respiratory depression. The depression begins to occur at alcohol blood levels of 0.20%; death occurs at approximately 0.40% to 0.50%. Death is also common from aspiration of vomitus and accidental injury, especially from automobile accidents. Gastrointestinal bleeding occurs most commonly in those patients who chronically abuse alcohol.

2 Correct answer—**D**

Head injury, drug overdose, and diabetic reactions can all mimic acute alcohol intoxication. Other disorders must also be considered, such as acute brain syndrome, meningitis, and psychiatric disorders. An accurate history and physical examination and appropriate diagnostic studies are necessary to arrive at the correct diagnosis.

3 Correct answer—**D**

The I.V. solution used for intoxicated patients should contain dextrose (e.g., D_5W or $D_{10}W$) to facilitate the metabolism of the alcohol. Diazepam and chlordiazepoxide are tranquilizers that may be helpful in controlling behavior. Strong sedatives should not be used, because they will increase the risk of respiratory depression. Diazepam is also indicated for seizure control. Thiamine maintains or restores neurologic function that may be impaired because of malnutrition and vitamin deficiency.

4 Correct answer—**B**

Delirium tremens typically begin 72 hours after alcohol is withdrawn and may continue for several days. However, the onset is unpredictable and it may begin as early as 6 hours after alcohol is withdrawn. It has a mortality of 10% to 15%. Adequate hydration and proper electrolyte balance are critical to maintain system functioning.

5 Correct answer—**D**

Antabuse–alcohol reactions mimic anaphylactic shock and should be managed in basically the same manner. Reactions may last up to several hours or as long as alcohol is in the bloodstream. Such reactions may occur up to 14 days after discontinuation of Antabuse, because the drug is slowly eliminated from the body.

6 Correct answer—**C**

The first message that must be conveyed is that the victim is in a safe, secure environment. Most sexual assaults occur in places known to the victim, and because the victim may even know the attacker, even familiar surroundings may be perceived as threatening. That sexual attacks commonly occur without warning contributes even more to the development of fear and sense of loss of control. The other messages may be conveyed after the patient's safety needs are met.

7 Correct answer—**B**

Clothing should not be shaken but should be folded inward by the patient, if possible, and placed in paper bags. This will retain evidence and prevent contamination of the clothing by staff members. Plastic bags should not be used, because they may retain moisture and alter the evidence. If the victim consents, all clothing and other belongings should be retained for evidence. Minute pieces of hair, clothing, semen, blood, leaves, and dirt provide concrete evidence that should be identified by a qualified laboratory.

8 Correct answer—**C**

Syphilis takes from 4 to 6 weeks to be detected serologically.

9 Correct answer—**D**

The victim's basic needs of food, shelter, and clothing must be met in order to begin reestablishment of control. Clear, concise, written instructions are necessary because the victim is unlikely to remember oral instructions. A list of referral telephone numbers is critical and should include at least one 24-hour resource.

10 Correct answer—**D**

Semen can be detected in urine and in a rectal swab specimen. In cases of oral assault, semen is likely to be found in oral secretions around the gum line. Evidence such as hair, blood, semen, and grass may be retained in clothing. The ultimate goal is to make sure that all evidence is collected and maintained to ensure its admission into court.

11 Correct answer—**A**

Infants, because they are defenseless, nonverbal, and difficult at times to manage, are most commonly injured.

12 Correct answer—**C**

In most cases, the abused child shows a wariness and distrust of adults, because they are the most common abusers. An abused child attempts to gain some control over the environment by wanting to know what will happen next and preparing for what may happen. Other children do not pose a threat to the patient, who may easily settle into the hospital environment.

13 Correct answer—**D**

Maltreatment is often noted in children who are mentally retarded. Children who are physically handicapped also have a higher incidence of maltreatment. In both cases, one of the contributing factors appears to be the increased difficulty in caring for these children. The increased incidence in premature children is attributed to the medical problems commonly encountered, financial stress, and interruption of the bonding process.

14 Correct answer—**C**

One of the most common hallmarks of chronic physical abuse is the appearance of ecchymotic lesions in various stages of healing. Initially, they are red to purple, then change to green (5 to 7 days), then yellow-brown (1 to 3 weeks), and disappear in 2 to 4 weeks. Symmetrical bruises on the knees of a 2-year-old child are common because of their tendency to fall on their knees. Lacerations are an uncommon physical finding in abuse of a 2-year-old child, especially one who then looks to the parent for support. Intentional burns are most often symmetrical and full thickness. This burn would most likely be from a 2-year-old child's natural curiosity or an accidental fall, which often results in burns to hands and forearms. The common areas intentionally burned are the feet and buttocks.

15 Correct answer—**C**

Head trauma is the most common cause of death; subdural hematoma is commonly seen. Abdominal trauma with bruising or rupture of abdominal viscera is the second most common cause of death in abused children. Asphyxiation does occur, but uncommonly. Malnutrition occurs but is rarely the cause of death, except for those children who are isolated from society.

16 Correct answer—**D**

All of the items listed are recognized forms of child abuse. Other categories include abandonment; nutritional, medical, and dental neglect; and inappropriate or insufficient clothing.

17 Correct answer—**C**

Sexually abused boys have greater difficulty in adjusting because abuse is usually more common for girls. For this reason, girls commonly receive more support. Incest that occurs and stops before adolescence causes less difficulty for the child, possibly because younger children are not as cognizant of society's norms. Children recover more easily if the abuser is outside the family, because they will not have to deal with the abuser on an ongoing basis. The family assumes a protective role if the abuser is a non-family member, but may not believe the child if the abuser is a family member.

18 Correct answer—**B**

Venereal disease in a young child indicates sexual abuse. Abuse of children can be present in many forms: physical, sexual, and emotional. Physical and behavioral indicators may be bruises, welts, burns, fractures, dislocations, lacerations, abrasions, dysuria, vaginal or penile discharge, wariness of physical contact with adults, feeding disorders, self-stimulation, withdrawal, or unusual sexual knowledge or behavior. Frequent accidents because of lack of adult supervision may indicate neglect. Pregnancy in early adolescence is indicative of sexual abuse; commonly, the child fails to disclose the paternal source. Excessive anger from a daughter directed toward the mother may be another indicator of child abuse; this results from the perceived failure of the mother to protect the daughter.

19 Correct answer—**C**

The abused child requires a constant care giver who provides acceptance and affection. Abused children may not readily return the acceptance and affection because their previous efforts were met by frustration, neglect, or abuse. As a result, the abused child does not easily establish a trusting relationship with an adult. The nurse must demonstrate affection while attempting to modify negative behaviors. Modeling, play therapy, and demonstration of alternative methods of interaction and discipline provide the child with appropriate ways to display anger and frustration. The abused child usually has little difficulty establishing peer relationships. Depending upon the nature and severity of the abuse, parental rights and contact may be terminated.

20 Correct answer—**A**

The nurse must examine personal feelings toward the parents and avoid expressing any negative feelings. As a result, the nurse who is primarily responsible for an abused child's care may not be the best person to develop a relationship and therapy program with the parents. Intervention should be focused on enhancing parental self-concept, establishing realistic expectations for the child, and promoting adequate parental problem-solving with appropriate discipline. In many cases, parents have unrealistic expectations for the child and thus need information about appropriate growth and development. Self-help groups may benefit abusive families by helping the parents gain personal insight and appropriate methods for releasing frustration. Crisis centers or hot lines may decrease the incidence of child abuse, but only in the short term. Poor peer relationships may be more common in the sexually abused child. Usually, the abused child adjusts to new environments and makes friends without difficulty. If foster care is necessary, the foster parents should be encouraged to visit the hospitalized child and participate in care. They must demonstrate affection and acceptance for the child to develop a sense of trust with the foster parents.

21 Correct answer—**C**

In many states, nurses are legally mandated to report all cases of suspected child abuse to an appropriate agency. The nurse is often the gatekeeper and must assume an active role in reporting and preventing child abuse. Because of the intimate nature of the nurse-patient relationship, the nurse may have more information to diagnose ineffective family-child relationships. The nurse may have the primary responsibility of case coordination and care of abusive families. Child abuse is multidimensional in nature and requires an interdisciplinary approach, in which the nurse may assume the central role. Direct confrontation is not recommended, because anger and fear will escalate and the parents may remove the child from the hospital before the proper authorities arrive.

22 Correct answer—**A**

Violence is viewed as an acceptable method of behavior modification in families who abuse or neglect children. Many factors contribute to this violence, such as mental or physical handicaps, low self-esteem, and poor coping mechanisms. These parents tend to be socially isolated and have minimal support systems. Most are not able to be self-sufficient, and this, together with the isolation, creates a very isolated nonsupportive environment. Studies have proven that child abusers have in many cases been the victims of abuse themselves.

23 Correct answer—**C**

The neglected child is often ignored; therefore, abuse is less likely to occur. An abusive parent or family tends to restrict the child's social interactions to minimize the risk of discovery. The parent or family in the neglectful situation allows the child to interact freely; this may actually place fewer demands on the parent, because the child's needs can be met elsewhere.

24 Correct answer—**C**

The family must be encouraged to expand its relationships, thereby improving support mechanisms. The child must be taught to express his needs directly, thus eliminating confusion and fostering realistic expectations. Helping the parents to understand themselves and fostering the sharing of power and responsibilities help to strengthen the family unit.

25 Correct answer—**B**

Barbiturates are noted for creating confusion along with lethargy, dysarthria, and emotional instability. Phencyclidine (PCP), amphetamines, and cocaine all usually create euphoria and increased activity.

26 Correct answer—**D**

The danger of respiratory depression is dose- and patient-related and may occur beyond 4 hours. Continuous assessment and serial toxicology levels are helpful in determining the patient's status.

27 Correct answer—**D**

Persons under the influence of PCP respond better to the least amount of stimulation. Contact should be limited to one person in a dimly lighted, quiet room. Phenothiazines are similar to PCP in clinical structure, and their administration may produce an anticholinergic crisis or potentiate the effects of PCP.

28 Correct answer—**C**

Methadone stays in a patient's system for approximately 48 hours. Depending on the patient's metabolism and drug history, withdrawal symptoms become evident in 24 to 36 hours.

29 Correct answer—**A**

Gastric lavage for overdose patients is achieved with 200-ml increments of warmed normal saline solution, which is drained off by gravity, intermittently. Iced normal saline solution causes local venous constriction and is effective for patients with gastrointestinal hemorrhage. The airway of an unconscious patient must be protected before gastric lavage; therefore, endotracheal intubation must be performed first. Magnesium sulfate is administered after the lavage is completed to enhance excretion. Activated charcoal may also be given at this time to increase adsorption of the toxin.

30 Correct answer—**D**

Tricyclic antidepressants are used chiefly to treat depression, which is usually manifested by mixed clinical signs of lethargy, insomnia, anorexia, or agitation. Tricyclic antidepressants produce excellent results in the treatment of nonorganic depression. However, as these patients are prone to self-destructive behavior, the use of tricyclic antidepressants is risky, because they are the drugs most often involved in potentially life-threatening overdoses.

31 Correct answer—**C**

Protection from aspiration holds the highest priority because it deals with airway maintenance. Definitive treatment for any overdose always begins with the ABCs of emergency care. All supportive care is based on the assessment and maintenance of these factors.

32 Correct answer—**A**

Evacuation of gastric contents has a very high priority. Tricyclic antidepressants slow peristalsis; significant amounts of ingested drugs can be found in the stomach several hours after intake. Gastric aspiration ensures removal of stomach contents; repeated lavage removes tricyclic antidepressant metabolites that are periodically released from the liver and gallbladder. Repeated charcoal administration has been recommended to deal with tricyclic antidepressant overdoses. The administration of quinidine will worsen the already toxic effects that produce a prolonged QRS complex and Q-T interval. Physostigmine administration may be required if anticholinergic symptoms develop. An indwelling (Foley) catheter may then be warranted to measure urine output.

33 Correct answer—**B**

The clinical manifestations of tricyclic antidepressant overdose do not include diaphoresis. These drugs mimic anticholinergic drugs and produce fever, agitation, dilated pupils, tachycardia, and dry mucous membranes. Many victims of tricyclic antidepressant overdose will show twitching that will progress to grand mal seizures.

34 Correct answer—**A**

The most effective and conservative treatment is to alkalize the blood to a pH of 7.5 using sodium bicarbonate. Studies indicate that tachycardia most commonly disappears at this pH; breaking the tricyclic antidepressant bonding with body protein is the proposed mechanism. Magnesium sulfate speeds the slowed peristalsis and hastens the elimination of drugs absorbed by charcoal. Diazepam (Valium) and phenytoin (Dilantin) are used to treat the seizure activity.

35 Correct answer—**D**

The condition of the hymen neither proves nor disproves penetration. The hymen may have been ruptured by various noncoital activities or accidents, or it may have enough elasticity for penetration without laceration. Nevertheless, the hymenal condition has legal significance and must be reported. The pelvic examination must be accomplished if penetration is suspected. Hair sampling and swabs for spermatozoa and gonorrhea must be obtained. A serologic test for syphilis is required and should be repeated 1 to 2 months after the initial examination. Procaine penicillin 100,000 units/kg I.M. for the child and 4.8 million units for the adolescent is recommended. After menarche, urine should be obtained for HCG to determine possible pregnancy.

Selected References

Alspach, J.G., and Williams, S. *Core Curriculum for Critical Care Nursing.* Philadelphia: W.B. Saunders Co., 1985.

American Medical Association Council on Scientific Affairs. "AMA Diagnostic and Treatment Guidelines Concerning Child Abuse and Neglect," *Journal of the American Medical Association* 254, August 9, 1985.

Mayhall, P.D., and Norgard, K. *Child Abuse and Neglect: Sharing Responsibilities.* New York: John Wiley & Sons, 1983.

Scipien, G., et al. *Comprehensive Pediatric Nursing,* 3rd ed. New York: McGraw-Hill Book Co., 1986.

Servonsky, J., and Opas, S. *Nursing Management of Children.* Boston: Jones and Bartlett Publishing, Inc., 1987.

Sheehy, S.B., and Budassi, J.B. *Emergency Nursing: Principles and Practice.* St. Louis: C.V. Mosby Co., 1985.

Whaley, L., and Wong, D. *Nursing Care of Infants and Children.* St. Louis: C.V. Mosby Co., 1987.

Chapter 16

Roles and Responsibilities of the Emergency Nurse Questions and Answers

You must begin with Question 1 of this chapter and progress in sequence. **Do not skip around.** Subsequent answers build on previous ones.

Carol A. Bottin, RN
Joanne Noone, RN, MSN, CCRN, CEN
Susan Schulmerich, RN, MS, MBA, CNA, CEN
Joanne Scotto, RN, BSN
Consultant: David Weaver, Esq.

1 Under what circumstances may a nurse use force against a patient?

A. Under no circumstances
B. To bring an emotionally distraught patient back to his senses
C. To assess an unconscious patient's level of reaction to physical stimuli
D. In self-defense, but only if the nurse has reasonable grounds to believe that she is being, or is about to be, attacked

2 An oral order given by a physician to a nurse:

A. Is legally valid alone but should be covered with a written order for professional safety
B. Is legally valid only when followed by a written order
C. Is legally valid only if made in the physical presence of a witness
D. Is never legally valid

3 If a patient does not understand the information just given by the physician during an informed consent, the nurse should:

A. Answer the patient's questions
B. Notify the supervisor
C. Notify the physician
D. Do nothing, as the consent is already signed

4 Giving a medication to a patient against his will is an example of:

A. False imprisonment
B. Negligence
C. Battery
D. Invasion of privacy

5 When witnessing an informed consent, the nurse is attesting that the:

A. Patient is informed about the procedure
B. Patient consents to the procedure
C. Patient is sufficiently alert and oriented to consent
D. Signature is that of the patient

6 Legally, besides being a witness to the informed consent, the nurse may also obtain:

A. The informed consent
B. The patient's signature
C. Telephone consents from the next of kin
D. Administrative consent

7 If a patient has questions regarding the correctness of treatment, the nurse should:

A. Inform the physician
B. Discuss other therapies
C. Refer the patient to other qualified physicians
D. Reinforce the appropriateness of the treatment

8 A nurse disagrees with the physician's judgment in ordering furosemide (Lasix) for a patient, feeling that, although Lasix is safe to give in this situation, dopamine (Intropin) would be more effective. If, after questioning the order, the nurse is told to give Lasix, she should:

A. Refuse to give Lasix
B. Give Lasix
C. Give Intropin
D. Ask another physician

9 In order for negligence to be committed:

A. The wrong therapy must be given
B. Injury must be incurred
C. A change in the patient's condition must be overlooked
D. An error in judgment must be made

10 Physical restraints should be used when there is:

A. A physician's order
B. A threat to the patient's safety
C. An uncooperative patient
D. Insufficient staff to watch the patient

11 The most appropriate way to legally document patient teaching is by:

A. Referring to it in the nurses' notes
B. Providing written instructions
C. Teaching with a witness present
D. Giving the patient a written examination

12 The most important goal of triage is:

A. Priority care for the most critically ill
B. Comprehensive patient assessment
C. Immediate patient assessment
D. Placement of patients in appropriate treatment areas

13 Which nursing action is inappropriate for the triage nurse to implement?

A. Initiating cardiopulmonary resuscitation
B. Intervening immediately in arterial bleeding
C. Splinting suspected or obvious fractures
D. Placing a Steri-strip over a minor laceration

14 The responsibilities of the triage nurse do *not* include:

A. Prevention of cross-contamination of suspected infectious patients
B. Complete and comprehensive patient assessment
C. Patient or family education
D. Fostering good public relations

SITUATION

The emergency department (ED) is notified by Emergency Medical Services (EMS) of a multiple-casualty accident involving a school bus and a truck carrying radioactive waste. The proximity of the accident to your facility suggests that your department will receive the bulk of casualties.

Questions 15 and 16 refer to the above situation.

15 Your first priority is to:

A. Designate a decontamination area
B. Notify the admitting office to clear five intensive care unit (ICU) beds
C. Clear the ED of all nonserious patients and move those awaiting admission to a holding area
D. Notify EMS of the number of casualties you can accommodate

16 Which support services would be especially needed to deal with this incident?

A. Laboratory and blood bank
B. Operating room
C. Pharmacy
D. Radiology

17 The objectives of quality assurance activity are to:

A. Monitor the quality of care
B. Identify actual or perceived problems
C. Identify educational or remedial needs
D. All of the above

18 Resources by which to identify patient care issues include:

A. Minutes of staff meetings and patient complaints
B. Staff suggestions and state regulations
C. Joint Commission on Accreditation of Hospitals (JCAH) guidelines
D. All of the above

19 Specific components of quality assurance monitoring are:

A. Problem identification, study or survey, results reporting, recommendations, and follow-up targets
B. Problem identification, study or survey, results reporting, recommendations, follow-up targets, and noncompliance consequences
C. The problem(s) must be retrospective; study or survey, recommendations, follow-up targets, and noncompliance consequences
D. The problem(s) must be concurrent; results reporting, recommendations, and follow-up targets

20 While you are on duty, you receive a phone call from an hysterical, nearly incoherent woman. You manage to calm her and determine that she has just been sexually assaulted. She asks what she should do. Appropriate advice includes:

A. Telling her to contact the police immediately
B. Telling her to contact the police and come to the hospital immediately with a change of clothes
C. Referring her to a rape crisis center
D. Obtaining her name, address, and phone number; telling her to call the police and come to the hospital immediately with a change of clothes

21 You answer the ED phone, and a woman states she has just moved into the area. She would like the name of a pediatrician. You should:

A. Give her the name of a pediatrician on staff
B. Give her the name of a new pediatrician who is just starting practice
C. Give her the number of the local medical society
D. Tell her to bring the child to the ED for evaluation and follow-up

22 The policy of your ED is to make follow-up phone calls after treatment. When you are making such a call, the patient tells you he thinks he is having a reaction to the prescribed antibiotic. You advise him to:

A. Decrease the dose and see if the reaction subsides
B. Continue taking the drug along with over-the-counter diphenhydramine (Benadryl)
C. Stop taking the drug
D. Stop taking the drug and return to the ED

23 In a police investigation, the law enforcement agency is entitled to:

A. A patient's name, address, age, and extent of injury
B. All patient information
C. A copy of the patient's medical record
D. None of the above without a court order

SITUATION

A prominent member of your community is brought to your ED after an attempted suicide. You receive a phone call from a newspaper reporter asking you to tell him about the incident.

Questions 24 and 25 refer to the above situation.

24 The correct nursing action is to:

A. Give the reporter the information requested because of the freedom of information act
B. Give the reporter the general patient information as dictated by hospital policy
C. Allow the reporter to interview the patient when condition permits
D. Notify the administrator or nursing supervisor

25 You allow the reporter to gain unauthorized access to the patient's chart. You are guilty of:

A. Breach of patient confidentiality
B. Malpractice
C. Professional misconduct
D. None of the above

SITUATION

An 18-year-old man is brought to the ED unresponsive, with shallow breathing and a rapid, weak pulse. His blood pressure is palpable at 80 mm Hg systolic. His friends state he "just slumped over." After stabilization, the patient's pockets are searched in an attempt to identify him. An envelope with white powder is discovered.

Questions 26 and 27 refer to the above situation.

26 The correct nursing action is to:

A. Replace the envelope and say nothing
B. Inform the physician
C. Inform the physician and secure the envelope
D. Inform the physician and notify the police

27 The nurse could be civilly liable in this situation for:

A. Illegal search and seizure
B. Invasion of privacy
C. Violation of constitutional rights
D. No civil liability exists

28 In any case, the integrity and security of evidence is known as:

A. The chain of evidence
B. Evidence integrity
C. Writ of evidence
D. Habeas corpus

29 "Emergency consents" are:

A. Informed consents
B. Administrative consents
C. Implied consents
D. All of the above

30 In the case of a minor who is suspected of being a victim of child abuse or neglect, the parent or legal guardian can:

A. Withdraw consent for treatment
B. Discharge the minor against medical advice
C. Be restrained by hospital personnel from taking the minor out of the hospital
D. Be restrained by police from taking the minor out of the hospital

31 One of the roles of the ED nurse involves air transport. The nurse is aware that air transport of patients may produce:

A. Change in vital signs and hypothermia
B. Pneumothorax and hypoxemia
C. Nausea and vomiting
D. All of the above

32 You work in an ED where most of the patient population does not speak English; however, discharge and patient instructions are in English. For a patient who does not speak English but is accompanied by a friend who does, you would:

A. Have the friend interpret for the patient
B. Determine if the friend understands the instructions, then have him/her interpret, and so document
C. Delay discharge until the hospital interpreter can be found
D. Tell the patient to go to his physician with the instructions so a medical person can interpret

33 The nurse's responsibility is to determine if a patient understands discharge instructions. To determine this, you should:

A. Have the patient repeat, verbatim, the instructions
B. Have the patient sign the ED record indicating the instructions were received
C. Have the patient explain the instructions to you, and so document
D. All of the above

34 Patient education is necessary for:

A. Medical and legal reasons
B. JCAH requirements
C. Professional responsibility
D. All of the above

35 Patient education is designed to:

A. Improve community relations
B. Decrease return visits to the ED for same or similar problems
C. Reinforce specific care instructions
D. All of the above

36 Discharge planning for the ED patient should be started by the nurse:

A. When a definitive diagnosis is made
B. When the patient is ready for discharge
C. As soon as the patient comes to the ED
D. When the patient indicates improvement and is able to participate in the planning

37 The goal of discharge planning is to:

A. Conform to JCAH requirements, prevent readmission for the same problem, and provide patient or family education
B. Conform to JCAH requirements, provide patient or family education, and enhance facility revenues
C. Prevent readmission and foster good public relations
D. Prevent patient or families from using the ED as primary care facility

38 Which statement regarding the offering of telephone advice in the ED is *incorrect?*

A. You cannot be sued for advice given over the telephone
B. Ascertain whether your professional liability insurance covers such activities
C. Ensure that your advice reflects current nursing practice
D. Avoid charging a fee for advice

39 Which situation does *not* constitute the establishment of a nurse-patient relationship?

A. At a party, a person asks you many questions about his health
B. When a neighbor inquires about her child's recent behavior, you check on the child the next day
C. A patient you have seen in the ED meets you in a supermarket and questions you about adverse effects of recently prescribed medications
D. A patient you have seen in the ED phones for a reexplanation of discharge instructions

40 Which statement reflects the legally correct action by a nurse when a person solicits medical advice?

A. The nurse must always refer the person to a physician
B. The nurse does not need to refer the person to a physician if she is convinced it is not necessary
C. If the nurse is in private practice without written physician's protocols, she may diagnose and treat the person without physician referral
D. The nurse must always follow up on the person's status a day or two later

41 A woman telephones the ED, stating that she is pregnant and bleeding vaginally. Which response by the nurse is *inappropriate* in this situation?

A. Asking the woman how many months pregnant she is, because the advice will vary each trimester
B. Asking the woman if she has had any prenatal care; if not, recommending that she come to the ED immediately to rule out placenta previa
C. Advising the woman to go to the nearest ED without soliciting any further information
D. Asking the woman to describe the amount of bleeding, in terms of the number of pads used in the last hour, to determine the bleeding's severity

42 A man who recently was discharged from the ED phones for advice about medication adverse effects. The most appropriate nursing response is to:

A. Check the *Physicians' Desk Reference (PDR)* or another valid resource, and tell the patient the adverse effects
B. Refer him to his physician
C. Refer him to a pharmacist
D. Ask him why he is concerned, relate to him the adverse effects, and refer him, if necessary, to a physician

43 Multiorgan donors are those patients who are:

A. Comatose
B. Brain dead
C. In a persistent vegetative state
D. All of the above

44 The word "tissue" usually refers to:

A. All organs
B. Organs, eyes, and bone
C. Skin only
D. Eyes, bone, skin, and heart valves

45 The responsibilities of a procurement coordinator include:

A. Managing the organ donor
B. Talking with the family of the deceased
C. Coordinating the organ retrieval
D. All of the above

46 Brain death is:

A. An irreversible cessation of the entire brain function, including brain-stem function
B. A very deep coma
C. A persistent vegetative state
D. Not necessary for organ retrieval

47 The patient should be declared brain dead:

A. Before removal of organs
B. Before discontinuing use of the ventilator
C. By two attending physicians
D. All of the above

48 The legal time of death is considered to be:

A. When the second brain death note is placed on the chart
B. When the ventilator is turned off in the operating room
C. When the first brain death note is placed on the chart
D. When the heart is removed during the retrieval process

49 Organ donors most commonly have died from:

A. Severe head injury
B. Cardiopulmonary arrest
C. Myocardial infarction
D. Respiratory arrest

50 Consent for organ donation must be given by:

A. The deceased before his death
B. The legal next of kin
C. Any member of the deceased's family
D. The physician

51 Kidney donations are usually accepted from persons:

A. Ages 2 to 60
B. Ages 15 to 50
C. Under age 95
D. Of any age

52 Effective organ retrieval requires all organ donors to have:

A. An intact heartbeat
B. Adequate blood pressure
C. Mechanical ventilator support
D. All of the above

53 The nurse would suspect a urinary output of greater than 100 ml/hour in a potential organ donor to be an indication of:

A. Fluid overload
B. Diabetes insipidus
C. Polyuric phase of renal failure
D. Adequate renal function

54 Which of the following conditions does *not* contribute to hypotension in organ donors initially:

A. Brain-stem herniation
B. Collapse of peripheral vascular resistance
C. Therapeutic dehydration
D. Disseminated intravascular coagulation

55 Which of the following cases would *not* fall under the jurisdiction of the medical examiner?

A. Deaths by homicide
B. Deaths by suicide
C. Deaths from accidental traumatic injury
D. Deaths by a witnessed cardiac arrest

56 What is the rationale for administering 1 g of methylprednisolone sodium succinate (Solu-Medrol) intravenously to an organ donor?

A. To decrease the body's inflammatory response
B. To stabilize the kidney membrane during the retrieval process
C. To help prevent infection
D. To prevent tissue rejection

57 An invalid criterion when considering organ recipients would be:

A. Urgency of need
B. ABO compatibility
C. Sex
D. Tissue matching

58 With few exceptions, people over age 65 cannot receive heart transplants because:

A. They are not within the age limit for organ recipients
B. Many of them have little or no insurance
C. Many have a preexisting poor health state
D. Their life expectancy will not be substantially increased

59 The physiologic criterion that is mandatory for transplanting all organs is:

A. Body size
B. Age
C. Tissue typing
D. Blood type compatibility

60 Who may be considered as a tissue donor?

A. Any patient who dies in a hospital
B. An individual referred within 6 to 12 hours after a cardiac death
C. Deceased patients of any age
D. All of the above

61 What are the age parameters for lung donors?

A. Newborn to age 40
B. Ages 2 to 50
C. Ages 4 to 60
D. Ages 12 to 40

62 The age parameters for bone donors are:

A. Ages 2 to 50
B. Ages 15 to 65
C. Ages 20 to 50
D. There are no age limits

63 The age parameters for eye donors are:

A. Newborn to age 65
B. Ages 6 to 55
C. Ages 10 to 90
D. There are no age limits

64 Prolonged hypotension in an organ donor may cause:

A. Cardiac death
B. Acute tubular necrosis in the transplanted kidney
C. Disseminated intravascular coagulation
D. All of the above

65 Norepinephrine (Levophed) and epinephrine should not be used as vasopressors in an organ donor because they:

A. Are extremely potent vasoconstrictors and may cause kidney and liver damage
B. Cannot be metabolized by a deceased patient
C. Are not effective in brain-dead patients
D. Cause donor reactions

66 The cost of the organ retrieval is paid by the:

A. Donor's family
B. Donating hospital
C. Transplant center
D. Federal government

67 Which conditions are *not* considered contraindications for organ donation?

A. Pneumonia, urinary tract infection, and intracranial cancer
B. Sepsis and I.V. drug abuse
C. Metastatic cancer
D. Positive HIV/HTLV-III test and heroin addiction

68 The goals of donor maintenance include:

A. Adequate ventilation
B. Hemodynamic stability
C. Infection prevention
D. All of the above

69 The explanation of organ donation to the donor family should include:

A. The recipients' names only
B. Details relating to the surgical procedure
C. The monetary value of the organs transplanted
D. The positive aspects of transplantation as well as answers to their questions about brain death

70 Prospective donor families should be provided with:

A. Time to accept the diagnosis of death, pastoral support, and a quiet place and time with the deceased
B. A statement of the charges relating to the retrieval
C. A complete copy of the chart, including the operative report
D. Access to the recipients after a 3-month time lapse

71 "Living related donor" is a term that concerns the:

A. Liver
B. Heart
C. Kidneys
D. Pancreas

72 Nursing interventions related to kidney donor maintenance include:

A. Maintaining systolic blood pressure of 100 to 110 mm Hg
B. Maintaining urinary output > 100 ml/hour
C. Maintaining adequate ventilation
D. All of the above

73 The organ procurement agency should be notified of all potential donors:

A. After consent is obtained
B. When the operating room is ready
C. As soon as a potential donor is identified
D. When the doctor says it is okay

74 Which of the following would *not* be a potential organ donor?

A. A 35-year-old with a positive HIV/HTLV-III test result and a self-inflicted gunshot wound to the head
B. A 2-year-old near-drowning victim with hypoxic encephalopathy
C. A 56-year-old man with a massive intraventricular hemorrhage
D. A 14-year-old boy with massive head injuries and chest trauma

75 A thorough medical history can prove invaluable because:

A. It can predict future organ function for the recipients
B. It can give important information to the recipients about the donor
C. It can help determine the existence of a disorder that may preclude organ donation
D. It is necessary for accurate record keeping

76 It is important for the donor family to understand that brain death:

A. Is irreversible
B. Is a very deep coma
C. Has no effect on cardiac or respiratory function
D. Means just the brain died and nothing else

77 Extended observation of potential organ donors under age 5 may be necessary because:

A. They have an increased resistance to brain damage and may recover
B. Federal law mandates it
C. It is comforting to the parents
D. Test results are more difficult to diagnose at that age

78 Which of the following temperature routes have been found to be as effective as the rectal route in preschool children?

A. Oral
B. Axillary
C. Esophageal
D. None of the above

79 What is the relationship between lunar phases and psychiatric admissions to the ED?

A. No relationship exists between lunar phases and psychiatric admissions to the ED
B. An increase in psychiatric admissions occurs during the full moon phase
C. An increase in psychiatric admissions occurs just before the full moon phase
D. A decrease in psychiatric admissions occurs during the full moon phase

80 Research studies have shown an increase in urinary tract infections in women who use which birth control method?

A. Intrauterine devices
B. Condoms
C. Diaphragms
D. Oral contraceptives

81 Research has found how much gastric lavage to be necessary in the treatment of tricyclic antidepressant overdose?

A. 500 ml
B. 1 liter
C. 5 liters
D. 10 liters

82 Which of the following statements is true regarding research on asymptomatic head-injured children with a positive Babinski's sign?

A. The child has an increased risk of permanent brain damage
B. The child should be monitored in the hospital for 2 to 3 days
C. The sign is a poor prognosticator in children over age 2
D. The child has not been found to have an increased risk of permanent brain damage

Answer Sheet

	A	B	C	D		A	B	C	D		A	B	C	D
1	○	○	○	○	31	○	○	○	○	61	○	○	○	○
2	○	○	○	○	32	○	○	○	○	62	○	○	○	○
3	○	○	○	○	33	○	○	○	○	63	○	○	○	○
4	○	○	○	○	34	○	○	○	○	64	○	○	○	○
5	○	○	○	○	35	○	○	○	○	65	○	○	○	○
6	○	○	○	○	36	○	○	○	○	66	○	○	○	○
7	○	○	○	○	37	○	○	○	○	67	○	○	○	○
8	○	○	○	○	38	○	○	○	○	68	○	○	○	○
9	○	○	○	○	39	○	○	○	○	69	○	○	○	○
10	○	○	○	○	40	○	○	○	○	70	○	○	○	○
11	○	○	○	○	41	○	○	○	○	71	○	○	○	○
12	○	○	○	○	42	○	○	○	○	72	○	○	○	○
13	○	○	○	○	43	○	○	○	○	73	○	○	○	○
14	○	○	○	○	44	○	○	○	○	74	○	○	○	○
15	○	○	○	○	45	○	○	○	○	75	○	○	○	○
16	○	○	○	○	46	○	○	○	○	76	○	○	○	○
17	○	○	○	○	47	○	○	○	○	77	○	○	○	○
18	○	○	○	○	48	○	○	○	○	78	○	○	○	○
19	○	○	○	○	49	○	○	○	○	79	○	○	○	○
20	○	○	○	○	50	○	○	○	○	80	○	○	○	○
21	○	○	○	○	51	○	○	○	○	81	○	○	○	○
22	○	○	○	○	52	○	○	○	○	82	○	○	○	○
23	○	○	○	○	53	○	○	○	○					
24	○	○	○	○	54	○	○	○	○					
25	○	○	○	○	55	○	○	○	○					
26	○	○	○	○	56	○	○	○	○					
27	○	○	○	○	57	○	○	○	○					
28	○	○	○	○	58	○	○	○	○					
29	○	○	○	○	59	○	○	○	○					
30	○	○	○	○	60	○	○	○	○					

Answer Sheet

	A	B	C	D		A	B	C	D		A	B	C	D
1	○	○	○	○	**31**	○	○	○	○	**61**	○	○	○	○
2	○	○	○	○	**32**	○	○	○	○	**62**	○	○	○	○
3	○	○	○	○	**33**	○	○	○	○	**63**	○	○	○	○
4	○	○	○	○	**34**	○	○	○	○	**64**	○	○	○	○
5	○	○	○	○	**35**	○	○	○	○	**65**	○	○	○	○
6	○	○	○	○	**36**	○	○	○	○	**66**	○	○	○	○
7	○	○	○	○	**37**	○	○	○	○	**67**	○	○	○	○
8	○	○	○	○	**38**	○	○	○	○	**68**	○	○	○	○
9	○	○	○	○	**39**	○	○	○	○	**69**	○	○	○	○
10	○	○	○	○	**40**	○	○	○	○	**70**	○	○	○	○
11	○	○	○	○	**41**	○	○	○	○	**71**	○	○	○	○
12	○	○	○	○	**42**	○	○	○	○	**72**	○	○	○	○
13	○	○	○	○	**43**	○	○	○	○	**73**	○	○	○	○
14	○	○	○	○	**44**	○	○	○	○	**74**	○	○	○	○
15	○	○	○	○	**45**	○	○	○	○	**75**	○	○	○	○
16	○	○	○	○	**46**	○	○	○	○	**76**	○	○	○	○
17	○	○	○	○	**47**	○	○	○	○	**77**	○	○	○	○
18	○	○	○	○	**48**	○	○	○	○	**78**	○	○	○	○
19	○	○	○	○	**49**	○	○	○	○	**79**	○	○	○	○
20	○	○	○	○	**50**	○	○	○	○	**80**	○	○	○	○
21	○	○	○	○	**51**	○	○	○	○	**81**	○	○	○	○
22	○	○	○	○	**52**	○	○	○	○	**82**	○	○	○	○
23	○	○	○	○	**53**	○	○	○	○					
24	○	○	○	○	**54**	○	○	○	○					
25	○	○	○	○	**55**	○	○	○	○					
26	○	○	○	○	**56**	○	○	○	○					
27	○	○	○	○	**57**	○	○	○	○					
28	○	○	○	○	**58**	○	○	○	○					
29	○	○	○	○	**59**	○	○	○	○					
30	○	○	○	○	**60**	○	○	○	○					

1 Correct answer—**D**

A nurse may legally use force against a patient in self-defense, but only if the nurse has reasonable grounds to believe that she is being, or is about to be, attacked. Everyone, including the nurse, has the legal right to self-protection as well as the right to work in a safe environment. When dealing with combative patients and at risk for harm, nurses have the right to defend themselves as long as the defense is reasonable and only to the extent necessary to defend themselves. This self-defense must not continue when the apparent danger has passed and the patient is no longer combative.

2 Correct answer—**A**

An oral order given by a physician to a nurse is legally valid alone but should be covered with a written order for professional safety. The problem lies in proving that the order was given if the physician later denies giving the oral order. The best solution is to obtain an oral order in the presence of a witness and to obtain a written order as soon as possible. Being aware of your hospital's policy regarding oral orders is also important. Some hospitals prohibit following oral orders; negligence could be charged if injury to a patient occurred because a nurse followed a prohibited oral order, since hospital policy was not followed.

3 Correct answer—**C**

If a patient does not understand the information just given by the physician during an informed consent, the nurse should notify the physician. The physician should return and answer the patient's questions. If the physician does not do so, the supervisor may need to be called and the procedure delayed until further explanations are rendered. The nurse should not answer the patient's questions because this would constitute assuming the role and expertise of the physician. If the patient has questions that the nurse is not at liberty to answer, an informed consent probably was not obtained.

4 Correct answer—**C**

Giving a medication to a patient against his will is an example of battery. Battery is an act that brings about harmful or offensive touching of one person by another. Assault, the threat of battery, is an act that creates a conscious, unreasonable apprehension in an individual of immediate, harmful, or offensive touching by another person. Giving a person medication or even a back rub against his will is battery. Assault and battery are examples of legal wrongs, or torts. The person who commits a legal wrong may be liable for damages in a legal action brought by the wronged person. Preventing a patient from signing out against medical advice is false imprisonment. Failing to secure side rails, which leads to a confused patient falling out of bed and fracturing a leg, is negligence. Failing to keep chart records confidential is invasion of privacy.

5 Correct answer—**D**

When witnessing an informed consent, the nurse is attesting that the signature is the patient's. The responsibility for obtaining consent lies with the physician and is part of the physician-patient relationship. Witnessing a consent does not mean witnessing the exchange of this information but that the signature is that of the particular patient.

6 Correct answer—**B**

Legally, besides being a witness to the patient's signature on an informed consent, the nurse may also obtain the patient's signature after the physician has informed the patient. Only a physician may obtain an informed consent. A nurse may be a witness if telephone consent is obtained. If the patient still has questions when the nurse attempts to secure the signature, it should not be obtained, and the physician should be notified. Individual hospital policy should be consulted about the nurse's role in obtaining the patient's signature, because it varies from institution to institution. Two physicians' statements are required to obtain administrative consent when the patient and family cannot.

7 Correct answer—**A**

If a patient has questions regarding the correctness of his treatment, the nurse should inform the physician, who should answer the questions. The nurse's role as a patient advocate in such situations is not clearly defined by state laws, so it is best to seek out the physician. Discussing other therapies and referring the patient to other qualified physicians have cost some nurses their jobs for interference in the physician-patient relationship. Reinforcing the appropriateness of the treatment does not minimize the patient's right to adequate information.

8 Correct answer—**B**

If the nurse disagrees with the physician's judgment in ordering a particular drug for a patient and thinks that another drug would be more effective, and if, after questioning the order, she is told to give the first drug, she should do so. A disagreement in judgment does not constitute permission for a nurse to act as a physician; for example, to prescribe one medication over another. In this situation, the nurse disagreed in theory with the choice of Lasix but did not question the safety of giving the medication. After questioning, the physician reaffirmed the order; the nurse should comply with the physician's wishes. If the nurse still feels uncomfortable giving the medication, the physician may be asked to administer it. Legally, the nurse cannot refuse to administer medication unless it is blatantly erroneous to do so.

9 Correct answer—**B**

For negligence to be committed, injury must be incurred. The breach of duty that occurs in the negligent act must be the proximate cause of the injury; that is, it must have occurred before and resulted in the injury. An error in judgment that results in an injury does not necessarily constitute negligence. If the judgment was made after careful assessment of the patient's condition and would have been made by any reasonable, prudent nurse in a similar situation, the resulting error and injury is unfortunate but not negligent. Giving the wrong therapy and overlooking a change in condition do not necessarily lead to injury.

10 Correct answer—**B**

Physical restraints should be used when there is a threat to the patient's safety. If a patient becomes confused and combative to the point of self-harm, reasonable restraint should be employed for safety only. Although a physician's order is necessary, do not wait to get the order, because harm may come to the patient during the interlude. Physical restraint should never be used as a replacement for nursing observation or as a method for dealing with confused or uncooperative patients who do not show signs of harming themselves; for example, by falling out of bed.

11 Correct answer—**B**

The most appropriate way to legally document patient teaching is by providing written instructions. The patient may dispute receiving oral instructions even if the incident is referred to in the nurses' notes. Nurses' notes are highly important, however, in legal actions. Written instructions should always accompany oral instructions and are also important if the information given is especially detailed. Patients and families can always refer to written instructions at home if they have any questions. Teaching with a witness present and giving the patients a written examination are impractical.

12 Correct answer—**C**

The most important goal of triage is immediate patient assessment so that critically ill patients get priority treatments. Triage is a French word that means sorting. The primary goal of triage is to sort patients into categories, identifying the urgency of care and appropriate treatment area. Comprehensive patient assessment is the responsibility of the care providers in the designated treatment areas.

13 Correct answer—**D**

Placing a Steri-strip over a minor laceration is an inappropriate action for the triage nurse. All other choices are appropriate functions. The triage nurse is responsible for providing immediate care or intervention for life-threatening or potentially life-threatening injuries or illnesses.

14 Correct answer—**B**

The triage nurse is not accountable for complete and comprehensive patient assessment. She is the first health care provider to identify potentially infectious patients and must take appropriate precautions in preventing contamination of other patients and personnel. The triage nurse also acts as a resource for patient or family education. Lastly, because the triage nurse is usually the first contact the patient or family has with hospital personnel, she is a significant representative of the hospital and thus is important in developing favorable public relations for the facility.

15 Correct answer—**C**

Your first priority is to clear the ED of all nonserious patients and move those patients awaiting admission to a holding area. Upon such notification, the ED must be prepared to receive casualties. In doing this, a decontamination area would be designated as patient care areas became available. Requesting the admitting office to clear ICU beds is inappropriate because the extent and number of casualties is unknown at this time. Notifying EMS of accommodations might be appropriate *after* preparing the ED.

16 Correct answer—**D**

Radiology and the radiation disaster planning coordinator are primary resources in this type of accident. Even if the hospital does not receive the driver of the truck carrying the radioactive waste, the victims and EMS personnel may be contaminated. Using these resources in radioactive incidents is important in the planning and management of the casualties and in preventing further contamination. The laboratory, blood bank, operating room, and pharmacy may be necessary in supporting roles.

17 Correct answer—**D**

The objectives of quality assurance are to monitor the quality of care, identify actual or perceived problems, and, as a result of monitoring activities, identify educational and remedial activities necessary to correct identified problems.

18 Correct answer—**D**

All are potential resources by which to identify patient care issues.

Additional resources include specific illnesses or injuries, the condition of patients upon arrival at the facility, and the response of support services to the ED. In short, anything having to do with the processing and care of patients in the ED can be developed into a quality assurance activity.

19 Correct answer—**A**

Problem identification, study or survey, results reporting, recommendations, and follow-up targets are the specific components of quality assurance monitoring as recommended by the JCAH. The absence of any one or more of these factors results in an incomplete quality assurance activity.

20 Correct answer—**D**

Obtain her name, address, and phone number; tell her to call the police and come to the hospital immediately with a change of clothes. Request the demographic information (name, address, and phone number) in case you become disconnected or for follow-up, if the patient does not arrive in the ED. As well as telling the patient to bring a change of clothes, you should instruct her not to change her physical appearance, shower, bathe, douche, urinate, or change her clothing. A brief explanation of why these things should not be done may be appropriate, depending upon the patient's emotional status.

21 Correct answer—**C**

Give the number of the local medical society to the caller. The society will give the mother the names, addresses, and phone numbers of pediatricians in her geographic area. This method is the most objective way of referring patients to physicians.

22 Correct answer—**D**

Advise him to stop taking the drug and return to the ED. This is the only appropriate answer, because any other answer could be construed as the nurse prescribing medications.

23 Correct answer—**A**

Name, address, and extent of injury are public information; the police are entitled only to this unless they have a valid court order, search warrant, or subpoena for information.

24 Correct answer—**D**

Notifying the administrator or nursing supervisor would be the most appropriate action in this situation. Under normal circumstances, the media is entitled to public information; however, because of the sensitivity of the diagnosis and the prominence of the patient, your first concern is to protect the patient's right to privacy.

25 Correct answer—**A**

You are responsible to secure and hold confidential a patient's chart and information. Failure to do so is a breach of patient confidentiality, regardless of how that breach occurred.

26 Correct answer—**C**

Inform the physician and secure the envelope. It is the nurse's responsibility to inform the physician of what has been discovered, because it may directly affect the care to be rendered to the patient. Securing the substance is within the nurse's purview because analysis of the contents may be necessary at a future time. Appropriate action for the staff nurse would be to inform the nursing supervisor or administrator at the hospital about the discovery.

27 Correct answer—**D**

No civil liability has occurred. The nurse was acting in good faith in attempting to make a positive identification or obtaining medical information necessary for the care of the patient.

28 Correct answer—**A**

The sequence of obtaining and securing evidence, known as the chain of evidence, is most important in a court of law. The integrity of the evidence is best assured by limiting the number of people who have access to it and by documenting how the evidence was obtained, where it was sent, and by whom it was received.

29 Correct answer—**C**

When the patient's condition requires immediate evaluation and intervention and the patient cannot give consent for treatment and a legal guardian or next of kin is not available, it is implied that the patient would agree to treatment if he could give consent. Consent is also implied when a patient presents to the ED; the implication is that the patient came to the ED expressly for evaluation and treatment. Even though consent is implied, it is imperative that an informed consent be obtained, when possible, before treatment. Administrative consents occur when two physicians agree that the procedure is required and the patient cannot consent because of his mental state.

30 Correct answer—**D**

In all 50 states, mandatory reporting laws exist for suspected or known child abuse or neglect. The law(s) identifies who must report cases of child abuse; responsible parties include registered nurses, licensed practical nurses, and other health care providers. Law enforcement agencies must investigate and, when necessary, place the minor in protective custody. The staff members of the hospital are not law enforcement agents; therefore, they do not have the power to restrain a parent in this situation. However, when the minor has been placed in protective custody, the hospital may not release the child to anyone other than a court-appointed guardian.

31 Correct answer—**D**

Air transportation can cause decreased blood pressure, hypothermia because of the decreased temperature at higher altitudes, pneumothorax and hypoxemia as a result of decreased barometric pressure, and nausea and vomiting from air sickness.

32 Correct answer—**B**

The nurse's responsibility is to determine whether the interpreter understands the instructions before translating for the patient. The documentation of who translated is most important to include on the ED record. If this situation occurs frequently, the discharge instructions should be translated into the most commonly encountered languages. Delaying discharge until a hospital interpreter can be found is impractical, since an interpreter is already available.

33 Correct answer—**C**

Part of discharge instruction is determining whether the patient understands the information or instructions given by you and the physician. The nurse's best choice is to make a concise statement on the record that the patient demonstrates understanding of the discharge instructions. Having the patient repeat the instructions or sign that he received them does not indicate understanding.

34 Correct answer—**D**

Patient education is a professional and legal responsibility of the nurse. JCAH standards, as well, state that patient education is a primary concern of the nursing and medical staff.

35 Correct answer—**D**

The goals of patient education are to improve patient well-being, to promote and foster good public relations, and lastly, to reinforce the prescribed medical regimen.

36 Correct answer—**C**

Planning should begin at the time of admission to facilitate the processing and discharge of the patient. Discharge planning with the patient is designed to enhance the care and disposition of patients.

37 Correct answer—**A**

The goal of discharge planning is to conform to JCAH requirements, prevent readmission for the same problem, and provide patient or family education. Discharge planning also identifies specific and individualized needs of the patient and incorporates a multidisciplinary approach to patient care. Discharge planning does not affect the use of the ED as a primary care facility.

38 Correct answer—**A**

Although these types of suits are rare, a nurse can be sued for giving incorrect information, especially when the information can be directly related to patient harm. You can best protect yourself by ascertaining that your malpractice insurance covers advice (given both on and off the job), ensuring that your advice reflects current nursing practice, and avoiding charging a fee for advice.

39 Correct answer—**A**

The person at a party asking you for advice has not indicated that he wishes to establish an ongoing nurse-patient relationship. An established nurse-patient relationship, such as in the other situations, obligates you to give the best nursing advice possible, which may include referral to a physician. Any misinformation could be considered, in a court of law, breach of contract. The issue of breach of contract may be a deciding factor in a malpractice suit.

40 Correct answer—**B**

A nurse does not need to refer a person soliciting advice to a physician if she is convinced it is truly not necessary. Nor does she need to follow up such advice, unless a nurse-patient relationship has been established. Even in private practice, a nurse can only diagnose and treat nursing problems, not medical ones, unless she is following standard orders.

41 Correct answer—**C**

Although sending the patient to a hospital, no matter what the prevailing condition, is safe advice legally, you can assess the patient's condition and prevent unnecessary trips to a health facility as well as unnecessary anxiety for the patient. For example, if a patient is 9-months pregnant with her first child, has had prenatal care, is staining and having mild contractions every half hour, you can advise her to come to the hospital when the contractions are 5 minutes apart and last 45 to 60 seconds, unless heavy bleeding begins. However, if the woman hasn't had prenatal care, recommend that she come to the ED immediately to rule out placenta previa. Find out how many months pregnant she is and how heavy her bleeding is (in terms of number of pads used in the last hour) to determine your advice to the woman.

42 Correct answer—**D**

Ask the patient why he is concerned, relate to him the adverse effects, and refer him, if necessary. Just supplying facts about adverse effects to the patient may cause him to discontinue the medication. Investigating his concerns may avoid this.

43 Correct answer—**B**

Multiorgan donors would include those patients who are brain dead. Neither comatose patients nor those patients in a persistent vegetative state would be considered for organ donation because these individuals still have brain-stem function. In brain death, all functions of the brain have ceased. In the persistent vegetative state, severe, irreversible damage has occurred to the higher centers of the brain, but the brain stem remains intact.

44 Correct answer—**D**

The word "tissue" usually refers to eyes, bone, skin, and heart valves when it concerns donation. Tissue transplantation does not require a heart-beating donor, whereas organ transplantation does.

45 Correct answer—**D**

The responsibilities of an organ procurement coordinator include managing organ donors, coordinating the organ retrieval, and speaking with the family of the deceased. Other responsibilities include public and professional education and the development of organ donation programs in hospitals.

46 Correct answer—**A**

Brain death is an irreversible cessation of the entire brain function, including brain-stem function. Clinical criteria for establishing brain death include the absence of all cortical brain-stem function, including cerebral responses to light, noise, motion, and pain; reflexes or muscle activity; spontaneous respirations; and cranial nerve reflexes and responses.

47 Correct answer—**D**

The patient should be declared brain dead before removal of the organs and before discontinuing the ventilator. Two attending physicians are necessary to declare a patient brain dead.

48 Correct answer—**A**

The legal time of death is considered to be the time that the second brain death note is placed on the chart. No notation or pronouncement of death should be made in the operative note. The donor must be declared dead before entering the operating room.

49 Correct answer—**A**

Organ donors most commonly have suffered severe head injury. The majority of multiorgan donors have succumbed to brain death. Patients who have sustained cardiopulmonary death are excluded from any type of donation except tissue.

50 Correct answer—**B**

Consent for organ donation must be given by the legal next of kin, including, in order of priority, the spouse, an adult brother or sister, the legal guardian of the deceased at the time of death, or a representative appointed by a court of competent jurisdiction who has ascertained that no person of higher priority exists who objects to organ donation.

51 Correct answer—**A**

Kidney donations are usually accepted from persons ages 2 to 60. Kidneys from donors under age 2 are not considered because they are not developed well enough; kidneys from donors over age 60 are not harvested because the incidence of kidney disease increases substantially with age.

52 Correct answer—**D**

Effective organ retrieval requires all organ donors to have an intact heartbeat, adequate blood pressure, and effective mechanical ventilator support. These criteria are necessary to maintain proper organ function and adequate tissue oxygenation and perfusion for effective organ procurement.

53 Correct answer—**B**

The nurse would suspect a urinary output of more than 100 ml/hour in an organ donor to be an indication of diabetes insipidus. This endocrine disorder commonly occurs in patients who have sustained severe head injury. The ensuing increase in intracranial pressure impairs the ability of the hypothalamus to produce antidiuretic hormone (ADH) or affects the posterior pituitary gland's secretion of ADH. Decreased or absent levels of this hormone prevent the kidneys from reabsorbing water back into systemic circulation. This causes an increase in urinary output, which is often greater than the patient's fluid intake.

54 Correct answer—**D**

Disseminated intravascular coagulation does not contribute to the development of hypotension in an organ donor initially. This syndrome commonly results from a prolonged hypotensive state rather than causes it, whereas brain-stem herniation impairs the vasomotor center in the medulla. Sympathetic tone to the body's blood vessels ceases and cardiovascular collapse ensues. Therapeutic dehydration may occur to intravascular depletion as evidenced by hypotension.

55 Correct answer—**D**

A witnessed cardiac arrest death would not fall under the jurisdiction of the medical examiner. Deaths that come under the jurisdiction of the coroner include those occurring from unknown causes or resulting from a suspected homicide, suicide, or accidental injury. Medical examiners usually give their consent for organ retrieval unless the removal of a particular organ may inhibit the investigation.

56 Correct answer—**B**

Solu-Medrol is given intravenously to the organ donor because it stabilizes the kidney membranes during the retrieval process. This medication should be given immediately before beginning organ procurement in the operating room.

57 Correct answer—**C**

Sex is an invalid criterion for considering organ recipients. The potential recipient's sex does not influence whether he or she is chosen. The most important factor governing recipient selection is urgency of need, followed by ABO compatibility and tissue matching.

58 Correct answer—**C**

With few exceptions, people over age 65 are not given heart transplants because of their preexisting poor health state. Since there is a tremendous shortage of organ donors, transplant candidates must be chosed carefully, with special consideration given to a person's overall health state. The person's ability to comply with changes in diet, drug regimens, and life-style also must be evaluated.

59 Correct answer—**D**

The physiologic criterion that is mandatory for transplanting all organs is blood type compatibility. Age is usually the second factor considered. In addition, body size is a necessary criterion for matching heart and liver recipients. Donor kidneys will adapt to the recipient's body size but require prior tissue typing.

60 Correct answer—**D**

An individual of any age who dies in a hospital or a person who is referred within 6 to 12 hours after a cardiac death may be considered as a tissue donor. If the tissue is not used for transplantation, it may be used for research.

61 Correct answer—**D**

The age parameters for lung donors are ages 12 and 40. This age range provides for lung maturity as well as for optimum lung health.

62 Correct answer—**B**

The age parameters for bone donors are ages 15 and 65. Bones are not taken from donors under age 15 because growth usually has not been completed. After age 65, bone strength deteriorates, particularly in women, from osteoporosis.

63 Correct answer—**D**

No age limit exists for the donation of eyes. If the tissue is not used for corneal transplantation, it may be used for research.

64 Correct answer—**D**

Prolonged hypotension in an organ donor may cause cardiac death, acute tubular necrosis in the transplanted kidneys, or the development of disseminated intravascular coagulation. Hypotension is the most commonly encountered complication during postmortem organ donor management.

65 Correct answer—**A**

Levophed and epinephrine should not be used as vasopressors in an organ donor because they are extremely potent vascoconstrictors and may cause kidney and liver damage. In cases of severe hypotension, they are used as a last resort. The extreme vasopressor action of these medications produces marked vasoconstriction, resulting in acute tubular necrosis of the kidneys, and severely decreases blood flow to the liver, causing irreversible organ engorgement.

66 Correct answer—**C**

The receiving transplant center is charged all expenses incurred in the retrieval of that particular organ. The donor's family, the donating hospital, and the federal government do not pay for organ donation retrieval.

67 Correct answer—**A**

Pneumonia, urinary tract infection, and intracranial cancer are not contraindications for organ donation. Patients with an intracranial cancer can be organ donors if the cancer is confined intracranially. If there is evidence of a urinary tract infection, the ureters can be cultured during the retrieval process and the recipient appropriately treated with antibiotics. Pneumonia is a contraindication for lung donations only. Such conditions as sepsis, I.V. drug abuse, positive HIV/HTLV-III test, and metastatic cancer are always contraindications for organ donation.

68 Correct answer—**D**

The goals of donor maintenance include adequate ventilation, hemodynamic stability, and infection prevention. All of these goals should be met for proper tissue perfusion and oxygenation. The recipients are already immunosuppressed and will be more so posttransplant with the severe regimen of antirejection drugs. They could not tolerate the introduction of microorganisms to their system.

69 Correct answer—**D**

The explanation of organ donation to the donor family should include the positive aspects of transplantation as well as answers to their questions about brain death. The organ recipients' names are kept strictly confidential. The families should not be concerned with surgical techniques or the monetary value of organs. They should understand that this is a donation and involves no cost or monetary compensation. The explanation should be made in clear, concise lay language, not in technical terms.

70 Correct answer—**A**

Prospective donor families should be provided with time to accept the diagnosis of death, pastoral support, and a quiet place and time with the deceased. One of the nurse's primary concerns should be that the donor's family receives support and has a clear understanding of organ donation.

71 Correct answer—**C**

"Living related donor" is the term used when a person donates one kidney to a blood relative, usually to a son, daughter, mother, father, sister, or brother.

72 Correct answer—**D**

Nursing interventions related to kidney donor maintenance include maintaining a systolic blood pressure of 100 to 110 mm Hg, a urinary output of greater than 100 ml/hour, and adequate ventilation. All these interventions should be met to ensure kidney perfusion and function and tissue oxygenation.

73 Correct answer—**C**

The organ procurement agency should be notified as soon as a potential donor is identified. The procurement coordinator is specially trained to assess the person and to approach the family tactfully.

74 Correct answer—**A**

The possibility of a positive HIV/HTLV-III test is reason enough to turn down this individual for organ donation. The other candidates would probably be suitable for one or all organs to be donated.

75 Correct answer—**C**

A thorough medical history can prove invaluable because it can help determine the existence of a disorder that may preclude organ donation. A good medical history can give evidence of chronic renal impairment, previous myocardial injury, or alcohol abuse, any of which could exclude the person as a kidney, heart, or liver donor.

76 Correct answer—**A**

The donor family must accept that brain death is irreversible and understand the concept of brain death before they can consider organ donation.

77 Correct answer—**A**

A child's brain is more resilient to brain damage and may recover even after brain function appears lost. EEGs and cerebral arteriograms may be necessary.

78 Correct answer—**B**

Axillary temperature has been found to be as effective as rectal temperature in determining the presence of fever in preschool children. When measured electronically, axillary and rectal temperatures had an average difference in readings of less than 1° F.

79 Correct answer—**A**

No relationship exists between psychiatric admissions and any of the four lunar phases: new moon, first quarter, full moon, or last quarter. Psychiatric admissions studied included alcohol intoxication, suicide attempts, and anxiety and depressive reactions.

80 Correct answer—**C**

A high incidence of urinary tract infections has been found in women who use the diaphragm as a birth control method. Gram-negative urinary tract infections are especially prevalent among diaphragm users, who should switch to another form of birth control if the problem recurs.

81 Correct answer—**C**

Five liters of gastric lavage fluid have been found to be effective in recovering most of the drug in tricyclic antidepressant overdose. Visible particulate matter in the return fluid should not be relied upon for determining overdosed drug recovery.

82 Correct answer—**D**

Research has found no increase in morbidity in asymptomatic head-injured children under age 16 who present with the lone sign of a positive Babinski's sign. These children don't need to be observed in the hospital; they can be monitored safely at home.

Selected References

Bennett, H.M. "Caring for Combative Patients," *Critical Care Nurse* 4:112, May/June 1984.

Bennett, H.M. "Informed Consent," *Critical Care Nurse* 1:31, May/June 1981.

Bennett, H.M. "Negligence—Part I," *Critical Care Nurse* 3:8, July/August 1983.

Brooks, D., and Harrold, A., eds. *Modern Emergency Department Practice.* London: Edward Arnold, 1983.

Creighton, H. *Law Every Nurse Should Know.* Philadelphia: W.B. Saunders Co., 1981.

Creighton, H. "Unruly Patients," *Nursing Management* 13:15-16, July 1982.

Dean, K.A. "Theory of Corporate Negligence," *Focus on Critical Care* 11:61-62, August 1984.

Documenting Patient Care Responsibly. Nursing Skillbook Series. Springhouse, Pa.: Springhouse Corp., 1978.

Gideon, M.D., and Taylor, R.B. "Kidney Donation: Care of the Cadaver Donor's Family," *Journal of Neurosurgical Nursing* 13:248, 1981.

Klaus, B.N. "What Every Nurse Should Know About Organ Donation," *Pennsylvania Nurse* 39:6, 1984.

Lanros, N. *Assessment and Intervention Emergency Nursing.* Bowie, Md.: Robert J. Brady Co., 1983.

Nashville Regional Organ Procurement Agency. *Organ Donation: A Reference Manual for Hospital Staff.* Nashville: Nashville Regional Organ Procurement Agency, 1985.

Rund, D., and Rausch, T. *Triage.* St. Louis: C.V. Mosby Co., 1981.

Simpson, H.H. "Understanding the Law: Organ Donation," *NursingLife* 5:24, 1985.

Chapter 17

Challenges in Dosage Calculations Questions and Answers

You must begin with Question 1 of this chapter and progress in sequence. **Do not skip around.** Subsequent answers build on previous ones.

Laura Gasparis, RN, MA, CCRN, CEN
June L. Olsen, RN, MS

SITUATION

A 50-year-old woman presents to the emergency department (ED) complaining of a severe headache. Her vital signs are blood pressure (BP), 220/130 mm Hg; pulse, 130 beats/minute; and respiratory rate, 26 breaths/minute. A diagnosis of hypertensive crisis is made. A continuous infusion of sodium nitroprusside (Nipride) is begun. The physician orders 250 ml dextrose 5% in water (D_5W) with 50 mg Nipride at 0.8 mcg/kg/minute. The patient weighs 144 pounds (65 kg).

Questions 1 to 4 refer to the above situation.

1 Preparation of the above solution would yield a Nipride concentration of how many mcg/ml?

A. 50
B. 150
C. 200
D. 250

2 What is the flow rate needed, in microdrops/minute, to infuse the Nipride solution at 0.8 mcg/kg/minute via an infusion system with a drip factor of 60 microdrops/ml?

A. 2
B. 8
C. 16
D. 52

3 If the dosage is increased to 0.9 mcg/kg/minute, the flow rate should be regulated at how many microdrops/minute?

A. 9
B. 18
C. 27
D. 58

4 Additional treatment for this hypertensive patient includes the administration of trimethaphan (Arfonad). A 500-mg ampule of Arfonad is diluted in 500 ml of D_5W. The physician orders 3 mg/minute of Arfonad. Which of the following is the appropriate flow rate in ml/hour?

A. 90
B. 150
C. 180
D. 250

SITUATION

A 19-year-old man with insulin-dependent diabetes mellitus is admitted in a diabetic ketoacidosis. His blood glucose level is 800 mg/dl; pH, 7.10; PCO_2, 28 mm Hg; and HCO_3^-, 15 mEq/liter. He appears severely dehydrated.

Questions 5 to 8 refer to the above situation.

5 An insulin drip at 8 units/hour is ordered. If 200 units of regular insulin are added to 250 ml of normal saline solution, the patient will receive how many ml/hour?

A. 8
B. 10
C. 18
D. 20

6 The physician orders 30 units NPH insulin subcutaneously. The label reads 1 ml = 100 units. How many milliliters will be administered to this patient?

A. 0.03
B. 0.3
C. 0.35
D. 0.75

7 Normal saline solution is to be infused at a rate of 40 drops/minute. Using an infusion system with a drip factor of 15 drops/ml, how much time will be required to deliver 1 liter of the saline solution?

A. 2 hours and 50 minutes
B. 3 hours and 30 minutes
C. 4 hours and 20 minutes
D. 6 hours and 15 minutes

8 Infusion of 1 liter of a 0.45% saline solution is started at 1 p.m. The flow rate is 42 drops/minute, and the drip factor is 10 drops/ml. At what time will the infusion be completed?

A. 4:05 a.m.
B. 4:58 p.m.
C. 5:30 p.m.
D. 5:42 p.m.

SITUATION

A woman is admitted to the ED with a pulmonary embolism. She is tachypneic. The physician plans to begin therapy with aminophylline and heparin.

Questions 9 to 13 refer to the above situation.

9 An order is written for 0.3 grams of aminophylline (Aminophyllin) to be administered by I.V. piggyback over 30 minutes. The label on the vial reads aminophylline 250 mg in 10 ml. How many milliliters should be administered?

A. 12
B. 14
C. 25
D. 30

10 The order reads: Add 25,000 units of heparin to 500 ml D_5W. Infuse 1,200 units per hour. What will the flow rate be in ml/hour?

A. 24
B. 60
C. 240
D. 600

11 Infusion of 1 liter of normal saline solution is started at 2 p.m. The flow rate is 40 drops/minute. The drip factor is 10 drops/ml. At what time will the infusion be completed?

A. 4:10 p.m.
B. 6:10 p.m.
C. 6:40 p.m.
D. 8:10 p.m.

12 The patient is to receive 50 mg of aminophylline (Aminophyllin) an hour. One gram of the drug is to be added to 500 ml D_5W. If the drip factor is 10 drops/ml, the patient will receive how many drops/minute?

A. 4
B. 8
C. 12
D. 14

13 One hundred ml of normal saline solution with 0.3 grams of aminophylline (Aminophyllin) is to be infused over 30 minutes. If the drip factor is 10 drops/ml, the patient will receive how many drops/minute?

A. 30
B. 31
C. 33
D. 42

SITUATION

A 54-year-old man is admitted to the ED with a massive anterior wall myocardial infarction. Cardiogenic shock is developing. He weighs 154 pounds (70 kg). All medications will be administered via an infusion system with a drip factor of 60 microdrops/ml.

Questions 14 to 19 refer to the above situation.

14 The physician orders 500 mg of dobutamine (Dobutrex) in 250 ml D_5W, infused at 10 mcg/kg/minute. What will be the flow rate in drops/minute?

A. 11
B. 14
C. 21
D. 42

15 If the order reads 250 mg dobutamine (Dobutrex) in 250 ml, infused at 4 mcg/kg/minute, the patient will receive how many ml/hour?

A. 16.8
B. 42
C. 168
D. 420

16 Nitroglycerin therapy is instituted with 50 mg diluted in 250 ml D_5W, infused at 10 mcg/minute. The patient will receive how many ml/hour?

A. 1
B. 3
C. 10
D. 90

17 If the dosage is increased to 30 mcg/minute, the flow rate will be how many ml/hour?

A. 9
B. 15
C. 50
D. 90

18 Sodium nitroprusside (Nipride) is then ordered at 0.5 mcg/kg/minute. If 50 mg Nipride is added to 250 ml D_5W, the patient will receive how many ml/hour?

A. 5
B. 11
C. 45
D. 110

19 If the dosage is increased to 0.8 mcg/kg/minute, the flow rate will be how many ml/hour?

A. 17
B. 20
C. 50
D. 140

SITUATION

A woman is found to have bleeding esophageal varices. Fluid replacement and administration of vasopressin (Pitressin) is initiated, and insertion of a Sengstaken-Blakemore tube is planned.

Questions 20 and 21 refer to the above situation.

20 The physician orders 200 ml of normal saline with 50 units vasopressin (Pitressin) infused at 0.5 units/minute. If the drip factor is 15 drops/ml, the patient will receive how many drops/minute?

A. 3
B. 5
C. 15
D. 30

21 The physician orders 1,000 ml of normal saline solution to be given I.V. over 4 hours. If the drip factor is 15 drops/ml, the patient will receive how many drops/minute?

A. 35
B. 63
C. 65
D. 240

Questions 22 to 30 refer to pediatric patients.

22 The usual adult dose of ampicillin (Amcill) is 500 mg. The appropriate dose for a 6-month-old infant is how many milligrams?

A. 0.2
B. 20
C. 30
D. 60

23 The adult dose of penicillin is 1,500,000 units. The appropriate dose for a 20-month-old child is how many units?

A. 10,000
B. 20,000
C. 100,000
D. 200,000

24 The usual adult dose of atropine sulfate is 1/150 grain. A 6-month-old infant should receive how many milligrams?

A. 0.016
B. 0.06
C. 0.16
D. 1.6

25 The usual adult dose of aspirin is 10 grains. A child weighing 20 kg should receive how many grains?

A. 2
B. 3
C. 6
D. 20

26 The usual adult dose of digoxin is 0.25 mg. An infant weighing 10 pounds should receive how many milligrams?

A. 0.0006
B. 0.01
C. 0.017
D. 0.03

27 The usual adult dose of digoxin is 0.25 mg orally. The appropriate dose for a child weighing 50 pounds is how many milligrams?

A. 0.08
B. 0.16
C. 0.18
D. 0.8

28 The usual adult dose of phenytoin (Dilantin) is 100 mg. A child weighing 65 pounds should receive how many milligrams?

A. 0.43
B. 4.3
C. 13
D. 43

29 The usual adult dose of meperidine (Demerol) is 100 mg. The appropriate dose for an 11-year-old child is how many milligrams?

A. 8.8
B. 26.4
C. 88
D. 92

30 The usual adult dose of cephradine (Velosef) is 1 gram orally. Which one of the following is the appropriate dose for a child whose body-surface area is 0.5 m^2?

A. 0.3 mg
B. 30 mg
C. 0.03 gram
D. 0.3 gram

Answer Sheet

	A	B	C	D
1	○	○	○	○
2	○	○	○	○
3	○	○	○	○
4	○	○	○	○
5	○	○	○	○
6	○	○	○	○
7	○	○	○	○
8	○	○	○	○
9	○	○	○	○
10	○	○	○	○
11	○	○	○	○
12	○	○	○	○
13	○	○	○	○
14	○	○	○	○
15	○	○	○	○
16	○	○	○	○
17	○	○	○	○
18	○	○	○	○
19	○	○	○	○
20	○	○	○	○
21	○	○	○	○
22	○	○	○	○
23	○	○	○	○
24	○	○	○	○
25	○	○	○	○
26	○	○	○	○
27	○	○	○	○
28	○	○	○	○
29	○	○	○	○
30	○	○	○	○

Answer Sheet

	A	B	C	D
1	○	○	○	○
2	○	○	○	○
3	○	○	○	○
4	○	○	○	○
5	○	○	○	○
6	○	○	○	○
7	○	○	○	○
8	○	○	○	○
9	○	○	○	○
10	○	○	○	○
11	○	○	○	○
12	○	○	○	○
13	○	○	○	○
14	○	○	○	○
15	○	○	○	○
16	○	○	○	○
17	○	○	○	○
18	○	○	○	○
19	○	○	○	○
20	○	○	○	○
21	○	○	○	○
22	○	○	○	○
23	○	○	○	○
24	○	○	○	○
25	○	○	○	○
26	○	○	○	○
27	○	○	○	○
28	○	○	○	○
29	○	○	○	○
30	○	○	○	○

1 Correct answer—**C**

The correct concentration is 200 mcg/ml. First, change the units into like equivalents; milligrams should be converted to micrograms. 1 mg = 1,000 mcg; therefore, 50 mg = 50,000 mcg. To determine the concentration of solution in 1 ml, divide the total solution (250 ml) into the total concentration (50,000 mcg).

$$\frac{50{,}000 \text{ mcg}}{250 \text{ ml}} = \frac{X \text{ mcg}}{1 \text{ ml}}$$

$200 \text{ mcg} = X$ Therefore, the solution would yield a concentration of 200 mcg/ml.

2 Correct answer—**C**

The flow rate is 16 microdrops/minute. First, multiply the dose desired (0.8 mcg) by the patient's weight in kilograms (65 kg) to yield the dose that will be delivered in 1 minute.
0.8 mcg x 65 kg = 52 mcg
Multiply the concentration (as calculated in Question 1) by the desired dose per minute by the drip factor, then

$$\frac{1 \text{ ml}}{200 \text{ mcg}} \times \frac{52 \text{ mcg}}{1 \text{ min}} \times \frac{60 \text{ microdrops}}{1 \text{ ml}} = \frac{3{,}120}{200} = 15.6,$$

or 16 microdrops/minute

The concentration of 200 mcg is the denominator in the first part of the equation, so the micrograms will cancel out.

3 Correct answer—**B**

The flow rate would be increased to 18 microdrops/minute.

0.9 mcg × 65 kg = 58.5 mcg/minute

$$\frac{1 \text{ ml}}{200 \text{ mcg}} \times \frac{58.5 \text{ mcg}}{1 \text{ min}} \times \frac{60 \text{ microdrops}}{1 \text{ ml}} = \frac{3{,}510}{200} = 17.55,$$

or 18 microdrops/minute

4 Correct answer—**C**

The flow rate to deliver 3 mg/minute of Arfonad is 180 ml/hour. Multiply the concentration of the solution by the dose desired, then by 60 minutes to determine the flow rate per hour.

$$\frac{500 \text{ ml}}{500 \text{ mg}} \times \frac{3 \text{ mg}}{1 \text{ min}} \times \frac{60 \text{ min}}{1 \text{ hr}} = 180 \text{ ml/hour}$$

5 Correct answer—**B**

The flow rate is 10 ml/hour.

$$\frac{250 \text{ ml}}{200 \text{ units}} \times \frac{8 \text{ units}}{1 \text{ hr}} = \frac{40}{4} = 10 \text{ ml/hour}$$

In this equation, you do not need to multiply by 60 min/hr because the order specified the amount to deliver per hour (8 units).

6 Correct answer—**B**

0.3 ml will deliver 30 units of insulin to the patient.

$$30 \text{ units} \times \frac{1 \text{ ml}}{100 \text{ units}} = 0.3 \text{ ml}$$

7 Correct answer—**D**

You will need 6 hours and 15 minutes to infuse a liter at 40 drops/minute using a drip factor of 15 drops/ml. Multiply the total amount of solution by the flow rate, then by the drip factor, and then by 60 minutes.

$$1{,}000 \text{ ml} \times \frac{1 \text{ min}}{40 \text{ drops}} \times \frac{15 \text{ drops}}{1 \text{ ml}} \times \frac{1 \text{ hr}}{60 \text{ min}} = \frac{250}{40} = 6.25,$$

or 6 hours and 15 minutes

Remember to invert the flow rate in order to cancel out the drops.

8 Correct answer—**B**

You will need 3 hours and 58 minutes to infuse the solution. If started at 1 p.m., the infusion will end at 4:58 p.m.

$$1{,}000 \text{ ml} \times \frac{1 \text{ min}}{42 \text{ drops}} \times \frac{10 \text{ drops}}{1 \text{ ml}} \times \frac{1 \text{ hr}}{60 \text{ min}} = \frac{1{,}000}{252} = 3.97$$

or 3 hours and 58 minutes

9 Correct answer—**A**

12 ml = 0.3 grams of aminophylline. Remember to convert to equivalent units: 0.3 grams = 300 mg.

$$\frac{10 \text{ ml}}{250 \text{ mg}} \times 300 \text{ mg} = \frac{300}{25} = 12 \text{ ml}$$

10 Correct answer—**A**

At a flow rate of 24 ml/hour, the patient will receive 1,200 units of heparin per hour.

$$\frac{500 \text{ ml}}{25{,}000 \text{ units}} \times \frac{1{,}200 \text{ units}}{1 \text{ hr}} = \frac{1{,}200}{50} \text{ or 24 ml/hour}$$

11 Correct answer—**B**

One liter of fluid administered at a flow rate of 40 drops/minute with a drip factor of 10 drops/ml will require 4 hours and 10 minutes for infusion. If started at 2 p.m., the infusion will end at 6:10 p.m.

$$1{,}000 \text{ ml} \times \frac{1 \text{ min}}{40 \text{ drops}} \times \frac{10 \text{ drops}}{1 \text{ ml}} \times \frac{1 \text{ hr}}{60 \text{ min}} = \frac{25}{6} \text{ or 4 hours and 10 minutes}$$

12 Correct answer—**A**

For the patient to receive 50 mg/hour of aminophylline at this concentration, the flow rate should be 4 drops/minute.

$$\frac{500 \text{ ml}}{1{,}000 \text{ mg}} \times \frac{50 \text{ mg}}{1 \text{ hr}} \times \frac{1 \text{ hr}}{60 \text{ min}} \times \frac{10 \text{ drops}}{1 \text{ ml}} = \frac{50}{12} = 4.17\text{, or 4 drops/minute}$$

13 Correct answer—**C**

To infuse 100 ml of fluid over 30 minutes with a drip factor of 10 drops/ml, the flow rate should be 33 drops/minute.

$$\frac{100 \text{ ml}}{30 \text{ min}} \times \frac{10 \text{ drops}}{1 \text{ ml}} = 33.3\text{, or 33 drops/minute}$$

14 Correct answer—**C**

For this 70-kg patient, 21 drops/minute is the flow rate at which to administer 10 mcg/kg/minute of dobutamine. First, we must determine the concentration of dobutamine in mcg/ml. 500 mg = 500,000 mcg.

$$\frac{500{,}000 \text{ mcg}}{250 \text{ ml}} = 2{,}000 \text{ mcg/ml}$$

The concentration of dobutamine is 2,000 mcg/ml.
10 mcg × 70 kg = 700 mcg/minute

The desired dose is 700 mcg/minute.

$$\frac{1 \text{ ml}}{2{,}000 \text{ mcg}} \times \frac{700 \text{ mcg}}{1 \text{ min}} \times \frac{60 \text{ drops}}{1 \text{ ml}} = 21 \text{ drops/minute}$$

15 Correct answer—**A**

At this concentration, 16.8 ml/hour will deliver 4 mcg/kg/minute to this patient.

250 mg = 250,000 mcg

$$\frac{250{,}000 \text{ mcg}}{250 \text{ ml}} = 1{,}000 \text{ mcg/ml}$$

The concentration of dobutamine is 1,000 mcg/ml.

4 mcg × 70 kg = 280 mcg/min
The desired dose is 280 mcg/minute.

$$\frac{1 \text{ ml}}{1{,}000 \text{ mcg}} \times \frac{280 \text{ mcg}}{1 \text{ min}} \times \frac{60 \text{ min}}{1 \text{ hr}} = \frac{840}{50} = 16.8 \text{ ml/hour}$$

16 Correct answer—**B**

At this concentration, 3 ml/hour will deliver 10 mcg/minute.

25 mg = 25,000 mcg

$$\frac{25{,}000 \text{ mcg}}{250 \text{ ml}} = 100 \text{ mcg/ml}$$

The concentration of nitroglycerin is 100 mcg/ml.

$$\frac{1 \text{ ml}}{200 \text{ mcg}} \times \frac{10 \text{ mcg}}{1 \text{ min}} \times \frac{60 \text{ min.}}{1 \text{ hr}} = \frac{600}{200} \text{ or } 3 \text{ ml/hr}$$

17 Correct answer—**A**

To deliver 30 mcg/minute, the flow rate must be increased to 9 ml/hour.

$$\frac{1 \text{ ml}}{100 \text{ mcg}} \times \frac{15 \text{ mcg}}{1 \text{ min}} \times \frac{60 \text{ min}}{1 \text{ hr}} = \frac{900}{100} \text{ or } 9 \text{ ml/hr}$$

18 Correct answer—**B**

A flow rate of 11 ml/hour will deliver 0.5 mcg/kg/minute of Nipride to this patient. 50 mg = 50,000 mcg.

$$\frac{50{,}000 \text{ mcg}}{250 \text{ ml}} = 200 \text{ mcg/ml}$$

The concentration of Nipride is 200 mcg/ml.
0.5 mcg/kg/min × 70 kg = 35 mcg/minute
The desired dose is 35 mcg/minute.

$$\frac{1 \text{ ml}}{200 \text{ mcg}} \times \frac{35 \text{ mcg}}{1 \text{ min}} \times \frac{60 \text{ min}}{1 \text{ hr}} = \frac{105}{10} = 10.5 \text{ or } 11 \text{ ml/hour}$$

19 Correct answer—A

A flow rate of 17 ml/hour will deliver 0.8 mcg/kg/minute of Nipride.
0.8 mcg × 70 kg = 56 mcg/minute

The desired dose is 56 mcg/minute.

$$\frac{1 \text{ ml}}{200 \text{ mcg}} \times \frac{56 \text{ mcg}}{1 \text{ min}} \times \frac{60 \text{ min}}{1 \text{ hr}} = \frac{168}{10} = 16.8 \text{ or } 17 \text{ ml/hour}$$

20 Correct answer—D

A flow rate of 30 drops/minute will deliver 0.5 units of Pitressin per minute.

$$\frac{200 \text{ ml}}{50 \text{ units}} \times \frac{0.5 \text{ unit}}{1 \text{ min}} \times \frac{15 \text{ drops}}{1 \text{ ml}} = 30 \text{ drops/minute}$$

21 Correct answer—B

To infuse 1 liter of fluid over 4 hours with a drip factor of 15 drops/ml, a flow rate of 63 drops/minute is required. First, convert hours into like equivalents of minutes: 4 hours = 240 minutes.

$$\frac{1{,}000 \text{ ml}}{240 \text{ min}} \times \frac{15 \text{ drops}}{1 \text{ ml}} = \frac{375}{6} \text{ or 63 drops/minutes}$$

22 Correct answer—B

For a 6-month-old infant, the appropriate dose of ampicillin is 20 mg. Be sure you know the safe adult dose before computing pediatric doses. When the pediatric dose is to be based on the child's age, an adult dose is equivalent to an age of 150 months. The pediatric dose is then calculated as follows:

$$\text{child's age in months} \times \frac{\text{adult dose}}{150 \text{ months}} = \text{pediatric dose}$$

$$6 \text{ months} \times \frac{500 \text{ mg}}{150 \text{ months}} = \frac{60}{3} \text{ or 20 mg}$$

23 Correct answer—D

The appropriate dose is 200,000 units of penicillin for a 20-month-old child.

$$20 \text{ months} \times \frac{1{,}500{,}000 \text{ units}}{150 \text{ months}} = 200{,}000 \text{ units}$$

24 Correct answer—**A**

A 6-month-old infant should receive 0.016 mg of atropine sulfate. The adult dose of atropine must first be converted from grains to mg. 1 grain = 60 mg.

$$\frac{1}{150} \times \frac{60 \text{ mg}}{1 \text{ gr}} = \frac{60}{150} \text{ or } 0.4 \text{ mg}$$

The adult dose of atropine is 0.4 mg.

$$6 \text{ months} \times \frac{0.4 \text{ mg}}{150 \text{ months}} = \frac{2.4}{150} \text{ or } 0.016 \text{ mg}$$

25 Correct answer—**B**

The appropriate dose for a 20-kg child is 3 grains of aspirin. Pediatric doses also can be calculated according to weight, again using the safe adult dose. The adult weight is equivalent to 150 pounds or 70 kg (depending on whether the child's weight is given in pounds or kg).

$$20 \text{ kg} \times \frac{10 \text{ gr}}{70 \text{ kg}} = \frac{20}{7} = 2.86, \text{ or } 3 \text{ grains}$$

26 Correct answer—**C**

A 10-pound infant should receive 0.017 mg of digoxin.

$$10 \text{ lb} \times \frac{0.25 \text{ mg}}{150 \text{ lb}} = 0.0166 \text{ mg or } 0.017 \text{ mg}$$

27 Correct answer—**A**

The correct dose of digoxin for a 50-pound child is 0.08 mg.

$$50 \text{ lb} \times \frac{0.25 \text{ mg}}{150 \text{ lb}} = \frac{0.25}{3} \text{ or } 0.08 \text{ mg}$$

28 Correct answer—**D**

A 65-pound child should receive 43 mg of Dilantin.

$$65 \text{ lb} \times \frac{100 \text{ mg}}{150 \text{ lb}} = \frac{130}{3} = 43 \text{ mg}$$

29 Correct answer—**C**

An 11-year-old child should receive 88 mg of Demerol. The child's age must first be converted to months. 11 years = 132 months. (Adult dosage is given when the patient's age is greater than 150 months.)

$$132 \text{ months} \times \frac{100 \text{ mg}}{150 \text{ months}} = \frac{264}{3} \text{ or } 88 \text{ mg}$$

30 Correct answer—**D**

The correct dose of Velosef for a child with a body-surface area of 0.5 m^2 is 0.3 gram. Body-surface area is derived from height and weight. The normal adult body-surface area is 1.7 m^2.

$$0.5 \text{ m}^2 \times \frac{1 \text{ g}}{1.7 \text{ m}^2} = 0.294, \text{ or } 0.3 \text{ g}$$

Selected References

Olsen, June Looby, et al. *Medical Dosage Calculations,* 4th ed. Reading, Mass.: Addison-Wesley Publishing Co., 1987.

Index

A

C

I

J

K

L

M

N

O

P

Q

R

S

T

U

V

W

Z